MAYO CLINIC
Guide to
Fertility and
Conception

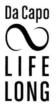

Da Capo

LIFE
LONG

A Member of the Perseus Books Group

IMAGE CREDITS

The individuals pictured in this book are models, and the photos are used for illustrative purposes only. There's no correlation between the individuals portrayed and the condition or subject discussed.

MAYO CLINIC

Medical Editors
Jani R. Jensen, M.D.
Elizabeth (Ebbie) A. Stewart, M.D.

Senior Editor
Karen R. Wallevand

Editorial Director
Paula Marlow Limbeck

Product Manager
Christopher C. Frye

Contributing Editors
Charles C. Coddington III, M.D.
Gaurang S. Daftary, M.D.
Shawna L. Ehlers, Ph.D., L.P.
Dean E. Morbeck, Ph.D.
Landon W. Trost, M.D.
Myra J. Wick, M.D., Ph.D.

Contributing Writers
Rachel A. H. Bartony
Alicia C. Bartz
Kelly M. Kershner
Jennifer Koski
Laura Hamilton Waxman

Art Director
Richard A. Resnick

Creative Director
Daniel W. Brevick

Illustration and Photography
Michael A. King
Jodi O'Shaughnessy Olson
Malgorzata (Gosha) B. Weivoda

Research Librarians
Amanda K. Golden
Deirdre A. Herman

Proofreading
Miranda M. Attlesey
Donna L. Hanson
Julie M. Maas

Indexing
Steve Rath

Administrative Assistant
Beverly J. Steele

Cataloging-in-Publication data for this book is available from the Library of Congress.

ISBN 978-1-56148-787-5

Published by Da Capo Press
A member of the Perseus Books Group
dacapopress.com

Note: The information in this book is true and complete to the best of our knowledge. This book is intended only as an informative guide for those wishing to know more about health issues. In no way is the book intended to replace, countermand, or conflict with the advice given to you by your own physician. The ultimate decision concerning care should be made between you and your doctor. Information in this book is offered with no guarantees on the part of the authors or Da Capo Press. The authors and publisher disclaim all liability in connection with the use of this book. The names and identifying details of people associated with events described in the book have been changed. Any similarity to the actual person is coincidental.

For bulk sales to employers, member groups and health-related companies, contact Mayo Clinic, 200 First St. SW, Rochester, MN 55905, or *SpecialSalesMayoBooks@Mayo.edu*.

Printed in the United States of America.

10 9 8 7 6 5 4 3 2 1

Introduction

Deciding to start or build your family is a life-changing decision. Maybe you recently decided to try to become pregnant or perhaps it's something you've been contemplating for a while. But once the decision is made, there's a whole new set of unknowns, including whether the journey will be easy or difficult.

You may already have a lot of questions: How can you increase your chances of becoming pregnant? What health and lifestyle changes should you make to have a healthy pregnancy? And if you're struggling to become pregnant, what medical treatments are available? Where can you get emotional support if you can't get pregnant or have had a miscarriage? And when is enough?

The fertility experts at Mayo Clinic are here to guide you through the process of trying for — and achieving — a successful pregnancy. *Mayo Clinic Guide to Fertility and Conception* is an easy-to-use yet comprehensive resource that provides answers and explanations to many common questions of couples hoping to have a baby. From lifestyle and dietary recommendations to understanding your ovulatory cycle to medications and procedures that can improve fertility, this book covers it all.

In the pages that follow, you will also hear from couples and individuals who have struggled to have a family. For a variety of reasons — health conditions, unexplained infertility or life circumstances — getting pregnant or deciding to have a family was difficult for them. These personal stories are to let you know that you're not alone in your journey, and to give you hope that with time and patience pregnancy is often possible.

A project of this scope requires the teamwork of many individuals. A special thanks to all of the people who helped make this book possible.

The Editors

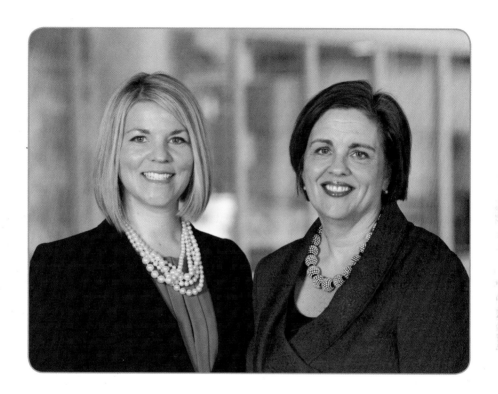

Meet the Editors

Jani R. Jensen, M.D., (left) is a specialist in the division of Reproductive Endocrinology and Infertility and the co-director of the In Vitro Fertilization Program at Mayo Clinic, Rochester, Minn. She is an assistant professor at Mayo Clinic College of Medicine and directs the Obstetrics and Gynecology Clerkship for medical students.

Elizabeth (Ebbie) A. Stewart, M.D., (right) is the chair of the division of Reproductive Endocrinology and Infertilty at Mayo Clinic, Rochester, Minn., and a professor of obstetrics and gynecology at Mayo Clinic College of Medicine. A noted researcher, author and clinician, Dr. Stewart's research interests focus on the epidemiology, diagnosis and treatment of uterine fibroids.

How to use this book

Mayo Clinic Guide to Fertility and Conception is a comprehensive medical reference that provides answers and explanations to questions and concerns related to fertility. To help you find what you're looking for, the book is divided into five sections.

Part 1: Getting Ready for Pregnancy
From exercise and eating right to medications and chronic illness, this section discusses daily habits and medical conditions that may affect your ability to become pregnant. Find out what steps you can take to prepare for pregnancy.

Part 2: How to Get Pregnant
Part 2 covers the intricacies of getting pregnant. In this section you learn how to determine when you're ovulating, when is the best time for sexual intercourse, and steps you can take to increase your chances of a successful outcome. You'll also read about early signs of pregnancy and of warnings of a possible problem.

Part 3: Common Fertility Problems
Sometimes infertility is the result of a specific health disorder. This section ad-dresses both common and unusual problems that can affect female and male fertility. There's also a discussion of age and pregnancy. With more women waiting longer to have their first child, understanding how age affects female fertility is important.

Part 4: When You Need Some Help
Here you'll learn about the latest in medical treatments to help you get pregnant. You'll find information on medications to improve fertility, as well as procedures such as intrauterine insemination. There's a detailed discussion of in vitro fertilization and other assisted reproductive technologies. You'll also learn about third-party reproduction, which may involve the use of donor sperm, eggs or embryos, or the assistance of a gestational carrier.

Part 5: Special Considerations
The last section of the book addresses unique situations — the options available and factors to consider. It also tackles the tough issue of moving forward when pregnancy is unobtainable.

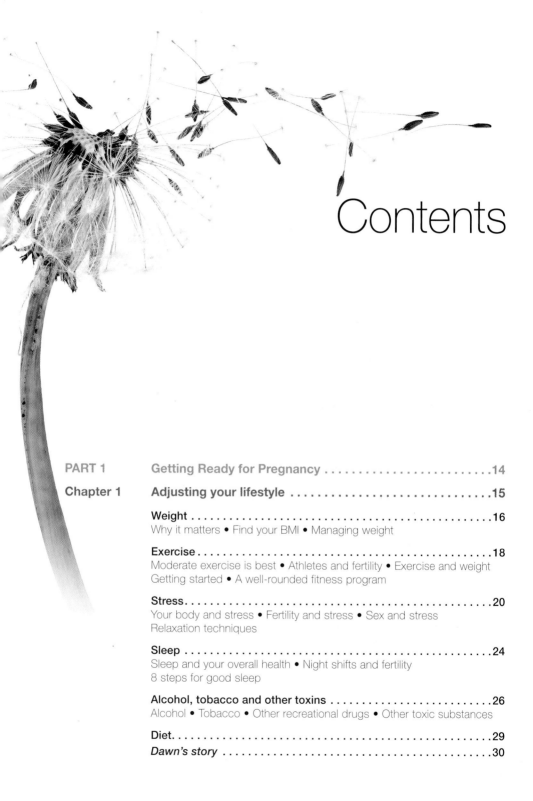

Contents

PART 1

Getting Ready for Pregnancy

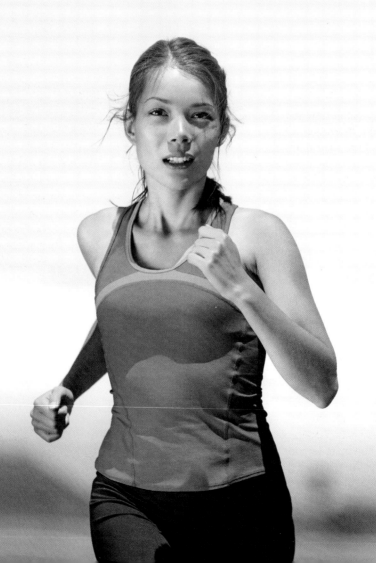

CHAPTER 1

Adjusting your lifestyle

Planning to have a baby is exciting. You may have thought about the possibility before, but now you're ready — ready to make it happen. Or at least try to. But hold on. Like many other women, until now you may have been more preoccupied with avoiding pregnancy than with getting pregnant. And now that you'd like to become pregnant, you're not quite sure that it's really all that easy! Sure, it can be simple — you have sex and you get pregnant. But it can also be more complicated than you might have thought. If that's the case, or if that's what you're worried about, this book is here to help.

The purpose of this book is to help you and your partner optimize your fertility so that you can conceive naturally and have a healthy pregnancy. If you have some questions — many couples do! — the information in the pages ahead will hopefully give you the answers you're looking for. Yes, sometimes there are bumps in the road, and it's possible you may need some medical assistance along the way. But bear in mind that most couples — 85 percent, in fact — do conceive within a year of trying and about half of the remaining couples will conceive naturally within a year after that. So it's rational to be optimistic.

We begin with taking a look at how your habits and surroundings — your everyday choices and encounters — affect your fertility. Some people become pregnant quite easily, regardless of their lifestyles or environments. But evidence suggests, and it makes sense, that healthy habits can boost your fertility. This doesn't mean you have to be exceptionally fit or in tremendous health to have a child, but if you're doing the right things to begin with, your chances of conception and having a healthy pregnancy are greater.

There's a lot you can do on your own to get ready to have a baby. For starters, there are obvious things such as staying away from toxic substances, including alcohol and cigarettes, which can decrease your chances of conception and create a harmful environment for a developing baby.

There are also plenty of other positive changes you can make to optimize your fertility. They include managing stress, getting enough sleep, exercising regularly and following a healthy diet. Tending to these aspects of your life can make you feel better in general and smooth the way for the intricate processes of conception and pregnancy. Ignoring these factors, on the other hand, can sometimes make it more difficult to get pregnant.

Take a minute to examine your daily habits. Then think about ways you might be able to improve your lifestyle. If you already practice a healthy lifestyle, you're one step ahead of the game. If you do need to make some changes, it doesn't have to be all at once. Sometimes, incremental changes work best and may, in fact, last the longest. And don't forget that this is a team venture! The advice and suggestions in this chapter apply both to you and your partner. You're both key players. Make the changes together and support one another along the way.

WEIGHT

Most women, regardless of their weight, don't have any problems becoming pregnant. But weight can sometimes be a factor in a couple's efforts to have a baby. Among women whose body mass index (BMI) puts them in the underweight or obese categories, their weight may affect the ovaries' ability to release an egg (ovulate) and, as a result, reduce chances of conception.

Why it matters Your pituitary gland, located in your brain, produces two hormones responsible for stimulating ovulation each month — follicle-stimulating hormone (FSH) and luteinizing hormone (LH). These hormones spur the growth and release of an egg in regular cycles each month. An unfertilized egg results in your monthly period; a fertilized egg, in pregnancy. Being at a weight that's on either extreme of the BMI chart can affect these hormones.

Being very thin — having a BMI less than 19 — can disrupt the cyclical production of FSH and LH, resulting in irregular or absent periods and lack of ovulation (anovulation). Although the ovaries can work well and produce normal eggs, the signals to start the egg maturation and ovulation process are missing or irregular.

Being at the other end of the chart — having a BMI of 27 or higher — can also interfere with ovulation and conception in general. Carrying too much weight may lead your body to overproduce insulin, which can then lead to production of too many androgens, hormones that can disrupt regular egg development and result in lack of ovulation. Other hormones may also affect ovulation and ovarian function.

But even women who experience regular periods may take longer to get

FIND YOUR BMI

Body mass index (BMI) is one measurement care providers use to evaluate your weight and your health. Use this chart to determine your BMI. Locate your height in the left column, and then scroll to the right until you find the weight closest to yours. Look above to see if that number falls within the normal, overweight or obese category.

	Normal		Overweight					Obese				
BMI	**19**	**24**	**25**	**26**	**27**	**28**	**29**	**30**	**35**	**40**	**45**	**50**
Weight in pounds												
4'10"	91	115	119	124	129	134	138	143	167	191	215	239
4'11"	94	119	124	128	133	138	143	148	173	198	222	247
5'0"	97	123	128	133	138	143	148	153	179	204	230	255
5'1"	100	127	132	137	143	148	153	158	185	211	238	264
5'2"	104	131	136	142	147	153	158	164	191	218	246	273
5'3"	107	135	141	146	152	158	163	169	197	225	254	282
5'4"	110	140	145	151	157	163	169	174	204	232	262	291
5'5"	114	144	150	156	162	168	174	180	210	240	270	300
5'6"	118	148	155	161	167	173	179	186	216	247	278	309
5'7"	121	153	159	166	172	178	185	191	223	255	287	319
5'8"	125	158	164	171	177	184	190	197	230	262	295	328
5'9"	128	162	169	176	182	189	196	203	236	270	304	338
5'10"	132	167	174	181	188	195	202	209	243	278	313	348
5'11"	136	172	179	186	193	200	208	215	250	286	322	358
6'0"	140	177	184	191	199	206	213	221	258	294	331	368
6'1"	144	182	189	197	204	212	219	227	265	302	340	378
6'2"	148	186	194	202	210	218	225	233	272	311	350	389
6'3"	152	192	200	208	216	224	232	240	279	319	359	399
6'4"	156	197	205	213	221	230	238	246	287	328	369	410

For most women, health risks begin with a BMI of 25. For Asian women, a BMI of 23 or higher is associated with increased health risks.
National Institutes of Health, 1998

pregnant if they're overweight. Obesity itself is associated with conditions in women that may undermine their ability to conceive, such as polycystic ovary syndrome, a hormonal disorder characterized by menstrual abnormalities, acne, excess facial and body hair, and other changes throughout the body.

And weight is not an issue just for women. Excess weight may also be a factor for men. The effect of a man's weight on fertility hasn't been studied as extensively as has a woman's, but some data suggests that the male partner's BMI does have an effect on the amount of time it takes to get pregnant. As with female hormones, excess weight may alter male reproductive hormone levels and affect chances of conception.

If both partners are overweight, the time to get pregnant may be even longer. Conception may also be elusive when one partner is overweight and the other underweight.

Managing weight The good news is that taking steps to achieve a more healthy body weight — within the BMI range of 19 to 26 — can improve the frequency and regularity of ovulation and the likelihood of getting pregnant. If you're overweight, even losing as little as 5 to 10 percent of your body weight can improve fertility. For many people, that amounts to 10 pounds or less. Being at a healthy weight is good for many reasons. Increasing your odds of pregnancy is one more reason you can add to the list! Shedding a few pounds is something that you and your partner can do together. Proven ways to lose weight include consuming fewer calories and exercising more. You can also ask your care provider to recommend a weight-loss program.

If you have a very low BMI, to help restore regular ovulation you may need to gain weight. But be careful to do this by consuming the right foods and beverages — those that improve your health, such as avocados, nuts, whole grains, fruits and vegetables, and other foods that are good for you. Also, try to maintain a schedule of regular meals.

Chapter 2 contains more information on eating healthy and how adjusting your diet may improve your fertility.

EXERCISE

Exercise. Just the thought of it makes some people groan. Maybe you're not a fan of exercise. But if you're thinking about having a baby and exercise hasn't been a regular part of your life, it may be time to rethink your response. Exercise can be very beneficial in a number of ways, including promoting fertility.

One of the most recent studies to investigate the relationship between exercise and fertility took place in Denmark. Over a period of 12 months, a group of investigators tracked more than 3,000 Danish women who were planning to conceive and who weren't using any fertility treatments. By way of an online questionnaire, the women responded to many lifestyle components, including the amount of time they spent being physically active and how strenuous their activity was. The researchers then tracked how long it took each woman to get pregnant.

Moderate exercise is best The investigators found that women who engaged in five hours or more of moderate physical activity a week, but not vigorous physical activity, had the shortest time to pregnancy. The effect wasn't huge, but it was enough to make a difference.

Like sleep, exercise is foundational to good health. It helps your body stay limber and mobile, protects against the effects of aging and chronic illness, and reduces stress and anxiety by promoting the release of "feel-good" endorphins. All of these things combined may give you just the edge you need to shorten the time it takes for you to conceive.

What is moderate physical activity? Brisk walking, leisurely bike riding and golfing are all considered moderately strenuous activities.

Athletes and fertility Although moderate physical activity can help promote fertility, too much exercise might have the opposite effect. Some research suggests that more than five hours a week of vigorous aerobic activity — such as running or fast cycling — can actually impair fertility. This may be due to changes in how your body uses its resources — increased demand placed by your musculoskeletal system may reduce the supply of resources to other systems, such as those regulating hormones.

While some studies have suggested that strenuous activity might impair fertility, other studies haven't been able to confirm this. In the Danish study, the more time women were engaged in vigorous physical activity, the longer it took for them to get pregnant. If you're a professional athlete or you engage in more than five hours of vigorous exercise during the week, there's no need to cut back entirely on exercise. But you might consider replacing some of your strenuous activities with more moderate ones. If you have any concerns, talk to your care provider. He or she can help you decide what's best for you.

Exercise and weight Perhaps the biggest effect that exercise has on fertility is when it comes to weight loss. Increasing evidence suggests a clear link between being overweight and problems with fertility, especially among women who are obese (see chart on page 17). Exercise is important to achieving and maintaining a healthy weight. Exercising regularly can help you shed excess pounds and come closer to a more fertility-friendly weight range. Losing even 5 to 10 percent of your body weight can help.

Interestingly, in the Danish study, among overweight or obese women, vigorous exercise was actually a good thing. Unlike women at a healthy weight in which vigorous exercise reduced fertility, among obese women vigorous physical activity did the opposite — it provided a slight fertility boost. If you've got weight to lose, the more you exercise, the more likely you are to benefit.

Getting started How much should you exercise? First of all, something is always better than nothing. So any amount of time you spend being physically active is better than doing nothing at all. Most health organizations generally recommend that healthy adults get 30 minutes of moderate aerobic activity most days of the week and engage in strength training exercises twice a week.

Starting a fitness program can be life changing, but it doesn't have to be overwhelming. By planning carefully and pacing yourself, you can make fitness a healthy habit that lasts a lifetime.

First, make it personal. Do something you like, so that it doesn't end up becoming a drudgery that you're always seeking to avoid. For example, if you hate running, don't jog. Instead, try swimming or taking part in an aerobics dance class at the gym. If you're not sure what to do, perhaps the best advice is to get out and walk for 30 minutes each day.

A WELL-ROUNDED FITNESS PROGRAM

Exercise comes in many forms, and different forms of exercise provide different results. Moderate exercise, no matter the type, may help improve fertility. However, specific forms of exercise may provide specific benefits, especially once you become pregnant. Whether you're a fitness novice or veteran, here are elements that you might want to include in your fitness routine:

Aerobic fitness Aerobic exercise causes you to breathe faster and more deeply, which maximizes the amount of oxygen in your blood. The better your aerobic fitness, the more efficiently your heart, lungs and blood vessels transport oxygen throughout your body and the easier it is to complete routine physical tasks. Aerobic exercise can help boost your strength and energy level during periods of fatigue that often accompany early pregnancy.

Aerobic exercise includes activities such as walking, jogging, biking, swimming, dancing and water aerobics. Try to get in 30 minutes most days of the week.

Strength training Strength training can help you maintain muscle mass while trying to lose weight to boost your fertility. Strength training also helps increase bone strength and muscular fitness. This is important because pregnancy can affect bone health and cause joints and ligaments to loosen and stretch.

Most fitness centers offer various resistance machines, free weights and other tools for strength training. But hand-held weights or homemade weights — such as

What you do isn't as important as doing it regularly. And make sure to involve your partner so that you both benefit.

One note of caution: If you haven't exercised for some time and you have health concerns, you may want to talk to your care provider before starting a new fitness routine.

STRESS

It's a fair question to ask: Can stress, especially high levels of stress, affect a couple's ability to get pregnant? You may be asking this question because you've overheard conversations in which a woman trying to become pregnant was told she was too stressed and anxious and that she should just "relax."

The truth is, stress won't keep you from getting pregnant. To date, there's no clear evidence that stress reduces fertility specifically. A study of women who were trying to conceive over a period of six months found no relationship between everyday stress levels and the ability to get pregnant. Similar results were found in a group of Danish men. But stress isn't good for your overall health, and anything you can do to reduce and manage stress is a good idea.

Your body and stress When you're under stress, your brain signals your body to release a burst of hormones to fuel your capacity to respond. Adrenaline in-plastic soft drink bottles filled with water or sand —work just as well. Do strength training exercises twice a week.

Core exercises Your core muscles are the muscles in your abdomen, lower back and pelvis that help protect your back and connect upper and lower body movements. Core exercises help train your muscles to brace your spine, enabling you to use your upper and lower body muscles more effectively. Having strong core muscles can help support an expanding uterus and growing baby and ease the demands of childbirth.

So what counts as a core exercise? It's any exercise that uses the trunk of your body without support, including abdominal crunches, better known as situps. You can also try various core exercises with a fitness ball.

Flexibility and stretching Stretching exercises increase flexibility and improve the range of motion of your joints. Regular stretching also promotes better posture and can even help relieve stress. Stretching exercises help prevent injuries during physical activity, and during pregnancy they help reduce aches and pains that may accompany body changes.

The best time to stretch is after you exercise — when your muscles are warm and receptive to stretching. If you don't exercise regularly, try to stretch at least three times a week to maintain flexibility. Activities such as yoga promote flexibility, too.

creases your heart rate, elevates your blood pressure and boosts energy supplies. Cortisol, the primary stress hormone, increases the availability of sugar (glucose) to your body while curbing nonessential functions, such as your digestive system.

After a stressful event is over, your body returns to its normal state. But if stress is chronic, your mind and body remain on a constant state of alert. The less control you have over potentially stress-inducing events and the more uncertainty they create, the more likely you are to feel stressed. The long-term activation of the stress-response system — and the body's overexposure to cortisol and other stress hormones — can disrupt normal processes. Chronic stress can increase

your risk of a variety of health concerns, including heart disease, sleep problems and depression.

Fertility and stress Even though studies haven't shown that stress itself reduces fertility, that doesn't mean that stress doesn't factor into the equation. The truth is that not being able to get pregnant can be stressful. Generally, the longer it takes to get pregnant, the more stress a couple begins to feel. Furthermore, it's a cycle that repeats itself every month. And if you're trying to time sexual intercourse to just the right moment before ovulation, you may be experiencing even more stress.

A survey of more than 120 couples being evaluated for infertility found that sexual problems and depression were common among the participants, both in the male and female partners. Men had a higher than expected incidence of erectile dysfunction and depressive symptoms. For the women, sexual difficulties arose from problems with desire, arousal and orgasm. In women, depression was highest among those who had been trying for two years or more, although these rates tended to subside as time went on. In addition, sexual problems experienced by one partner increased the likelihood of sexual difficulties in the other partner.

From this study, the investigators concluded that the stress of not being able to get pregnant may cause sexual difficulties and depression. These conditions can make it even more difficult to get pregnant.

Sex and stress If you find that stress is disrupting your sexual life so that intercourse isn't fun, then it may be time to step back and assess your situation. If you need to, seek medical guidance. The bottom line is that you want to find ways to make your sexual encounters something you enjoy and look forward to. That may mean not worrying so much about becoming pregnant — putting aside the thermometers and ovulation predictor kits — and spending more time enjoying the moment. Yes, when you've got dreams of a baby on your mind this can be difficult to do. But remember you can have your cake and eat it, too! You can have an exciting sex life and still conceive a baby.

It's also important that you try not to bring daily stresses to bed with you. If your job is demanding, perhaps you can reduce your obligations at work or say no a little more often to protect your time alone or with your partner. It's important to find time to decompress from the pressures of everyday life. Other stress management strategies include getting regular exercise, getting plenty of sleep and eating a healthy diet (more on these in a moment), practicing relaxation techniques, fostering healthy and supportive friendships, seeing the humorous side of life, and seeking professional help when you need it.

Although stress may or may not affect fertility directly, managing your stress in a positive way can make you feel better about yourself and your circumstances and give you a positive frame of mind.

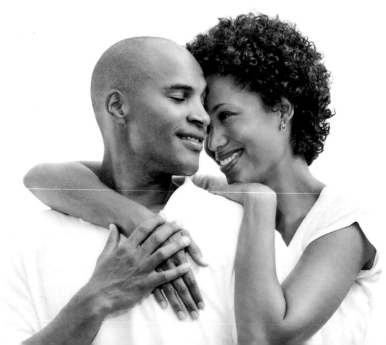

RELAXATION TECHNIQUES

There are a variety of methods you can use to reduce stress. They include massage therapy, yoga and meditation, to name just a few. You can go to a gym or a class and learn from an instructor how to practice these techniques. But you can also learn some of them on your own. To get the most benefit, practice relaxation techniques daily and incorporate them with other healthy habits such as exercising, eating well and getting enough sleep.

In general, relaxation techniques involve refocusing your attention on something calming and increasing your awareness of your body. It doesn't matter which relaxation technique you choose. What matters is that you pick one or two that you're willing to practice regularly.

Positive self-talk It's easy to lose objectivity when you're stressed. One negative thought can lead to another, and soon you've created a mental avalanche. Be positive. Instead of thinking, "Something is wrong with me, and I'll never be able to get pregnant," say to yourself, "It hasn't happened yet, but it will. We'll get through this together."

Progressive muscle relaxation Use this technique after a long day or if your muscles are feeling tense and bunched up. With this method, you focus on slowly tensing and then relaxing each muscle group, so that you can feel the difference between muscle tension and muscle relaxation. Start by tensing and relaxing the muscles in your toes and progressively working your way up to your neck and head. You can also start with your head and neck and work down to your toes. Tense your muscles for at least five seconds, relax for 30 seconds, and repeat.

Visualization With this technique, you form mental images that allow you to take a visual journey to a peaceful, calming place. During visualization, try to use as many senses as you can, including smell, sight, sound and touch. If you imagine relaxing at the ocean, for instance, think about such things as the smell of salt water, the sound of crashing waves and the warmth of the sun on your body. You may want to close your eyes or sit in a quiet spot.

Present moment awareness This technique can be quite simple and can have a great impact if you practice it regularly. The idea is to cultivate awareness of what's going on right here and right now. It's easy to become so preoccupied with what might happen in the future, or what has happened in the past, that you forget to enjoy the present. The next time you rush to do a task, slow down and take in the little things around you. Notice the soothing sound of water coming from the faucet when you fill up a glass, the shadows in the room when you turn off a light or the smoothness of the sheets as you climb into bed. Focusing your awareness onto the present helps to dissipate stressful thoughts about the future or the past.

SLEEP

Sleep is good for you. It provides your body with the opportunity to renew its defenses against illness and reset its internal clock. Getting a good night's rest keeps you in good overall health, helps reduce stress and helps to regulate key hormone cycles in your body, including those related to fertility.

You may think that you can get away with just a few hours of sleep here and there, but sooner or later lack of sleep takes its toll.

Sleep and your overall health If you've ever pulled an all-nighter, you know the immediate effects of not getting enough sleep: You feel moody, irritable, unfocused and slow. Or try making it through a busy workweek with only a few hours of sleep a night — it's a recipe for stress.

Lack of sleep not only makes a difference in how you feel but also can make a difference in whether you get sick. During sleep, your immune system releases proteins called cytokines, some of which help promote sleep. Certain cytokines need to increase when you're fighting an infection or inflammation, or when you're under stress. Sleep deprivation can decrease production of these protective cytokines and make it difficult to fight infection.

Research also suggests that continued lack of sleep over time can increase your risk of obesity, diabetes, and heart and blood vessel (cardiovascular) disease, conditions that can present their own challenges if you're trying to get pregnant.

How much sleep do you need to stay healthy? The optimal amount for most adults is seven to eight hours of quality sleep each night. See the opposite page for suggestions on how to sleep well.

Night shifts and fertility If you work nights, you may have wondered if your work and sleep schedule might be affecting your chances of becoming pregnant. You could be right. A number of studies suggest that women who regularly work night shifts may be at higher risk of infertility than women who don't work nights. How does this happen?

Humans are naturally wired to be awake during the day and asleep at night. This innate tendency is tied to your body's circadian rhythms, which act as an internal clock, guiding such things as your sleep-wake cycle, metabolism and body temperature. Shifts in your circadian rhythms, which can result from sleeping during the day and working at night, can affect the regulation of your reproductive hormones and they may affect the regularity of your menstrual cycles. Working a rotating shift schedule for months at a time has been associated with very short (less than 21 days) or very long (more than 40 days) menstrual cycles, as well as irregular cycles. This can affect fertility.

The relationship between circadian rhythm shifts and disruption of reproductive hormones isn't exactly clear. It may be linked to altered production of melatonin, a hormone that makes you feel sleepy and is normally released during dark hours. Or it may be that altered sleep-wake patterns directly affect the release of luteinizing hormone (LH), which plays a prominent role in regulating your monthly cycles.

If you want to become pregnant, working the night shift may not be ideal. But sometimes night shifts can't be avoided. If you do work the night shift, try to get enough sleep when you're not working. It may be difficult to sleep during the day and tempting to run errands during your off hours, but it's important that you get adequate rest.

8 STEPS FOR GOOD SLEEP

If you're having trouble getting a good night's rest, consider these sleep tips:

1. **Pay attention to what you eat and drink.** Don't go to bed either hungry or stuffed. Your discomfort might keep you up. Caffeine and alcohol deserve caution, too. Their stimulating effects can wreak havoc with quality sleep.
2. **Stick to a sleep schedule.** Go to bed and get up at the same time every day, even on weekends, holidays and days off. Being consistent reinforces your body's sleep-wake cycle and helps promote better sleep at night.
3. **Create a bedtime ritual.** Do the same things each night to tell your body that it's time to wind down. This might include taking a warm bath or shower, reading a book, or listening to soothing music — preferably with the lights dimmed. Relaxing activities can promote better sleep by easing the transition between wakefulness and drowsiness. Be wary of watching TV, checking email or using other electronic devices before bedtime. Sometimes they can be more stimulating than soothing.
4. **Get comfortable.** Create a room that's ideal for sleeping. Often, this means cool, dark and quiet. Your mattress and pillow can contribute to better sleep, too. Choose what feels most comfortable to you and make sure you have enough room to stretch out.
5. **Limit daytime naps.** Long daytime naps can interfere with nighttime sleep — especially if you're struggling with insomnia or poor sleep quality at night. If you nap during the day, limit yourself to about 10 to 30 minutes and make it during the midafternoon. If you work nights, you'll need to make an exception to the rules about daytime sleeping. In this case, keep your window coverings closed so that sunlight — which adjusts your internal clock — doesn't interrupt your daytime sleep.
6. **Include exercise in your daily routine.** Regular physical activity can promote better sleep, helping you to fall asleep faster and to enjoy deeper sleep. Timing is important, though. If you exercise too close to bedtime, you might be too energized to fall asleep. If this seems to be an issue for you, exercise earlier in the day.
7. **Manage stress.** When you have too much to do — and too much to think about — your sleep is likely to suffer. To help create peace in your life, consider healthy ways to manage stress. Start with the basics, such as getting organized, setting priorities and delegating tasks. Before bed, jot down what's on your mind and then set it aside for tomorrow.
8. **Know when to contact your doctor.** Nearly everyone has an occasional sleepless night — but if you often have trouble sleeping, talk to your care provider. Identifying and treating any underlying causes can help you get the better sleep you deserve.

You may also need to adjust how you check for evidence of ovulation. For example, basal body charting may be less accurate when you sleep irregular hours, but ovulation predictor kits that detect a pre-ovulatory LH surge could still be useful (see Chapter 6 for more information). You might also need to rethink when you have intercourse — perhaps before you go to work in the evening rather than when you're exhausted after your shift is done.

ALCOHOL, TOBACCO AND OTHER TOXINS

If you're accustomed to a glass of wine or a bottle of beer on a regular basis, or if you're a smoker, it may be tempting to think that you can get away with these habits while trying to conceive. But the truth is that these substances do pose a risk, both in terms of increasing the time it takes to get pregnant as well as experiencing a healthy pregnancy.

Will one drink or cigarette ruin your chances of becoming a parent? Probably not. But we do know that alcohol and tobacco aren't safe during pregnancy, so it would be hard to say where you should draw the line. Plus, it isn't always easy to stop. Your best bet is to avoid alcohol and tobacco altogether while trying to conceive, but especially during pregnancy.

In addition to alcohol and tobacco, take stock of other toxic substances you may encounter during your day. If you or your partner work with pesticides or other hazardous materials, there are certain precautions you may want to take.

Alcohol If you're trying to get pregnant, it's generally best to avoid alcohol. One of the big reasons is that alcohol exposure can cause birth defects in the early weeks of your pregnancy, before you may know you're carrying a child. It doesn't matter if you drink beer, wine or other forms of liquor — if you drink alcohol, so does your baby. Once in your bloodstream, alcohol passes through the placenta to your baby. Sustained drinking during pregnancy increases your risk of miscarriage, fetal death and severe birth defects. Children whose mothers drink even moderately may be born with some of these problems.

Q. WHAT IF I HAD SOME ALCOHOL BEFORE I KNEW I WAS PREGNANT? DID I HARM THE BABY?

A. It's best to avoid alcohol when you're pregnant because it's clear that heavy drinking can be dangerous to the baby. Studies, however, have not found occasional consumption — one drink at a holiday celebration or an "accidental drink" before you knew you were pregnant — to cause problems. So, you can relax and let go of your guilt. It's highly unlikely the small amount of alcohol you drank before realizing that you were pregnant did any harm to your baby. But now that you know you're pregnant, it's best to avoid alcohol. Because it's difficult to determine exactly how much alcohol might be OK to consume during pregnancy, the safest bet is simply to stay away from it altogether.

WAYS TO QUIT SMOKING

It's not always easy to quit smoking. Many people try several times before they succeed. So don't give up. If one method doesn't work for you, try another. Or talk to your care provider about using a combination of methods to help you quit. Here are some examples of methods that successful quitters have used:

- ▶ Cold turkey method (setting a quit date and stopping abruptly)
- ▶ Smoking cessation medications
- ▶ Individual or group counseling
- ▶ Hypnotism
- ▶ Treatment program

The method you use to quit isn't as important as finding a technique that works — something that will help you stop smoking for good. Enlist support from friends and family and remind yourself regularly of the benefits of quitting, including a better chance of becoming pregnant!

In addition, alcohol can also interfere with conception. Most studies show that women who drink moderate to heavy amounts of alcohol take longer to get pregnant than do women who drink less. Moderate intake typically equates to three to 13 drinks a week, while heavy intake is usually defined as more than 14 drinks a week. In men, heavy alcohol use is associated with reduced testosterone production, impotence and decreased sperm production.

Tobacco If you smoke, you likely know how hard it is to quit. But there's no question that tobacco is harmful to your health. And studies of thousands of women have consistently shown that smoking can significantly decrease fertility. Substances found in cigarette smoke are known to damage ovarian follicles — tiny sacs carrying immature eggs — and to cause premature aging of the ovaries. Tobacco can also decrease male fertility by reducing sperm quality and altering hormone levels.

In addition, smoking during pregnancy increases your risk of stillbirth, of your baby being born too early or too small, and of sudden infant death syndrome (SIDS) after birth. It may even damage your baby girl's ovaries, causing decreased fertility in your daughter, or reduced sperm production in your baby boy.

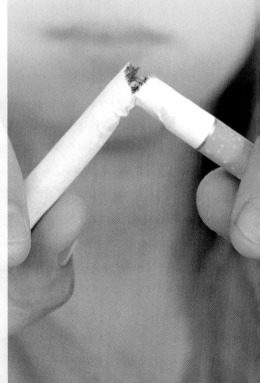

Cigarette smoke contains literally thousands of harmful chemicals. Two toxins especially — carbon monoxide and nicotine — can reduce the flow of oxygen to the developing baby. And nicotine, which causes your heartbeat and blood pressure to increase and your blood vessels to constrict while smoking, can also decrease the supply of nutrients that pass through the placenta.

Fortunately, quitting smoking improves your overall health, as well as your chances of conceiving and delivering a healthy baby. If you're ready to break the habit, ask your care provider for help. He or she can help you weigh the benefits and risks of various smoking cessation products and provide support.

Other recreational drugs Marijuana is the most commonly used illicit drug among women of reproductive age. There's been limited research into the effects of marijuana use in regard to fertility and pregnancy, but it's strongly recommended that couples trying to become pregnant avoid it.

Marijuana use has been linked to decreased fertility in both men and women. In females, there's evidence marijuana may disrupt normal menstrual and ovulation cycles. In men, marijuana is thought to decrease sperm quality and testosterone levels. It's also thought to decrease the ability of sperm to move quickly and has been linked to sperm abnormalities. These factors can make it difficult for a woman to become pregnant.

Other recreational drugs, such as anabolic steroids and cocaine, also can affect fertility, producing menstrual irregularities in women and sperm and semen abnormalities in men.

Other toxic substances Though not common, it's possible that the environ-ment that you work in may be hampering your efforts to become pregnant. Think about your daily routine and whether you encounter any substances on a regular basis that may be harmful. Some examples include lead, mercury, ionizing radiation (X-rays), drugs used to treat cancer, nitrous oxide and mixed solvents.

If you work in a manufacturing or health care setting, you may be exposed to some of these substances. Industries in the United States are required by federal law to have material safety data sheets on file that report hazardous substances in the workplace and to make this information available to employees. Generally, though, if you and the company you work for follow established safety protocols for handling or working around toxic substances, your risk of being harmed is low.

Tell your care provider about any part of your job that exposes you to chemicals, drugs or radiation. Also tell your care provider about any equipment you use to minimize your exposure. This may include gowns, gloves, masks and ventilation systems. Your care provider can use this information to determine whether a risk exists and, if so, what can be done to eliminate or reduce it.

Some women also are concerned about exposure to certain chemicals used in plastics, such as bisphenol A (BPA) and phthalates. BPA is used to make hard, polycarbonate plastics, which are often used in water bottles. It's also used in the waxy coating applied to some canned goods. Phthalates are used to make soft, flexible plastic containers and polyvinyl chloride (PVC) products. These chemicals have received a fair amount of attention because of studies suggesting they may pose health risks and specific risks to a developing baby in the uterus.

Investigations on the relationship between these substances and reproductive health and pregnancy have yet to reach firm conclusions. Many manufacturers now produce containers and bottles that are free of BPA. But there are certain precautions you can take to avoid being exposed to these substances, such as:

- Avoid using containers that have No. 7 on the bottom, since they may contain BPA, or No. 3, which may be made with phthalates.
- Don't microwave food in plastic containers. Use glass instead.
- Reduce your use of canned foods.
- Opt for glass, stainless steel, porcelain or BPA-free plastics to store food or liquids.

DIET

Another important aspect of your lifestyle that's important to good health and that may have an effect on your chances of becoming pregnant is your diet. While there's no such thing as a "fertility diet," there is some evidence that certain foods may help boost fertility. Undoubtedly, eating a balanced diet is essential to good health and it can help you lose weight, which itself is likely to improve your ability to conceive more than any particular food. But certain foods may be worth a try, too.

In the next chapter, you'll learn more about the best foods to eat and drink and those you might want to avoid as you and your partner get pregnancy-ready.

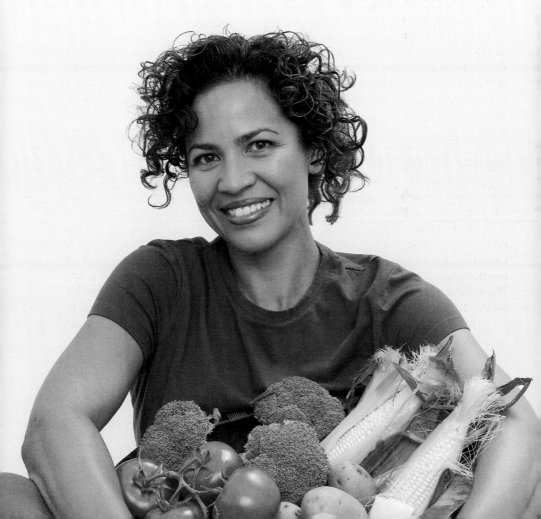

Dawn's Story

When my husband and I got married in our mid-20s, we were eager to start a family.

Sure, I'd been told I had polycystic ovary syndrome when I was in college — a hormonal disorder that can make it difficult to conceive a baby. But I had no time to worry about that because we became pregnant almost instantly. I delivered a baby boy just 13 months after our wedding.

We wanted to have our children close together, so when our son was 15 months old, we started trying for another baby. We expected to get pregnant as easily as we did the first time, but this time it wasn't so easy.

Month after month after month went by, and still we weren't pregnant. Initially, I just chalked it up to stress. After all, I was working full time as a nurse while going to school to get my Bachelor of Science degree in nursing — in addition to taking care of our son. But then we found out that my polycystic ovary syndrome had kicked in. I wasn't ovulating or getting my period.

After 10 months without success, my gynecologist prescribed clomiphene citrate (Clomid), a drug that helps stimulate ovulation. My husband and I were optimistic that Clomid was our ticket to a baby … but we still didn't get pregnant.

What made it even harder was that it seemed like everywhere we looked people were having babies. A month didn't go by that friends weren't announcing their pregnancies. Some, who married around the same time we did, had already had three children. It seemed so unfair.

A year and a half after we started trying for our second child, and after six months on Clomid, my gynecologist referred us to a specialist in reproductive medicine.

By this time, I was pretty depressed — not to mention stressed out. What I soon learned was that with all I had going on in my life, I had quit taking care of myself and had started packing on the pounds. The weight had crept up on me so gradually that I hadn't even realized it, but the signs were undeniable — even my work scrubs were getting too tight.

When I stepped on the scale for the first time in a long time, I was shocked to learn what I weighed. I figured I'd gained about 30 pounds, but clearly I was in denial. I had gained 70 pounds. The doctor told me I was nearly morbidly obese.

"Before we can do anything," she said, "you have to lose some weight."

I was devastated. I thought, "What have I done?" All I'd wanted was to have another child, and instead I'd damaged my chances. I was so upset at myself for making it even harder to conceive.

I had my pity cry. I let myself feel the anger and the sorrow. And then I decided to do something about it. I met with a nutritionist, who worked with me on setting and meeting goals. She taught me that if I could meet my short-term goals, I could get to my long-term goal: Losing enough weight to get pregnant.

I started incorporating healthy habits into my daily life. I wrote down everything I ate. I learned to follow the food pyramid when planning my meals, preparing more vegetables than starches.

I stopped drinking calories: Instead of buying 400-calorie cups of flavored coffee, I started brewing my own without the cream. I portioned out serving sizes of snacks into baggies — three cookies, eight crackers — so that I wouldn't eat more than I should.

I also found opportunities in my busy day to move more. I worked on the seventh floor, so instead of taking the elevator all the way up, I started by walking up two flights of stairs, and then getting on the elevator. My husband made the commitment to getting healthier, too. He took up refereeing basketball.

At the time, losing weight felt like a terribly slow process. But just over five months later, I'd lost nearly 70 pounds. I was at the weight I'd been when we conceived our son — and just 10 pounds from my goal weight.

When I visited my doctor in November of that year, she said, "Make it through the holidays and you can start trying Clomid again in January."

I was ecstatic. I made it through the holidays without any setbacks. I completed an evaluation with my doctor in December, and then in January I was given Clomid.

By this point, we'd been trying to get pregnant for more than two years. But now, with my weight in check, we had more options than ever. After starting the Clomid, we also chose to do intrauterine insemination (IUI) with my husband's sperm. I had many hopes for this procedure and high expectations that this would be the month that we would finally get pregnant.

My doctor told me that I could take a pregnancy test two weeks after the insemination procedure. I didn't sleep the whole night before. I just kept thinking, "I can take a pregnancy test tomorrow!" Finally, at 4 a.m., I couldn't wait any longer. I went to the bathroom, took the test and started crying. I ran back into our room and jumped on my husband.

"Wake up! Wake up!" I yelled. "It's positive!"

Nine months later — and almost three years after we'd started trying to have another baby — I delivered a little boy. When he turned 16 months old, I became pregnant again, this time with a girl.

My husband and I have continued living a healthy lifestyle, only now we share our personal goals with our children. We've maintained our weight loss and, as a family, we stay active. Our two boys play basketball, and my husband coaches. We play football or baseball or tag together. We live on a bike path and go on rides together. We adopted a large dog into our family so that we're committed to daily walks.

We know that this lifestyle made it possible for us to have our family — and we want to stay healthy for many years to come.

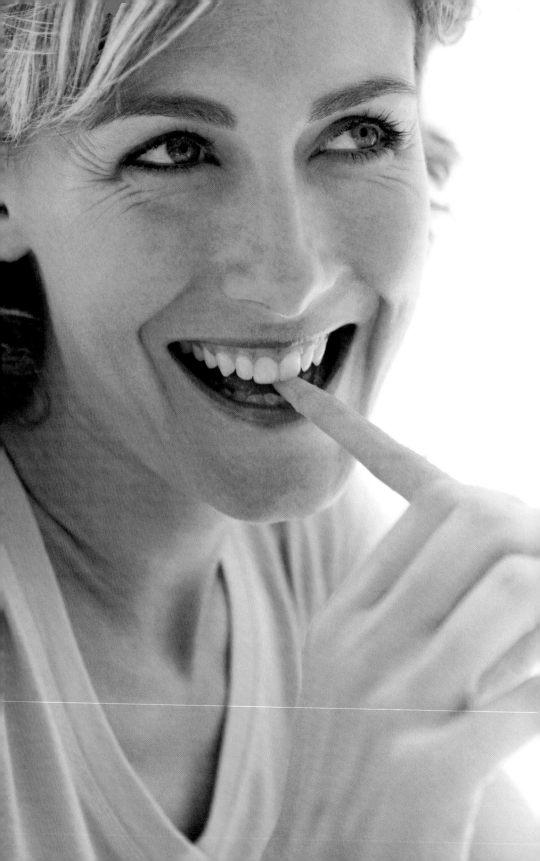

Eating to conceive

As you might guess, what you put into your body matters. Like other aspects of life, what you eat and drink on a daily basis can have a big impact on your health. And, as it turns out, it may even affect your fertility. Although there's no silver bullet when it comes to food and fertility, there are certain groups of nutrients that may influence the process of ovulation in your favor. And there are other nutrients that may do the opposite, impede fertility.

The largest body of evidence to the effects of diet on fertility so far comes from a longstanding group of studies related to women's health started in the mid-1970s. They are known collectively as the Nurses' Health Study. Every couple of years investigators collect questionnaires filled out by hundreds of thousands of registered nurses answering questions related to oral contraceptive use, pregnancy history, menopausal status, diet, smoking and other lifestyle factors. So far, three groups of women (cohorts) have been established.

A group of investigators, led by Dr. Walter Willett from the Harvard School of Public Health, developed a plan to study how diet might affect fertility in women participating in the second round of the Nurses' Health Study. About 18,000 women in the study said they were trying to conceive. Over the next eight years, the researchers found that most of these women had no trouble getting pregnant, but some of them did experience problems, including several hundred who had problems with ovulation. This group was described as having "ovulatory infertility." By comparing the dietary habits of the women who got pregnant quite easily with the dietary habits of women who had ovulation difficulties, the researchers were able to draw some interesting conclusions.

Note: A few study results are also emerging for the relationship between nutrition and male fertility. You can read more about improving male fertility in Chapter 4.

With few exceptions, eating to conceive looks much the same as eating for good health. So if you already eat a healthy diet, you're well on your way to paving the road for conception. And if you need to make some changes to the way you eat, you'll be doing your heart, blood vessels, brain and other body systems plenty of good, in addition to your reproductive system. Plus, eating a healthy diet can help you reach a healthy weight if you have weight concerns, which can further improve your chances of conception. What's not to like? Read on to find out what Dr. Willett and his colleagues discovered.

CARBOHYDRATES: NATURAL, NOT PROCESSED

Carbohydrates have gotten a bit of a bad rap in the last decade or so, especially when it comes to weight loss. A number of popular diets emphasized eating very few carbs or no carbs at all. Carbs aren't all bad, though. In fact, most of the time, they're your body's main source of energy.

But when it comes to optimizing your chances of getting pregnant — and really, your health in general — not all carbs are created equal. Based on results from the Nurses' Health Study, some types of carbs appear to be kinder to your fertility than others.

Carbs explained Carbohydrates are a macronutrient found in many different foods and beverages. When you consume carbs, your body uses them to make blood sugar (glucose), the fuel that travels through your bloodstream to give your body the energy it needs to function.

There are two basic types of carbohydrates: complex and simple. Complex carbs include foods containing starch and dietary fibers, such as starchy vege-

tables, legumes and whole-grain products — foods made with the whole grain still intact as opposed to refined. Think whole wheat versus white bread. Simple carbs include naturally occurring sugars found in fruits, some vegetables and milk, as well as sugars added during food processing and refining.

Carbs and blood sugar Carbs can also be classified by the way they affect your blood sugar levels (glycemic index). Simple carbs that are easily absorbed and quickly converted to glucose — especially those that are highly processed, such as white bread, candy, cake and many breakfast cereals — are high on the glycemic index. These kinds of carbohydrates cause an abrupt and often sharp increase in your blood sugar.

Carbs that are low on the glycemic index generally are of the more complex variety. They contain more fiber, take longer to be digested and provide energy over a longer period of time. These include foods such as oatmeal, barley, brown rice, vegetables, fruits, chickpeas, lentils and beans.

Two hormones from your pancreas help regulate your level of blood sugar. The hormone insulin moves sugar from your blood into your cells when your blood sugar level is high. The hormone glucagon helps release the sugar stored in your liver when your blood sugar level is low. This process helps keep your body fueled and ensures a natural balance in blood sugar.

If you eat too many carbs that are high on the glycemic index you may be more prone to large spikes in your blood sugar level or to chronically high blood sugar levels. When your blood sugar and insulin levels stay high, or cycle up and down rapidly, your body has trouble responding and over time this can contribute to insulin resistance. In this condition, your pancreas still produces insulin but your body doesn't respond to normal amounts and your blood sugar level stays high. The pancreas continues to make more insulin until the body catches up and then blood sugar levels can come crashing down. Insulin resistance is associated with a number of health problems, including type 2 diabetes and heart disease, but it may also be associated with fertility problems.

Carbs and fertility The Nurses' Health Study found that the total amount of carbohydrates women took in didn't make a difference in terms of fertility. But women who consumed primarily simple and refined carbohydrates — a diet with a high glycemic load — were at greater risk of not ovulating than were women whose diets registered a lower glycemic load. These women were described as having a greater risk of ovulatory infertility. On the other hand, women who ate mostly low-glycemic foods were at a lower risk of ovulation problems.

This may have to do with increased insulin resistance and its effects on reproductive hormones. Using computer models of the women's diets, however, the investigators also discovered that consuming refined carbs at the expense of naturally occurring fats — substituting a bag of chips for a handful of nuts, for example — also increased the risk of ovulatory infertility. So it may be that natural fats, particularly unsaturated ones, improve ovulation, as well. More on that in a minute.

What's the bottom line? Whenever you can, skip the french fries, cookies, and oversized portions of pasta or rice in favor of whole grains, veggies, whole fruits and beans. This might mean packing a lunch more often or making differ-

ent choices at your favorite restaurant, but the payoff may just be worth it. The latter group of foods will provide your body with healthy, long-lasting fuel, keep your blood sugar in balance and your hormones running smoothly, and potentially make it easier for you to conceive.

DIETARY FATS: GO FOR GOOD FATS

When it comes to fats and fertility, there's a particular villain: trans fat. In the Nurses' Health Study, the research team found that neither total fat intake nor the intake of specific fats, such as saturated, monounsaturated or polyunsaturated fat, had any bearing on ovulatory function.

But they did find that consuming trans fat in place of healthier unsaturated fat led to a significant increase in the risk of ovulatory infertility. Specifically, replacing just 2 percent of calories from monounsaturated fat with 2 percent from trans fat more than doubled the risk of ovulatory infertility. That's potentially a big deal.

Phasing out trans fat Fortunately, getting trans fat out of your diet will soon become easier. The Food and Drug Administration (FDA) has announced it will require the food industry to gradually phase out all trans fat in foods, calling the fat a public health threat. This is good for your health and your fertility.

Although trans fats occur naturally in some foods, most are made during food processing through partial hydrogenation of unsaturated fats. This process creates fats that are easier to cook with and less likely to spoil than are naturally occurring oils. These fats are called industrial or synthetic trans fats.

Scientists aren't sure exactly why, but the addition of hydrogen to oil increases your cholesterol more than do other types of fats. Research studies show that synthetic trans fat can increase unhealthy low-density lipoprotein (LDL) cholesterol and lower healthy high-density lipoprotein (HDL) cholesterol. This can increase your risk of cardiovascular disease.

Look at the label Commercial baked goods, such as crackers, cookies and cakes — and many fried foods, such as doughnuts and french fries — often contain trans fat. Shortenings and stick margarines also are sources of trans fat.

In recent years, trans fat has been showing up less in food products due to its health risks, and now the fat is being banned. Until the phase-out deadline, you can check for trans fat by looking at the nutrition label.

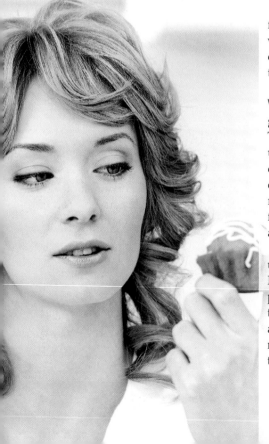

It doesn't take much to get you to levels research suggests is bad for fertility. Consider that 2 percent of total calorie intake for someone eating 2,000 calories a day equates to 200 calories, or roughly 4 grams, of trans fat.

What does that mean in real terms? Food manufacturers in the United States and many other countries list the amount of trans fat a food contains on the product's nutrition label. But when it comes to deciphering nutrition labels, things can get a little tricky. In the United States, if a food has less than 0.5 grams of trans fat per serving, the food label can read 0 grams trans fat. Though that's a small amount of trans fat, if you eat multiple servings of foods with just a little less than 0.5 grams of trans fat, you could get to 4 grams pretty fast. A little margarine on your toast, a few cookies made with shortening, an order of fries and a doughnut — it adds up.

An easy way to find out whether a food contains trans fat is to look for the words *partially hydrogenated* vegetable oil in the ingredients list. That's another term for trans fat.

What should you eat? OK, so you've got the message — no more doughnuts. The truth is an occasional doughnut is unlikely to do you much harm. But you do want to avoid a regular diet of foods containing trans fat or partially hydrogenated vegetable oil. Plus, these types of foods are usually packed with calories and not a lot of nutrition.

Instead, go for fats that are found naturally in foods, especially plant foods. Monounsaturated fat — found in olive, peanut and canola oils — is a healthy option for cooking. Nuts and avocados are also good choices because they contain monounsaturated fats. Research shows that monounsaturated fats may benefit

GOOD FATS

Monounsaturated fat	Polyunsaturated fat
Olive oil	Soybean oil
Canola oil	Corn oil
Peanut oil	Safflower oil
Avocados	Fatty fish (salmon, mackerel, albacore tuna)
Nuts	Soy milk

BAD FATS

Saturated fat	Trans fat (being phased out)
Fatty cuts of meat	Packaged snack foods (chips, crackers)
Chicken with the skin	Cookies, cakes and pastries
Butter	Fried foods
Cheese	Frozen pizza
Ice cream	Stick margarine

insulin levels and blood sugar control, which as mentioned previously, may help improve ovulatory fertility. Polyunsaturated fats are another healthy alternative. Sources of polyunsaturated fats include fish and soy products and a variety of vegetable oils.

Here are some tips to help you make over the fat in your diet:

▶ Read food labels and ingredient lists and avoid products with partially hydrogenated vegetable oil listed among the first ingredients.

▶ Sauté with olive oil instead of butter.

▶ Use olive oil in salad dressings and marinades. Use canola oil when baking.

▶ Use egg substitutes instead of whole eggs when possible.

▶ Sprinkle slivered nuts or sunflower seeds on salads instead of bacon bits or croutons.

▶ Snack on a small handful of nuts rather than potato chips or processed crackers. Unsalted peanuts, walnuts, almonds and pistachios are good choices. Air-popped popcorn also is a healthy choice, provided it's not loaded with butter and salt.

▶ Try nonhydrogenated peanut butter or other nonhydrogenated nut-butter spreads. Spread them on celery, bananas or whole-grain toast.

▶ Add avocado slices, rather than cheese or mayonnaise, to your sandwich.

▶ Prepare fish such as salmon and mackerel instead of meat twice a week. Limit sizes to 4 ounces of cooked seafood per serving.

PROTEIN:
EAT MORE BEANS AND NUTS

Where's the beef? Or pork or chicken or turkey! Meat and poultry are a big part of the American diet. And they provide your body with a key nutrient — protein. Proteins are naturally found within your body. They form the building blocks of all your cells, tissues and organs. They also repair body structures, produce body chemicals, carry nutrients and regulate body processes. These hard-working proteins are not permanent, however. They're constantly being broken down.

To replace them, your body uses protein obtained from your diet.

Meat and poultry are important sources of protein, but they're not the only ones. Seafood, eggs, beans and peas, soy-based foods, nuts, and seeds also are good sources of protein. And if you're goal is to get pregnant, you might want to pay attention to some of these other protein-rich foods, especially the plant-based ones. Because while there's nothing wrong with enjoying a juicy steak on occasion, it does appear that getting most of your protein from animal sources can put you at a fertility disadvantage when compared with getting more from plant sources.

One of the dietary factors the women in the Nurses' Health Study reported on was protein intake. When evaluating their responses — and after accounting for other factors that might affect fertility such as body weight, smoking and physical activity — researchers noticed that the women who reported the highest intake of protein were more likely to have ovulation problems than were women who came in at the lowest end. Researchers also noted that adding one serving of meat (mostly chicken and turkey among these particular women) a day, while keeping calorie intake constant, was as-sociated with a 32 percent greater risk of ovulatory infertility.

The research team then plugged the data in to a set of computer models to see what would happen if you started substi-tuting one source of energy (calories) for another. Consuming 5 percent of total energy intake from meat or poultry in-stead of carbohydrates was associated with a 19 percent greater risk of ovulatory infertility. On the other hand, getting 5 percent more energy from vegetable pro-teins instead of carbohydrates resulted in a 43 percent lower risk of ovulatory infer-tility. And choosing vegetable proteins over animal proteins yielded an even lower risk of ovulatory infertility — more than 50 percent. These last two substitu-tions were especially true for women older than 32 years of age.

A protein plan If you're like many Americans, meat probably plays a big role at mealtimes. And it's not always easy to change eating patterns, especially if you're cooking for others beside your-self. Plus, you're often cooking in a hurry and you may not have time to dream up new recipes.

But making small changes here and there can add up. It helps to think ahead. At the beginning of the week, make a

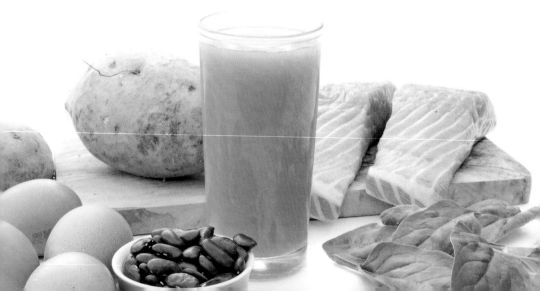

Q. HOW MUCH PROTEIN DO I NEED?

A. In general, it's recommended that women age 19 and older get around 46 grams of protein a day. To give you an idea of the protein content of food, here are some examples:

- 1 ounce almonds (24 nuts) = 6 grams protein
- 1 cup milk = 8 grams protein
- 1 bagel = 8 grams protein
- 8-ounce container yogurt = 12 grams protein
- 1 cup black beans = 15 grams protein
- 3 ounces cod fish = 15 grams protein
- ½ boneless, skinless chicken breast = 26 grams protein

meal plan for the next several days that includes more sources of vegetable protein and fewer sources of animal protein. Planning ahead also allows you to arrive at the supermarket armed with a list, so you don't get distracted and buy foods that are unhealthy.

For your meal plan, you might think about instituting one meatless dinner a week, for example. And get into beans and peas. These are often referred to as legumes, which essentially refer to a large family of plants whose seeds develop inside pods and are usually dried for easy storage. (Green beans and green peas don't fall under legumes; they're considered a different type of vegetable.) Legumes are high in protein and make excellent substitutes for animal sources of protein. They're also versatile and inexpensive.

Common types of legumes include:
- White and navy beans
- Lima beans
- Pinto and black beans
- Black-eyed peas
- Split peas
- Brown and red lentils
- Chickpeas (garbanzo beans)

There are lots of ways that you can incorporate legumes into everyday meals.

Here are just a few suggestions:
- Feature beans, peas or lentils in soups, stews or casseroles, or pair them with rice.
- Add chickpeas or black beans to salads.
- Use pureed beans as a base for dips and spreads.

Eggs, milk and milk products also are sources of protein. Nuts provide protein as well as healthy unsaturated fats. Soy products are another source and include foods such as tofu and miso.

DAIRY PRODUCTS: CREAMIER IS BETTER

Wouldn't it be great if there were at least some kind of perk to this whole trying to get pregnant thing? Funny you should ask. Because when it comes to milk and other dairy products, you might be surprised to find out that the richer and creamier, the better for conception. Based on data from the Nurses' Health Study, whole-fat dairy products seem more likely to improve your chances of conception than do low-fat and no-fat varieties.

CAFFEINE AND CONCEPTION

If you're like the vast majority of American women, caffeine has a definite place in your daily diet. Whether it's in your morning coffee or tea, or in a soda or energy drink, caffeine is there to pick you up and help you make it through the day. Advice on caffeine as part of a healthy diet has gone back and forth in the past. And because limits on caffeine are generally recommended during pregnancy, many women who are trying to conceive wonder if it might be affecting their chances of getting pregnant.

To date, there's no real evidence that having a cup or two of coffee a day has any harmful effect on fertility. A few studies observed a decrease in fertility associated with caffeine intake, especially at high levels of consumption (more than 5 cups of coffee a day). But subsequent studies, including ones that accounted for other factors that might also affect fertility, haven't found a similar link. Other research has found decreased odds of conception in women who consumed sodas but increased fertility in women who drank tea. So it isn't always easy to determine whether caffeine itself, free of other confounding factors, has any kind of effect on the ability to get pregnant.

Despite the lack of definitive data, most reproductive experts recommend limiting your consumption of caffeine to about 200 to 300 milligrams a day if you're trying to conceive. And keep in mind what you take with your coffee or tea. Nondairy creamers often contain partially hydrogenated oils (trans fats) that can have their own set of harmful effects on your heart health and possibly your reproductive health. (See page 35 for more on trans fats.)

Coffee may be the most popular source of caffeine, but it's not the only one. And even within the coffee category, amount of caffeine content varies according to roast, brewing method and portion size. One large coffee from Dunkin' Donuts or a venti coffee from Starbucks is enough to put you well over the recommendation of 200 to 300 milligrams. The roast also is important. Light roast coffee beans actually have more caffeine in them than do dark roast beans. The longer the beans are roasted, the more caffeine is lost.

Other beverages and even foods can contain caffeine, and they may add up to give you more caffeine than you think. Check the chart on caffeine content to see where you fall in terms of your caffeine consumption.

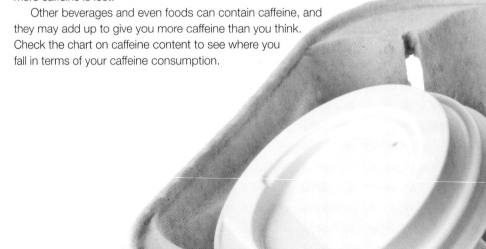

Caffeine amounts

Food or beverage	Size	Caffeine (mg)
Dunkin' Donuts coffee	Large, 20 oz.	436
Starbucks coffee	Venti, 20 oz.	415
Starbucks coffee	Grande, 16 oz.	330
Starbucks coffee	Tall, 12 oz.	260
Dunkin' Donuts cappuccino	Large, 20 oz.	151
Starbucks latte or cappuccino	Grande, 16 oz.	150
Keurig coffee K-Cup	1 cup, 8 oz.	75-150
McDonald's coffee	Large, 16 oz.	133
Brewed coffee (at home)	8 oz.	102-200
Starbucks Tazo chai tea latte	Grande, 16 oz.	115
Black tea	8 oz.	30-80
Green tea	8 oz.	35-60
Mountain Dew	20-oz. bottle	90
Diet Coke	20-oz. bottle	78
Pepsi	20-oz. bottle	63
5-hour Energy drink	1.9 oz.	208
Monster Energy drink	16 oz.	160
Red Bull	8.4 oz.	80
Cold Stone Creamery mocha ice cream	12 oz.	52
TCBY coffee frozen yogurt	Large, 13.4 oz.	42
Hershey's Special Dark chocolate bar	1.5 oz.	20
Excedrin Migraine	2 tablets	130
Midol Complete	2 caplets	120

Center for Science in the Public Interest

As with protein and carbs, total intake of dairy products didn't appear to affect the risk of ovulatory infertility either way. But the researchers did observe a significant pattern when it came to low-fat versus high-fat dairy foods. After accounting for other factors that might affect fertility, they noted that eating a lot of low-fat dairy products, such as low-fat milk and yogurt, was linked to a greater risk of ovulatory problems. The opposite was true when it came to high-fat dairy products, such as whole milk, ice cream and cheese. Eating these foods actually reduced the risk of ovulatory problems.

If you're thinking, "This is the opposite of what I thought I was supposed to do," you're right. Nutrition experts recommend sticking with low-fat dairy products and skim milk once you reach the age of 2! This advice is mostly to help people avoid consuming unnecessary calories, since you can get the same amount of calcium and other nutrients from low-fat dairy products as you can from the high-fat ones.

But it takes only one cup of whole milk a day — while remembering to keep total daily calories constant — to potentially reduce your risk of ovulatory disorders. Likewise, eating ice cream once or twice a week may help improve fertility.

Before you splurge on a pint of your favorite ice cream, though, bear in mind that you want to keep your total calorie intake constant. Gaining weight can have its own set of fertility problems. We're talking small servings of full-fat dairy products that are substituted for other sources of energy in your diet. For example, you might consider eating less meat at dinner and having a half-cup of ice cream or some cheese and fruit for dessert. Or ask for whole milk in your latte and skip the muffin.

Once fertility is no longer a concern for you, you can switch back to low-fat dairy products. And if you don't like milk or dairy products, don't sweat it. There are other ways to enhance fertility.

FOCUS ON YOUR HEALTH

It's tempting to say that if you follow the dietary suggestions discussed in this chapter, you'll definitely increase your chances of getting pregnant. But you also have to remember that fertility is a complex process. Your fertility is affected by a broad range of factors in addition to your diet. These include other aspects of your lifestyle, your genes, the environment, and other factors that may be out of your control. Also, the suggestions represented here are based on results from just a few studies, which although well-designed, still need to be confirmed by other independent research studies.

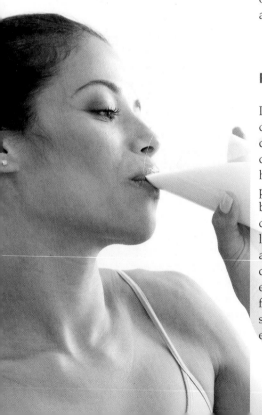

FERTILITY FOODS THROUGHOUT HISTORY

Twenty-first century researchers aren't the first ones to explore possible connections between food and fertility. Since ancient times, people have searched for foods that might enhance sexual performance and conception.

Between the first and seventh centuries A.D., varieties of orchid bulbs, arugula and the flesh of a North African lizard called a skink were considered reliable aphrodisiacs. Other popular ingredients included anise, basil, carrots, pistachio nuts, turnips and river snails. Dill, lentils and lettuce, however, were believed to have the opposite effect.

Mandrake root was perceived to have fertility-enhancing powers in the Near East and is mentioned in the book of Genesis. Mandrake root does, in fact, have physiological effects but mostly on the lethal side!

A cure for infertility supposedly prescribed in a tale from *The Book of the Thousand Nights and One Night* involved a concoction of opium, skink meat, frankincense and coriander mixed with honey, which was to be consumed after a meal of spicy mutton and pigeon.

Spanish fly (cantharides), a powder made from bright green beetles from North Africa, was banned from sale in Moroccan markets in the 1990s because of its harmful properties, but it remains the stuff of tales and anecdotes related to male potency.

Herbal preparations became popular in the 16th and 17th centuries in Europe, accompanied by long lists of ingredients and specific instructions on preparation. The sweet potato was often cited as an ingredient in 17th century European aphrodisiac recipes and the plain potato as well.

Oysters have been featured in literature and folklore as aphrodisiacs. Beer and wine have been noted as aphrodisiacs, although even in the Middle Ages excess consumption of alcohol was considered to reverse sexual potency.

Some have likened the search for true aphrodisiacs and fertility foods to trying to find the pot of gold at the end of the rainbow. Probably so. Yet it's also worth noting that Hippocrates' proposal for a healthy lifestyle still fits today: "exercise, food, drink, sleep and the pleasures of sex, all in moderation."

Nonetheless, with the exception of the recommendations on dairy products perhaps, most of these findings fall in line with the general health recommendations that are made to almost everyone — eat more fruits, vegetables and whole grains; stick with healthy fats; choose a variety of protein sources, including plant-based ones; and try to keep your calorie intake within a healthy range.

If you focus on these general rules of good eating, in addition to exercising regularly and not smoking, you'll be doing your health one of the biggest favors possible. And as an added bonus, you may also be giving your fertility a boost.

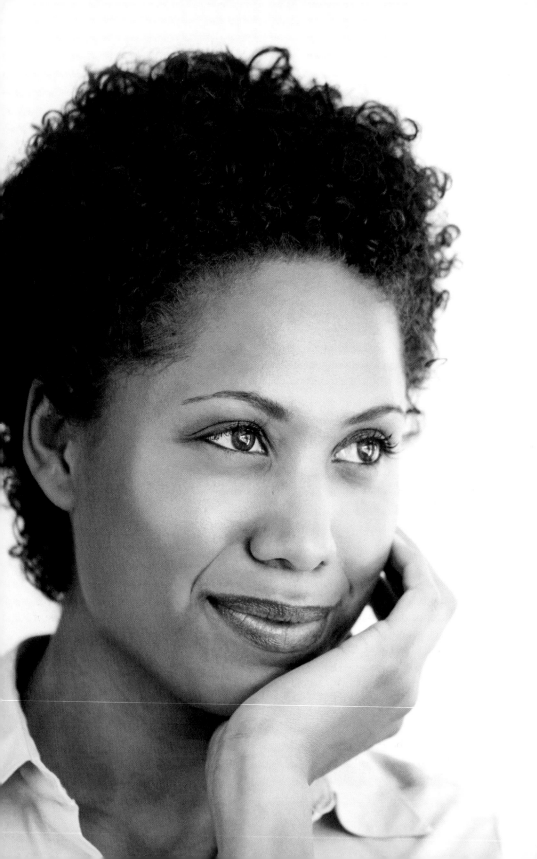

CHAPTER 3

Additional preparations

In the first two chapters, we talked about lifestyle changes that can help improve your fertility so that you're at maximum health when you're ready to try to have a baby. In this chapter, we look at some final steps to prepare your body for conception. In general, a healthy mom plus a healthy dad equals a healthy baby. Your first step toward making sure that both of you are "a go" is scheduling an appointment with your doctor or other health care provider, whether it be your family doctor, obstetrician-gynecologist, nurse practitioner or a midwife. A preconception visit gives you and your care provider a chance to identify any potential risks to a healthy pregnancy and establish ways to minimize those risks.

Ideally, both partners should attend the preconception visit. It's important to understand early on that both of you are in this together. A man's health and lifestyle can be just as important as a woman's when it comes to conception and the health of the baby. Here are some of the topics your care provider is likely to discuss with you at that initial visit.

GOING OFF BIRTH CONTROL

Perhaps you thought it would take a while after stopping your birth control pills before you could become pregnant. You may be surprised. If you've been taking birth control pills, ovulation is possible as soon as two weeks after you stop taking the pill — although it can take longer for some women. The same is true for the birth control patch or ring.

Unlike what you may have heard or read, you don't need to take a pill-free break before trying to conceive. However, it's typically easier to estimate when you ovulated and when your baby is due if you have at least one normal period before conceiving. If you want to wait a few months, use a backup form of birth control, such as a condom, a contraceptive sponge or natural family planning, until the time is right.

If you've been taking the daily continuous form of the pill — the kind you take every day with no break for a period to happen — the facts are basically the same. Recent studies show that when women stop taking this type of birth control, they return to normal cycles within a month or so.

If you've been using certain types of long-acting birth control — such as progestin implants or injections — your return to fertility might take a little longer. Implants need to be removed and injections need time to wear off. Still, most women are back to their normal menstrual cycles within three to five months regardless of the birth control they used. Those trying to get pregnant usually conceive within 12 months of stopping any type of reversible birth control. If you have an intrauterine device (IUD), fertility is generally restored immediately after the device is removed.

MEDICATIONS AND SUPPLEMENTS

If you use any types of medications, creams or other products — prescription or nonprescription — it's a good idea to talk with a care provider at your preconception visit about what you should continue to take. Depending on the product and your overall health, your care provider might recommend changing doses, switching to something else or stopping the product before you conceive.

Not all pills are bad, and some serve a very important purpose. But as you probably know, some medications can cause birth defects. Common examples include thalidomide (Thalomid), prescribed for multiple myeloma and other diseases, and isotretinoin (Amnesteem, Claravis), for severe acne. These drugs can cause serious problems for an unborn baby, such as malformed limbs, heart disease, mental retardation and other irreversible conditions. People who take these drugs are often required to follow a strict pregnancy avoidance plan.

For most medications people take on a regular basis, it's difficult to say what their effects are on pregnancy. A big reason is that pregnant women are almost always excluded from drug trials to avoid any possible harm to the fetus. Based on the evidence that's available, the stage of the pregnancy also plays an important role in how a medication can affect the baby. The first eight weeks of pregnancy, when the baby's organs and limbs are forming, can be a particularly vulnerable time, which is why it's so important to review your medications before you conceive.

When it comes to prescribing medications to women who are pregnant or hoping to become pregnant, most doctors try to weigh the potential harm the medication might cause to the baby against the drug's possible benefits for the mom. For example, if you take medication to keep your asthma under control, your doctor will most likely have you continue with your treatment plan to keep you healthy prior to and throughout your pregnancy.

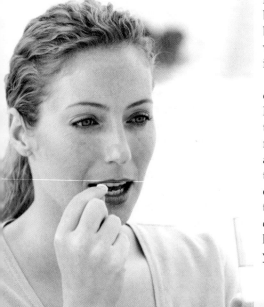

Q. WHAT IF I TAKE ANTIDEPRESSANTS?

A. Women who are on antidepressant medications and considering pregnancy are often concerned about their situation. They worry the medications they take may harm the baby. Maybe this is you. If you're taking antidepressants and are trying to get pregnant, it may be tempting to go off of them for the baby's sake. But while taking any sort of medication carries a certain amount of risk for the baby, you also need to consider what can happen if you don't take the drug.

The physical changes and influx of hormones associated with pregnancy can have a strong impact on mood and emotions — which can deliver a double whammy to women with a history of depression or anxiety. In a large study of the use of antidepressants during pregnancy, investigators found that depression relapse was fairly common among all of the pregnant participants, but it was significantly more common among women who discontinued their medications just before conception or in early pregnancy. Risk of relapse was also higher among women who opted to decrease their doses. Untreated depression during pregnancy and after delivery poses its own set of risks:

Mom	Baby
Worsening of symptoms	Inadequate growth during pregnancy
Not practicing good self-care	Low birth weight
Inadequate weight gain	Developmental delay after birth
Weight loss	Cognitive impairment after birth
Preterm labor	
Difficulty bonding with newborn	
Inability to cope with stress of parenting	

Research on the effects of antidepressants on an unborn baby suggests the risks are low. Most women who take antidepressants during pregnancy have roughly the same outcomes as women who aren't on antidepressants. Potential risks to the baby may range from temporary problems after birth, such as mild tremors or rapid breathing, to more serious lung problems or heart defects. But the jury is still out on many of these possible complications, and more research is needed to make firm conclusions.

Most experts believe the benefits of maintaining treatment of moderate to severe depression in the mom-to-be outweigh the risks of antidepressant exposure to the baby. However, your care provider may suggest a change in medication. While many medications that treat depression work similarly, some are preferred over others. Paroxetine (Paxil), for instance, generally isn't recommended during pregnancy.

If you have mild depression, talk to your care provider about nonmedication therapies. Examples include cognitive behavioral therapy, which focuses on modifying distorted beliefs and behaviors, or interpersonal therapy, which helps you better express your emotions and communicate with others.

Don't forget to discuss with your care provider any over-the-counter drugs that you're currently taking or that you take on occasion — such as pain relievers or antihistamines. Your care provider can help you determine which are best for you. Generally, acetaminophen (Tylenol) for pain and cetirizine (Zyrtec) for seasonal allergies are considered safe during pregnancy. Keep in mind, though, that all medications, herbs and supplements carry risks. If you don't need it, you're probably better off not taking it.

PRENATAL VITAMINS

When you visit with your care provider one thing you'll likely be advised to do right away as you prepare for pregnancy is start taking prenatal vitamins. In fact, it's best to start taking prenatal vitamins three months before conception. Prenatal vitamins can help ensure you're getting enough folic acid, calcium and iron — essential nutrients during pregnancy.

Here's why these nutrients are so important:

▶ *Folic acid helps prevent neural tube defects.* These defects are serious abnormalities of the brain and spinal cord. A baby's neural tube, which becomes the brain and spinal cord, develops during the first month of pregnancy — perhaps before you even know that you're pregnant. Prepping your body beforehand with folic acid gives your baby his or her best shot at avoiding neural tube defects.

▶ *Calcium promotes strong bones and teeth for both mother and baby.* Calcium also helps your circulatory, muscular and nervous systems run normally.

WHICH PRENATAL VITAMIN IS BEST?

At your preconception visit, your care provider may recommend that you take a specific brand of prenatal vitamin or he or she may leave the choice up to you. Multiple kinds of prenatal vitamins are available over-the-counter (OTC) in pharmacies, ranging from generic store brands to a variety of name brands. You can also get prenatal vitamins by way of a prescription. So what does this mean? Are some better than others?

The truth is there's no single "best" prenatal vitamin. And for most women, less expensive generic versions are just as good as the brand-name ones.

In general, look for a prenatal vitamin that contains:

▶ Folic acid: 400 to 800 micrograms
▶ Calcium: 250 milligrams
▶ Iron: 30 milligrams
▶ Zinc: 11 milligrams
▶ Vitamin B-6: 2 milligrams
▶ Vitamin C: 85 milligrams
▶ Vitamin D: 600 international units

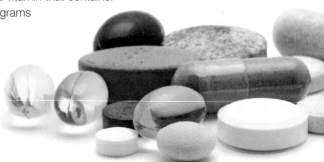

- *Iron supports the development of blood and muscle cells for both mother and baby.* Iron helps prevent anemia, a condition in which blood lacks adequate healthy red blood cells.
- *Prenatal vitamins may improve birth weight.* Some research suggests that prenatal vitamins decrease the risk of low birth weight.

If your prenatal vitamins make you feel queasy, try taking them at night or with a snack. Chewing gum or sucking on hard candy right after may help, too. If they seem to make you constipated, drink plenty of water, and include more fiber in your diet and physical activity in your daily routine. Also, ask your care provider about using a stool softener.

If these tips don't seem to help, ask about other options. Perhaps taking another type of prenatal vitamin or taking the nutrients separately may work better.

VACCINATIONS

In your quest to be as healthy as you can be as you prepare for pregnancy, one thing you want to be up to date on are your vaccinations. Certain infections — such as chickenpox (varicella), German measles (rubella) and hepatitis B — can be dangerous for an unborn baby. If your vaccinations aren't complete or you're unsure about your immunity to specific infections, your care provider may recommend you receive certain vaccines.

For some vaccinations, particularly rubella and varicella, you should avoid becoming pregnant for at least four weeks after getting immunized.

If you're planning on traveling abroad, your care provider may recommend other vaccines — such as hepatitis A, meningococcal or pneumococcal vaccines

Remember, prenatal vitamins are a complement to a healthy diet — not a substitute for good nutrition. They won't necessarily meet 100 percent of your vitamin and mineral needs, so it's important that you eat well. In addition, your care provider might suggest higher doses of certain nutrients depending on your circumstances.

Prescription vs. OTC

Some women require a higher dose of folic acid than is available in OTC prenatal vitamins, so their care providers may recommend a prescription version containing greater amounts of folic acid. Prescription prenatal vitamins usually contain 1 milligram (1,000 micrograms) of folic acid. In some circumstances, such as in the case of a woman who previously had a baby with a neural tube defect, the daily folic acid requirements are even higher.

If your care provider recommends that you get that much folic acid every day, it's safer to take one prescription pill than to attempt to take multiple over-the-counter pills to achieve the same dose. By trying to maximize your folic acid intake, you don't want to accidentally overdose on other vitamins or minerals.

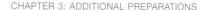

GUIDE TO VACCINATIONS AND PREGNANCY

Vaccine	Protects from	Before pregnancy	During pregnancy
Hepatitis A (inactivated)	Liver disease caused by hepatitis A virus, spread most often by fecal-contaminated food or water	Yes, if at risk	Yes, if at risk
Hepatitis B (inactivated)	Liver disease caused by hepatitis B virus, spread most often through body fluids; can become chronic	Yes, if at risk	Yes, if at risk
Human papillomavirus (HPV)	Common types of genital HPV that cause cervical cancer and genital warts	Yes, if under 26 years of age	No, under study
Influenza LAIV (live)	Seasonal flu and H1N1 (swine) flu	Yes, but avoid conception for four weeks	No
Influenza TIV (inactivated)	Seasonal flu and H1N1 (swine) flu	Yes	Yes
Meningococcal - polysaccharide (inactivated) - conjugate (inactivated)	Meningococcal infection caused by bacterium that can lead to brain infection (meningitis)	If indicated	If indicated

— to protect you from certain infections. If you traveled to a place where vaccinations are required, when you return home you may want to wait a few weeks before becoming pregnant to be certain you didn't pick up an infection.

Check the chart above to see which vaccines are appropriate before pregnancy and which ones are OK to receive during pregnancy.

Vaccines during pregnancy The best time to catch up on your vaccinations is before you get pregnant. Some vaccines are safe during pregnancy; others carry a potential risk. Generally, vaccines that contain killed (inactivated) viruses can be given during pregnancy because the risk to the baby is low. But vaccines that contain live viruses aren't recommended for pregnant women because the risk that the baby may become infected can't be ruled out.

Two vaccinations are almost always recommended during pregnancy because of their importance to mom and baby.

Flu (influenza) shot. The Centers for Disease Control and Prevention (CDC) recommends seasonal flu shots for anyone who will be pregnant during flu season — typically early October through late March — unless you have a severe allergy to eggs or you've had a severe

Vaccine	Protects from	Before pregnancy	During pregnancy
MMR	Measles, mumps and rubella (German measles)	Yes, but avoid conception for four weeks	No
Pneumococcal polysaccharide (inactivated)	Pneumococcal disease, a potentially serious infection; examples include pneumonia and meningitis	If indicated	If indicated
Tdap, one dose only (toxoid/ inactivated)	Tetanus, diphtheria and pertussis (whooping cough)	Yes, preferred	Yes, preferred
Tetanus/ diphtheria (Td) (toxoid)	Tetanus and diphtheria, a respiratory disease	Yes, Tdap preferred	Yes, Tdap preferred; optimal timing between 27 and 36 weeks of gestation
Varicella (live)	Chickenpox	Yes, but avoid conception for four weeks	No

Centers for Disease Control and Prevention

reaction to a previous flu vaccination. If you're trying to conceive, this vaccine is for you, too.

Pregnancy puts extra stress on your heart and lungs. Pregnancy can also affect your immune system. These factors increase the risk not only of getting the flu but of developing serious complications of the flu, such as pneumonia and respiratory distress. Flu complications may lead to miscarriage, premature labor or other pregnancy complications. A seasonal flu shot can help prevent these potential problems.

Better yet, a flu shot during pregnancy helps protect your baby after birth. Infants are at high risk of complications from the flu, but childhood flu vaccines can't begin until a baby is 6 months old. If you have a flu shot during pregnancy, the antibodies you develop will pass through the placenta to help protect your baby from the flu.

If you're uncertain whether you're pregnant, request the flu shot and not the nasal spray vaccine. The flu shot (influenza TIV) is made from an inactivated virus, so it's safe for both mother and baby during any stage of pregnancy. The nasal spray vaccine (influenza LAIV) is made from a live virus, which makes it less appropriate during pregnancy. Both the flu shot and the nasal spray vaccine are OK before pregnancy, but conception should be avoided for four weeks after vaccination with the nasal spray.

Each year, the Food and Drug Administration (FDA) determines the viruses to be used in the season's flu vaccine. The decision is based on which flu viruses were circulating the previous year and which vaccine viruses would offer the best protection against the circulating viruses. After 2010, the flu vaccine was formulated to include protection from both H1N1 flu (swine flu) and seasonal flu.

Tdap vaccine. One dose of tetanus toxoid, reduced diphtheria toxoid and acellular pertussis (Tdap) vaccine is recommended during each pregnancy to offer protection from whooping cough (pertussis), tetanus and diphtheria, regardless of when you had your last Tdap or tetanus-diphtheria (Td) vaccination. Whooping cough can be dangerous — even life-threatening — for infants. Getting the Tdap vaccine during pregnancy can help protect you from the infection and might also help protect your baby after birth.

CHRONIC MEDICAL CONDITIONS

If you have a chronic medical condition, it's natural that you may be concerned whether the condition will in any way affect your ability to become pregnant or affect your baby. Relax, and try not to worry. Having a medical condition — such as diabetes, asthma, epilepsy, depression or high blood pressure — doesn't mean you can't get pregnant or have a healthy baby. It just means that you and your care provider may need to monitor your health a little more closely to create the best conditions possible for making a baby. In particular, you'll want to work with your care provider to make sure your condition is under control and that you're as healthy as possible before you conceive.

In many cases, this means continuing with the treatment plan you're on. In fact, planning for pregnancy is a great time to place even greater emphasis on the healthy lifestyle components of your treatment plan, such as exercising regularly and eating a balanced diet. Simple steps such as these can improve your own health as well as your chances of conceiving and delivering a healthy baby.

The main thing is that you don't stop taking your medications without talking to your care provider. Together, the two of you can discuss your best options. He or she might recommend adjusting your medication or switching to a different

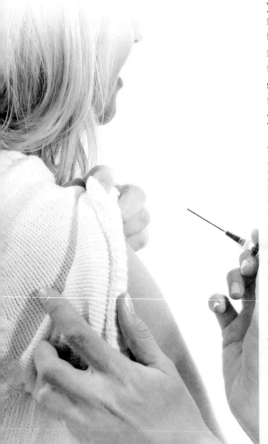

Q. CAN I STILL BECOME PREGNANT IF I'VE LOST AN OVARY?

A. Yes. If you've had surgery to remove one of your ovaries, perhaps for an ovarian tumor, your chances of conception may be diminished, but it's still possible to have children.

Although research on women who become pregnant after a single ovary removal is limited, existing data suggests that almost 50 percent of women in this category are able to conceive. Most of the pregnancies are likely to occur naturally, without the need for reproductive assistance. Some women, however, may have had reason to remove an ovary that's linked to decreased fertility.

Age may play a role in defining your odds. The younger you are, the more eggs you're likely to have in an ovary. But age alone shouldn't stop you from trying. Number of ovaries aside, most of the recommendations in this book apply to you as well as any woman seeking to become pregnant.

---

drug to minimize any risks related to conception or pregnancy. Your care provider will also explain any special care you might need during pregnancy. To minimize drug exposure during sensitive times of fetal development, he or she may recommend:

▶ Using the fewest medications and lowest doses possible while still providing you with effective treatment
▶ Choosing the least risky medications
▶ Avoiding newer or experimental drugs for which little information exists regarding their effects on pregnancy

If your condition is mild and the benefits of medication aren't enough to warrant exposing the baby to it, you and your doctor may decide to discontinue using the drug before becoming pregnant. With mild high blood pressure, for example, some doctors forgo antihypertensive drugs while closely monitoring the pregnancy, especially in the first trimester when blood pressure tends to decrease anyway. For some medications, doctors recommend tapering off the drug slowly rather than stopping it abruptly.

GENETIC TESTS

It's understandable that a discussion on genetic testing may not exactly be your topic of choice. Not many parents-to-be want to hear or read about potential genetic problems they could pass on to their children. Don't be frightened, though, by the subject matter. Of all the babies born in the world, most are born healthy with no problems.

Genetic screening may be discussed at your preconception visit so that you can determine if it's something you and your partner should consider. Why? Some people have a genetic makeup that increases their risk of having a child with health problems. Genetic carrier screening tests are available that offer parents-to-be an opportunity to explore some of the risks that genetics may pose for their unborn children.

For example, if you or your partner has a family history of a genetic disorder, such as cystic fibrosis, you may choose to have carrier testing before you have children. The tests can determine if you or your partner carry an altered gene that

POPULATION-BASED SCREENING

Certain racial and ethnic groups are at higher risk of specific disorders than are others. If you belong to one of these groups, talk to your care provider or a genetic counselor about your risks of being a carrier and the screening process. Typically, you're considered at increased risk if you carry at least 25 percent of the ethnic group in your background.

With genetic carrier tests, the testing is often done in one partner. If the screening is normal, the second partner isn't tested. If the screening in the first partner finds an abnormality, then it's recommended that the other partner be tested as well.

Racial or ethnic group	Genetic disorder
Eastern European (Ashkenazi) Jews	Bloom syndrome, Canavan disease, cystic fibrosis, familial dysautonomia, Fanconi anemia, Gaucher's disease, mucolipidosis IV, Niemann-Pick disease, Tay-Sachs disease
French Canadians, Cajuns	Cystic fibrosis, Tay-Sachs disease
Blacks of African descent, Hispanics, Italians, Greeks	Sickle cell disease
Chinese, Southeast Asians (Cambodians, Filipinos, Laotians, Vietnamese), Asian Indians, Pakistanis, Bangladeshis, Middle Easterners	Beta-thalassemia
Chinese, Southeast Asians, Mediterraneans	Alpha-thalassemia
Non-Hispanic whites	Cystic fibrosis

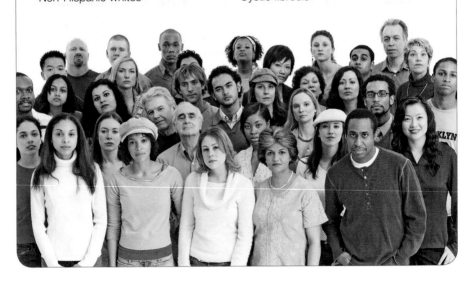

would put your child at risk of inheriting the disorder.

The risks of inherited disease are often misunderstood. Some people feel they're highly likely to develop a condition that may run in the family, such as familial breast cancer or Huntington's disease, when in fact their risk may be lower than they think. Genetic testing may reveal whether you or your partner has inherited a defective gene. Testing can also determine the odds of passing on a defective gene to your offspring.

You might consider talking to a genetic counselor, a person with specialized training in medical genetics and counseling, if:

▶ You or your partner has a family history of a particular genetic disease.
▶ You're from an ethnic group that has a higher carrier frequency for certain disorders. For example, people of Eastern European Jewish (Ashkenazi Jewish) descent are at increased risk of several genetic disorders, including Tay-Sachs disease and cystic fibrosis. People of Asian, Middle Eastern and Mediterranean descent are at risk of thalassemia. See the chart on the opposite page for additional populations at increased risk.
▶ You're older than age 35. A mother's age, and sometimes that of the father, can affect the chances of a genetic defect in the baby.
▶ You already have a child with an inherited disorder.
▶ You've had previous problems with pregnancy or recurrent miscarriages.
▶ You're concerned that your job, lifestyle choices or medical history may pose a risk to your pregnancy.
▶ You and your partner aren't aware of any increased genetic risks, but you want to learn more about screening options.

Genetic counselors typically work as members of a health care team to provide information and support to families who may be affected by an inherited condition. A genetic counselor can help you:

▶ Understand if your potential future child is at risk of birth defects or hereditary disorders
▶ Decide whether screening is right for you and how you will use the screening results
▶ Interpret test results
▶ Understand how a specific disease may affect your child
▶ Make decisions that are consistent with your values and beliefs

TAKE HEART

If all of the information you've read so far seems like a lot to take in, don't worry. In practice, it's not as overwhelming as it may seem in print. The main thing to focus on is becoming as healthy as you can be — a worthy goal in any scenario but especially when you're trying to conceive.

Your care provider is best positioned to help you and your partner achieve that goal. Together you can work out a wellness plan that's tailored to your specific circumstances. Some of it can even be kind of fun, such as exercising with your partner or trying out new, healthier foods.

So take a positive approach. The steps you take now toward better health will almost certainly come to benefit you in the future.

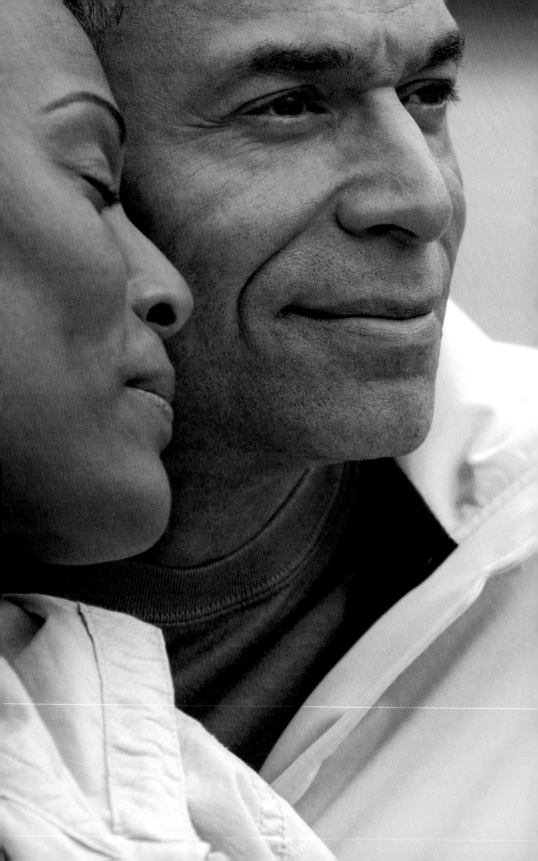

CHAPTER 4

Producing healthy sperm

When it comes to having a baby, it seems that women get all the attention. Because the woman is the one who carries the pregnancy for nine months, the connection is pretty obvious. But when it comes to actually making the baby, the man's role is equal in importance to the woman's. Enter the sperm. To fertilize a female egg, one lucky sperm must navigate its way through the woman's reproductive system, find the egg and make its way inside so that the two cells can be united.

This is no small feat. Of the millions of sperm released into the vagina during a single ejaculation, only a few thousand ever make their way to the fallopian tube, the site of the waiting egg. The path is also littered with obstacles — acidic fluid in the vagina, heavy mucus in the cervix, defensive cells on guard against foreign invaders. Finally, chemical barriers around the egg itself allow only one sperm to penetrate. To conceive, you need strong, healthy sperm that can complete the journey.

Healthy sperm aren't always a given. Still, there are ways you can help your sperm be top performers. Start by knowing what makes a healthy sperm, and then see what things you can do to improve your fertility.

SPERM HEALTH AND FERTILITY

A man's reproductive system is all about the manufacture, storage and transport of sperm, the microscopic cells that contain half the genetic material a baby will need. The key male reproductive organs include the testicles, epididymides, vasa deferentia, prostate gland, seminal vesicles, urethra and penis.

Reproduction begins in the testicles. Coiled within each testicle is a delicately interwoven mass of tubules (seminiferous tubules) where waves of sperm cells are produced. Within these tubules, regular-shaped, round cells called spermatogonia divide first into spermatocytes and then into spermatids. The spermatids grow into young sperm. As sperm matures, each

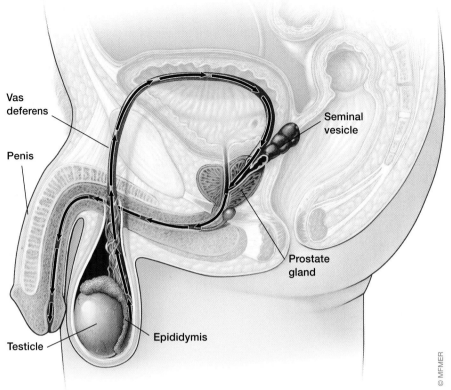

Vas deferens

Penis

Seminal vesicle

Prostate gland

Epididymis

Testicle

© MFMER

Sperm are produced in the testicles and migrate to the epididymides where they mature while they're stored. During ejaculation, sperm are expelled from the epididymides into the vasa deferentia. In the prostate gland, the vasa deferentia join with the seminal vesicles to form the ejaculatory duct, which empties into the urethra. Sperm travel through the urethra and are expelled from the penis.

develops its distinctive shape: a head (which contains the genetic material of the cell), a body and a tail to propel it.

Developing sperm aren't very good at moving around. They only become functional once they leave the testicle and move to the epididymis, a long, coiled tube attached to each testicle. While traveling through the epididymis, sperm go through changes that help them mature. Complete, waiting sperm are stored in each epididymis for the moment of ejaculation, when they're carried out of the body in a white, sticky fluid called semen.

After ejaculation occurs, sperm undergo a final phase of development while in the female reproductive tract called capacitation. It allows them to fertilize an egg.

From first division to maturation, a cycle of sperm production takes about two to three months, meaning any changes you make to your overall health may take several months to improve your fertility. Typically, there are several cycles going on at once, generating waves of sperm at various stages of development within the testicles and epididymides. So there's always some sperm on the assembly line, which helps to ensure that a man is fully ready to reproduce.

When it comes to sperm and fertility, quantity, structure and movement are important, with quantity and movement being most important.

Quantity Normally, millions of sperm are contained in a single ejaculation. Too little sperm in an ejaculate may make it more difficult to get pregnant because there are fewer candidates available to fertilize the egg. So the more sperm there are, the better.

Structure Normal sperm have oval heads and long tails, which work together to propel them forward in a straight, speedy line. Irregularly shaped heads or sharply angled tails may indicate underlying problems that can make it more difficult for sperm to navigate the female reproductive tract and penetrate an egg. The more sperm you have with a normal shape and structure, the more likely you are to be fertile. Another term for structure is morphology.

Movement To reach and fertilize an egg, sperm must travel a long distance — wriggling and swimming through a woman's cervix, uterus and fallopian tubes. This is known as motility. You want most of your sperm on the move. If fewer than 40 percent of your sperm are moving, this may be contributing to decreased fertility.

While sperm are definitely important, it also pays to remember that each man is different and sperm characteristics vary

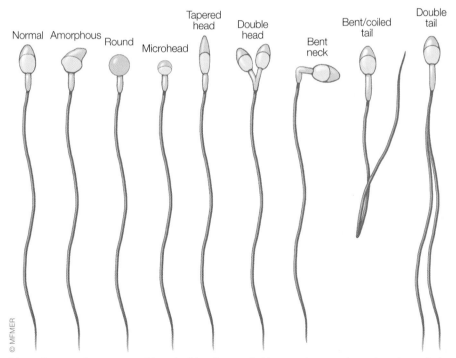

Normal sperm have an oval head with a long tail. Abnormal sperm have head or tail defects, such as a large or misshapen head or a bent or double tail. These defects may affect the ability of the sperm to reach and penetrate an egg.

even within the same man from one ejaculation to the next. Each sperm characteristic may enhance or decrease fertility, but it won't guarantee that you'll be fertile or infertile. It's also true that your health can have an impact on your sperm. In general, the healthier you are, the better the quality of your sperm.

HOW TO IMPROVE SPERM HEALTH

Although not a lot of research has been done on how to improve male fertility, a small but increasing amount of evidence suggests that there are some things you can do that might help. These include maintaining a healthy weight, eating a healthy diet, staying physically active and managing stress. Practicing these habits won't guarantee that you and your part-

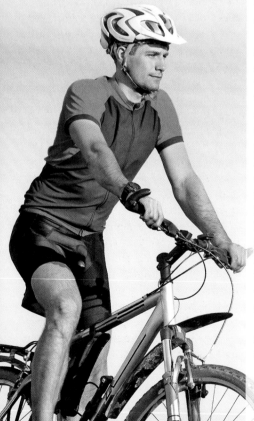

ner will get pregnant, but they may help. And, just as importantly, they won't harm you. In fact, making these kinds of choices can help you become more healthy overall, which is an important goal in optimizing your fertility, both for yourself and as a couple.

Maintain a healthy weight Some research suggests that obesity can hinder fertility in men. For example, a few studies have found that increasing body mass index, or BMI, (see page 17) in the male partner may cause infertility or increase the time it takes to achieve pregnancy. Studies examining the effect of weight on male fertility have shown that increasing BMI is associated with decreasing sperm counts, testosterone levels and successful live births and an increased need for assisted reproductive technology (ART). This was true even after accounting for other factors such as reproductive diseases and smoking. A high BMI may also affect the ability of sperm to move well.

How excess weight might affect sperm quality isn't clear, but the effects are most likely due to more than one factor, including hormone changes and alterations to sperm DNA. As with women, carrying around excess pounds can alter the way in which the body produces reproductive hormones. In men, being too heavy can lead to a decrease in the production of androstenedione and testosterone, primary male hormones, and an increase in estrogen, a primarily female hormone but which men produce in smaller quantities. This and other types of hormone changes can affect the production of sperm as well as sexual function — obesity has also been tied to erectile dysfunction.

On the bright side, losing weight may reverse these hormonal changes. Studies also suggest that being lean and physically active reduces your risk of sexual dysfunction. Eating a healthy diet is key to attaining a healthy weight. Exercising regularly can help you keep the pounds off as well.

If you need to lose weight but are unsure how to begin, talk with your care provider. He or she can help you come up with a plan that's tailored to your needs. And enlist the help of your partner. Working out together and cooking simple, healthy meals can be a bonding experience as well as a way to enhance your combined fertility.

Eat a healthy diet A balanced, nutritious diet is good for your overall health and it can help you achieve and maintain a healthy weight. When it comes to enhancing your fertility, two things stand out: eating plenty of fruits and vegetables and steering clear of saturated fats.

Studies have found a "prudent" diet high in fish, chicken, fruit, vegetables, whole grains and legumes improves sperm mobility compared with a Western diet high in red meat, processed foods and sweets. A balanced diet also helps avoid vitamin deficiencies associated with infertility.

Splurge on fruits and veggies. One reason fruits and vegetables are desirable is because they're rich in antioxidants, substances that help combat the effects of free radicals on your cells.

Free radicals are byproducts of your metabolism, formed when your body converts food to energy or when you exercise. Your body can also absorb free radicals from things in the environment, such as cigarette smoke, air pollution and sunlight. The production of sperm itself generates a small amount of free radicals.

If too many free radicals begin to float around, though, excess free radicals begin to damage healthy cells, including sperm, in a process called oxidative stress. Oxidative stress can inhibit sperm's ability to move and function, damage a sperm cell's DNA, and over time contribute to infertility.

Enter antioxidants as the good guys. They scavenge and dispose of free radicals, working to counteract the effects of oxidative stress and to protect sperm and other cells from damage. For example, in a study comparing the food intake of fertile versus infertile men, researchers found that men who had a higher intake of lettuce, tomatoes and fruits such as peaches and apricots — foods high in antioxidants — also had better sperm quality.

Bottom line: Next time you're at the grocery store, throw some salad fixings in your cart along with some fresh fruit. It'll help your heart and your sperm!

Limit saturated fat. The same study that reported that men who ate lettuce, tomatoes and fruit had stronger sperm also observed an association between poor sperm quality and eating processed meats and dairy products high in saturated fat.

A second study, conducted in a general population of young Danish men, supported these results. The men, who were undergoing a physical exam required by the country's military drafting process, volunteered a semen sample and agreed to complete a food intake questionnaire.

The researchers categorized the men according to their daily intake of different types of fat, including saturated fat, polyunsaturated fat and monounsaturated fat. After accounting for other variables that might affect sperm quality — such as BMI, alcohol consumption and smoking — they found that sperm concentration and total sperm count decreased as the

SUPPLEMENTS FOR BETTER SPERM?

No doubt you've noticed there's no shortage of vitamins and supplements advertising their powers to increase your sperm production, improve your fertility and generally increase your overall virility. Take care when considering these products, however. Many are overpriced and fail to deliver as promised.

The best way to get your daily dose of nutrients, including antioxidants, is by eating whole foods. Science is great, but it still hasn't figured out how exactly the vitamins and minerals found in fruits, vegetables and other foods benefit your body. Isolating nutrients into supplements may inadvertently skip complex interactions found in the total package of an orange or a blueberry, thus minimizing the full benefits.

Investigators are looking into specific nutrients that might help improve male fertility. Some evidence has shown limited benefits with selected supplements, including alpha-lipoic acid, anthocyanin, L-arginine, astaxanthin, beta carotene, biotin, acetyl-L-carnitine, L-carnitine, cobalamin, coenzyme Q10, ethyl cysteine, pentoxifylline, polyunsaturated fatty acids, selenium, vitamins A, C, D, E and zinc, among others.

While eating a balanced diet is best, the use of antioxidant supplements in men with decreased fertility is worth consideration. The right supplements may improve the likelihood of achieving pregnancy, particularly among couples undergoing assisted reproductive technology (ART).

Given their low rate of side effects, routine use of nutrient supplements in couples trying to conceive is generally reasonable and safe. However, it's best to check with your care provider before taking any supplements to review the risks and benefits and the recommended dosages. Some supplements taken in high doses (megadoses) or for extended periods of time may be harmful to sperm and your overall health.

percentage of energy (calories) from saturated fat intake increased. Several other foods may be associated with impaired fertility, including foods high in trans fats and sugar-sweetened beverages.

At this point, nothing has been proven when it comes to diet. So what do you do? Think of your diet in terms of general trends rather than specifics. There's no need to swear off certain foods or beverages; just consider eating foods high in saturated fat, trans fat or sugar in smaller portions. It's better for your overall health and probably better for your sperm, too.

Exercise Regular exercise is on everyone's list of things that are good for you. And well it should be. If there ever was an elixir of life, exercising or even just being physically active is surely a top candidate. Engaging in regular exercise reduces your risk of chronic conditions, such as heart disease, diabetes, lung and kidney disease, Alzheimer's disease, and some cancers. Maintaining physical fitness can also extend your life span by several years and increase your quality of life.

The science is less abundant when it comes to the effects of exercise on male fertility. The few findings scientists have uncovered generally pertain to men who exercise intensely for at least five hours a week — in other words, professional or semiprofessional athletes. In these men, evidence suggests that intense sports such as competitive cycling or endurance running may lower testosterone levels and reduce sperm concentration, as well as reduce the total number of motile sperm.

But for most men, moderate exercise doesn't appear to cause any damage. In fact, it can increase levels of powerful antioxidant enzymes, which can help protect sperm. Regular amounts of moderate exercise can also help you maintain a healthy weight, increase your testosterone levels, decrease stress and make you feel better. And let's face it, sex — the key to having a baby — is generally more enjoyable when you're relaxed and feeling good about yourself.

What constitutes moderate exercise? Walking at a brisk pace, hiking, recreational cycling, using a punching bag or a rowing machine with moderate effort, lifting weights, dancing, playing doubles tennis, shooting hoops, and golfing are all examples of moderate exercise. Aim for at least 30 minutes a day most days of the week, the amount recommended by the American College of Sports Medicine and the American Heart Association.

Manage stress Something else you can do to improve your overall health and possibly enhance your fertility is to reduce and manage stress. The hormones produced while your mind or body is under stress can alter the delicately balanced regulatory mechanisms that coordinate testosterone and sperm production.

The effects are complex, though. They can fluctuate or be temporary. This makes it hard to draw a straight line from chronic daily stress to impaired fertility. A number of studies have observed an association between stress and decreased male fertility, but others have not.

As discussed earlier, not being able to get pregnant as quickly as you would like can be very stressful. Some studies have shown that the stress of being evaluated for infertility can negatively affect semen quality, creating a potentially vicious cycle. Furthermore, stressing out about not getting pregnant can rub off on your partner and your sex life. The point is that stress is unlikely to be helpful and it may even make it more difficult to conceive. So reducing stress makes sense.

There are many steps you can take to ease your mind and relax your body, starting first and foremost with daily basics such as regular exercise, adequate sleep and a balanced diet. Having good friends and being involved in volunteer, sports, church or other activities also can be a big help. If you feel you might benefit from professional help, don't hesitate to contact your care provider or a counselor. They are trained to help you find ways to reduce stress and anxiety, or at least they can refer you to someone who is. Chapter 1 has more information on stress and fertility, as well as specific relaxation techniques.

Prevent and treat infections Another factor associated with male fertility is a genitourinary infection, such as infection or inflammation of the testicles (orchitis) or of the epididymides (epididymitis). These infections may be acquired through sexual or nonsexual transmission and are commonly due to organisms such as gonorrhea bacteria, the human immunodeficiency virus (HIV) and the mumps virus. Epididymitis or orchitis may also result from noninfectious causes and it may be recurrent or chronic in nature.

Signs and symptoms of a genitourinary infection may include pain, swelling, discomfort or tenderness when sitting, and penile discharge outside of sexual intercourse. Sometimes, the infection is only detectable on laboratory results.

Damage from orchitis or epididymitis may result in temporary or permanent infertility through generation of reactive oxygen species, obstruction of the ducts transporting sperm, development of antibodies against sperm, or permanent scar formation.

The best way to deal with these infections is to prevent them through safe sex practices and vaccination. But early recognition and treatment may potentially reduce long-term effects. If you suspect that you may have a genitourinary infection, discuss this with your care provider. He or she may perform an examination or additional laboratory tests.

WHAT TO AVOID

In addition to adopting healthy habits to promote your fertility, there are some things you're better off avoiding to improve your chances of conception. Sperm can be especially vulnerable to certain environmental factors, from cigarettes to lubricants. To protect your fertility:

▶ *Don't use tobacco.* Men who smoke cigarettes or chew smokeless tobacco are more likely to have low sperm counts. Tobacco use may also decrease sperm movement and cause sperm to be misshapen. And if you smoke around your partner, you may be affecting her fertility as well. The good news is that within a year of quitting you can reverse the damage caused to sperm production. Quitting can be tough, but you can do it. Ask your care provider for help.

LAPTOPS, HOT TUBS AND SPERM PROBLEMS

Did you know that temperatures in your scrotum are generally a few degrees cooler than your normal body temperature? The purpose of this thermoregulation is to provide a healthy environment for the production of sperm in the testicles. The testicles are purposefully enclosed in a dangling scrotum away from the abdomen in order to protect them from excessive body heat. The scrotum's thin skin and abundant sweat glands also make it easier to release heat when it's hot out.

Increases in scrotal temperature of just a few degrees are known to disrupt the production of sperm. A number of sources of genital heat have been hypothesized to affect sperm production. Some examples include using saunas and hot tubs, placing your laptop on your lap for hours at a time, sitting for long periods (professional drivers, for instance), prolonged biking, extensive use of heated car seats, wearing tight clothing, or working with welding irons or hot ovens.

It makes sense that you wouldn't want to overheat that particular area, especially if you're trying to conceive. However, science has yet to offer definitive support for this type of conclusion. In any event, it probably won't hurt to avoid excessive heat in the scrotal area whenever possible — skip the hot tub, take breaks from sitting and put your laptop on a table, at least for now.

BOXERS VS. BRIEFS

Some men may worry that the type of underwear they prefer is actually keeping them from conceiving. Boxers have been recommended over briefs and other tightfitting underwear because theoretically they allow for greater air movement and less heat retention. This is considered desirable because heat can have a detrimental effect on sperm production.

Scientific studies have been conducted on the matter. Some have found that tightfitting underwear does increase scrotal temperature, while others have found no difference between boxers and briefs. A link between tightfitting underwear and decreased sperm quality has been even harder to prove.

In the grand scheme of things, whether you wear boxers or briefs is probably fairly negligible in terms of your fertility. For example, smoking is likely to have a stronger impact on your sperm than is wearing briefs.

▶ *Limit the amount of alcohol you drink.* Heavy drinking can lead to reduced testosterone production, impotence and decreased sperm production. If you drink alcohol, do so in moderation, meaning no more than one to two drinks a day.

▶ *Steer clear of illegal drugs.* Using marijuana, cocaine or methamphetamines can alter hormones, decrease sperm movement and cause sperm to be misshapen.

▶ *Avoid anabolic steroids.* Using testosterone, human chorionic gonadotropin and other anabolic steroids can significantly lower your sperm count. It may take several years for it to return to normal levels.

▶ *Avoid lubricants during sex.* Information on the effect of lubricants on fertility is incomplete and conflicting. In general, it's better to avoid lubricants during intercourse, if possible. If a lubricant is needed, try hydroxyethyl cellulose-based products, baby oil (mineral oil) or canola oil instead of skin lotions, K-Y jelly and similar products.

▶ *Talk to your care provider about medications.* Calcium channel blockers, tricyclic antidepressants, anti-androgens, opioids and various other medications can contribute to fertility issues. Chemotherapy drugs and radiation treatment for cancer can sometimes cause permanent infertility. If you need one or more of these medications, ask your care provider about their impact on your fertility — or the possibility of retrieving and storing sperm before treatment.

▶ *Watch out for toxins.* Exposure to pesticides, solvents, lead and other toxins at work or home can affect sperm quantity and quality. Whether you're affected typically depends on how you were exposed, how much of the hazard you were exposed to, for how long and other factors. If you must work with toxins, do so safely. For example, wear protective clothing and equipment, and avoid skin contact with chemicals. To protect your partner, avoid bringing contaminated clothing or other objects home.

PART 2

How to Get Pregnant

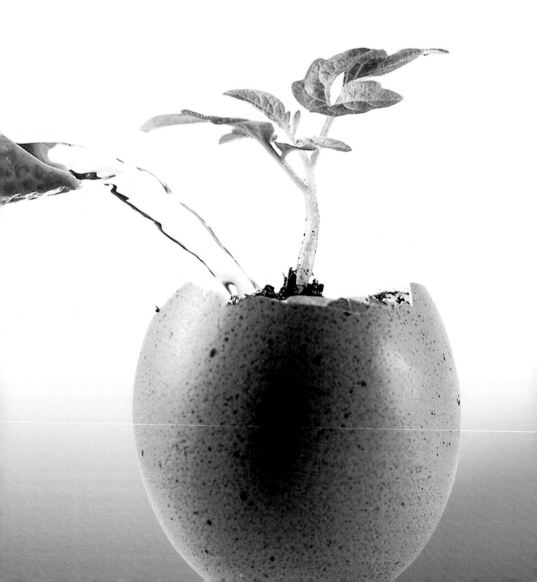

CHAPTER 5

How babies are made

It seems like a fairly straightforward process: Egg and sperm meet and you have a baby (egg + sperm = baby). That's the basic formula, but consider it the simplified version. In reality, there's more to baby-making then just having sexual intercourse. Within the female body, many events take place that make it possible for female and male sex cells to unite.

This chapter walks you through the basics of ovulation and conception. By knowing a bit more about these processes, you'll understand why timing and patience are often key components to the baby equation.

REPRODUCTIVE ORGANS

You likely learned about the female and male reproduction systems in health class in school. To a naive 10- or 11-year-old, it can be a memorable classroom experience! We're not going to take you back to your childhood and repeat your elementary or junior high health lesson, but in discussing ovulation and fertility, it may help to brush up on the roles of a few key organs and processes.

Female organs The female reproductive system is made up of these internal organs: vagina, uterus, fallopian tubes and ovaries.

▶ *Vagina.* The vagina is a muscular, hollow tube that extends from the vaginal opening to the uterus.
▶ *Uterus.* The uterus connects with the vagina at the cervix and is shaped like an upside-down pear. It has a thin lining and muscular walls. The lining of the uterus thickens in response to hormone signals to make a good place for a pregnancy to develop. If no pregnancy occurs during that particular cycle, the lining sheds during menstruation.
▶ *Fallopian tubes.* At the upper corners of the uterus are the fallopian tubes. The fallopian tubes serve as pathways from the ovaries to the uterus. Each

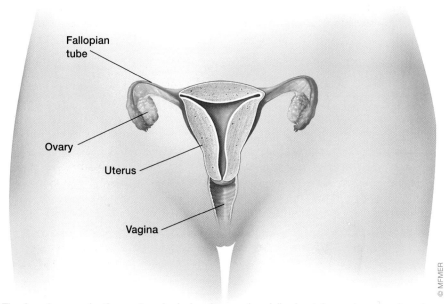

The female reproductive system includes the ovaries, fallopian tubes, uterus and vagina.

fallopian tube is about 4 inches long and the opening inside is about as wide as a piece of spaghetti. The tubes open into the abdominal cavity, where they pick up an egg released from an ovary.

▶ *Ovaries.* The oval-shaped ovaries measure about 1½ to 2 inches in an adult woman. They store eggs and release a mature egg each month. The ovaries also produce hormones. When a baby girl is born, her ovaries contain hundreds of thousands of immature egg cells (ova) — her lifetime supply. The eggs remain inactive until the girl reaches puberty.

Male organs The male reproductive system includes the testicles, duct system, accessory glands and penis.

▶ *Testicles.* The two male testicles make and store millions of tiny sperm cells. Unlike women, who are born with a lifetime supply of eggs, men make sperm throughout life. The testicles also produce hormones.

▶ *Duct system.* The duct system includes the epididymis and vas deferens. The epididymis is a coiled tube — there are two, one for each testicle — where sperm cells from the testicles mature and are stored. Attached to each epididymis is a long, muscular tube called the vas deferens. It transports fluid containing sperm (semen) to the urethra. Each vas deferens is just less than 12 inches long.

▶ *Accessory glands.* The accessory glands include the seminal vesicles and the prostate gland. They provide additional fluid to lubricate the duct system and transport and nourish sperm.

▶ *Penis.* At the end of the penis is a small opening through which semen exits the body. During intercourse, the semen travels down the urethra and is ejected from the penis into the female vagina. Both semen and urine travel through the same passageway — the urethra — but not at the same time.

OVULATION

Ovulation is the process in which a mature female egg is released from an ovary into the abdominal cavity, where it is picked up by one of the fallopian tubes. The female body has two ovaries, but in any given menstrual cycle, ovulation usually occurs from just one of them.

Ovulation is a coordinated effort involving two parts of the brain — the hypothalamus and the pituitary gland — and the ovaries. The hypothalamus, which is in charge of maintaining hormone levels, sends signals to the pituitary gland to coordinate production of a hormone called follicle-stimulating hormone (FSH). This hormone causes a small group of immature eggs within the ovaries to begin maturing. Development of the eggs takes place within small sacs in the ovary called follicles. As the follicles mature, they release the hormone estrogen. High levels of estrogen signal back to the hypothalamus and pituitary gland that the developing eggs are almost mature and ready for ovulation.

At the same time, the pituitary gland is producing another hormone called

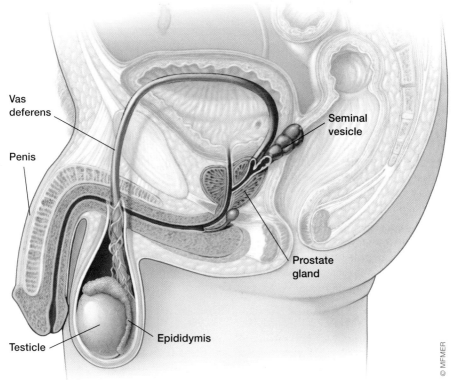

Vas deferens

Penis

Seminal vesicle

Prostate gland

Epididymis

Testicle

© MFMER

The male reproductive system is composed of the testicles, duct system (epididymides and vas deferentia), accessory glands (seminal vesicles and prostate gland) and the penis.

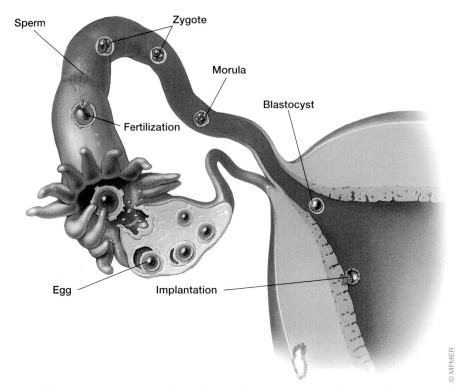

As a fertilized egg moves through a fallopian tube, it continues to divide — the number of cells doubling about every 12 hours. Four to five days after fertilization, it reaches the uterus where it implants itself.

luteinizing hormone (LH). Production of this hormone reaches its highest level shortly before ovulation. At that time — in what's often referred to as an LH surge — large amounts of the hormone cause one of the developing eggs within an ovary to undergo final maturation steps and release from the follicle, a process known as ovulation (see the illustration above). The other developing follicles stop maturing and the eggs they contain don't ovulate.

After the egg is released, the ruptured follicle begins to produce the hormone progesterone, in addition to estrogen. Progesterone causes the lining of the uterus to thicken and prepare for a possible pregnancy.

The released egg, meanwhile, moves into one of the fallopian tubes — the ovaries are adjacent to but not actually attached to the fallopian tubes — and it slowly travels down the tube to the uterus. Because the ovaries and fallopian tubes are close together, sometimes the left fallopian tube can pick up an egg from the right ovary and vice versa. Finger-like structures at the opening of the fallopian tube (fimbriae) catch the egg and place it on the proper course.

The egg is viable — meaning it's able to be fertilized — for about 12 to 24 hours after it's released from the ovary. If you have intercourse shortly before or during this time, you can become pregnant. If fertilization doesn't occur, the egg will dissolve and the lining of your uterus will be shed during your menstrual period. Following menstruation, estrogen and progesterone levels are low, triggering the hypothalamus to once again release follicle-stimulating hormone, beginning the cycle again.

FERTILIZATION

Fertilization is the process in which a woman's egg and a man's sperm unite to form a single cell — the starting point for a baby. The process begins when you and your partner have sexual intercourse. When your partner ejaculates, he releases into your vagina semen that contains millions of sperm cells. Unlike a female, who comes complete at birth with all of the eggs she'll ever need, a man isn't born with ready-made sperm. The male body makes new sperm continuously.

Each sperm has a long, whip-like tail that propels it toward your egg. Millions of these sperm swim up through your reproductive tract. They travel from your vagina, up through the lower opening of your uterus (cervix), through your uterus and into your fallopian tubes. Male sperm can live for a few days in the female reproductive tract, but many are lost along the way. Only a fraction reach the fallopian tube containing the egg.

The female egg is covered with a layer of nutrient cells called the corona radiata and a gel-like shell called the zona pellucida. To fertilize your egg, your partner's sperm must penetrate this covering. At this point, the egg is about $\frac{1}{200}$ an inch in diameter, too small to be seen. Hundreds of sperm may try to penetrate the gel-like shell of the egg, and several may begin to enter the outer egg capsule. But in the end, only one succeeds and enters the egg itself. After that, the membrane of the egg changes and all other sperm are locked out.

As the sperm penetrates to the center of the egg, the two sex cells merge to become a one-celled entity called a zygote.

BOY OR GIRL?

For men who may feel a little left out of the baby-making process, remember it's the male partner who makes one of the key decisions in pregnancy — whether the child will be a boy or a girl!

The sex of a baby is determined by whether that one sperm that made its way into the egg cell contains an X or a Y sex chromosome. The female egg cell always carries an X chromosome. If the sperm cell contains a Y chromosome, the baby will be a boy (XY pair). If it contains an X chromosome, the baby will be a girl (XX pair). It's always the father's genetic contribution that determines the sex of the baby.

Now, you may be wondering — perhaps because you've read about it in magazines or gotten "advice" from friends — are there things you can do during intercourse to increase your chances of having a boy or a girl? For your answer, see Chapter 7.

The zygote has 46 chromosomes — 23 from you and 23 from your partner. These chromosomes contain many thousands of genes. This genetic material is like a blueprint, determining your baby's sex, eye color, hair color, body size, facial features and — at least to some extent — intelligence and personality. Fertilization is now complete.

IMPLANTATION

Once an egg is fertilized, there's no taking a break. All sorts of things begin to happen very quickly. The next step in the process is cell division. Within about 12 hours after fertilization, the one-celled zygote divides into two cells. The cells continue to divide as the zygote moves through the fallopian tube to the uterus. Within about three days after fertilization, it becomes a cluster of 12 to 32 nonspecialized cells resembling a very tiny raspberry. At this stage, the developing baby is called a morula. It now leaves the fallopian tube and enters the uterus.

Within four to five days after fertilization, the developing baby — now made up of a few hundred cells — reaches its destination inside the uterus. By this time, it has changed from a solid mass of cells to a group of cells arranged around a fluid-filled cavity and is called a blastocyst. The inner section of the blastocyst is a compact mass of cells that will develop into the baby. The outer layer of cells, called the trophoblast, will become the placenta, which will provide nourishment to the baby as it grows.

Once inside the uterus, the blastocyst clings to the uterine surface for a time. It releases enzymes that slowly dissolve the lining of the uterus, allowing the blastocyst to embed itself there. This typically happens about a week after fertilization. By the 12th day after fertilization, the blastocyst is firmly embedded in its new home. It adheres tightly to the lining of the uterus, called the endometrium, and there it receives nourishment from the mother's bloodstream.

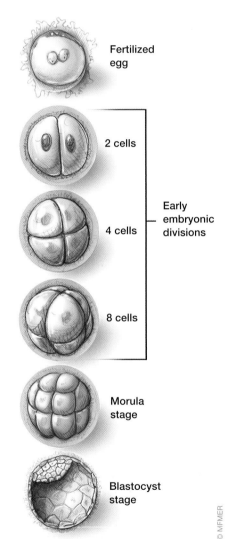

Fertilized egg

2 cells

Early embryonic divisions

4 cells

8 cells

Morula stage

Blastocyst stage

© MFMER

After fertilization, the one-celled zygote divides into two cells. Those two cells then each split into two, and so on, with the number of cells doubling every 12 hours.

Once the pregnancy is connected to the mother's bloodstream, the hormones produced by the pregnancy enter into the mother's circulation. That's why you can get a blood pregnancy test about two weeks after ovulation; the pregnancy makes a hormone called human chorionic gonadotropin (HCG) that can be detected in the mother's circulation.

Also within about 12 days after fertilization, the placenta begins to form. Tiny projections sprout from the wall of the blastocyst. From these sprouts, wavy masses of tiny blood-vessel-filled tissue develop and take shape, eventually forming the placenta.

PREGNANCY

At this point, when the blastocyst has attached itself to the uterus, you are considered pregnant. It may be a couple more weeks, however, until you miss your period and suspect that a baby may be in your near future.

At 14 days after fertilization, or about four weeks from your last menstrual period — about the time you first suspect a possible pregnancy — the fetus is about the size of a poppy seed and is divided into three different layers, from which all tissues and organs will eventually develop:

▶ *Ectoderm.* This top layer will evolve into a groove along the midline of the baby's body, called the neural tube. The baby's brain, spinal cord, spinal nerves and backbone will develop here.

▶ *Mesoderm.* This middle layer of cells will form the beginnings of the baby's heart and a primitive circulatory system — blood vessels, blood cells and lymph vessels. The foundations for bones, muscles, kidneys, and ovaries or testicles also will develop here.

▶ *Endoderm.* This inner layer of cells will become a simple tube lined with mucous membranes. It's from this tube that the baby's lungs, intestines and urinary bladder will develop.

This is the beginning of months of growth and change. It is also a delicate period in a pregnancy. If a miscarriage is going to occur, it's generally within the next couple of weeks that it happens. Up to 30 percent of pregnancies result in miscarriage, sometimes before a woman even realizes that she's pregnant. But don't let this frighten you. Early miscarriages usually can't be prevented. If you're feeling a little scared, remind yourself that most pregnancies are successful. And don't forget that most women who have a miscarriage often go on to experience a healthy pregnancy.

MULTIPLE BABIES

Occasionally, ovulation and fertilization veer from the normal course and follow a slightly different path. Instead of one egg and one sperm uniting to form one baby, there may be two babies, or even more. There are different ways this can happen.

Identical twins, also known as monozygotic twins, occur when a single egg, fertilized by a single sperm, splits into two identical halves. Two separate babies with identical DNA are formed. Identical twins are always the same sex and blood type. They almost always share the same placenta but may also have two separate placentas. The timing of when the egg splits generally determines if identical twins will share the same placenta.

Fraternal twins, also known as dizygotic twins, result when two separate eggs are fertilized by two separate sperm. Biologically, the babies have no more in common than do nontwin siblings. Fraternal twins can be the same sex or they may be different. They may or may not have the same blood type. They always have separate placentas, but it's possible for their placentas to fuse together during the course of pregnancy and appear as one at birth. Fraternal twins are more common than are identical twins.

Triplets can occur in several ways. In most cases, three separate eggs are produced by the mother and fertilized by three separate sperm. Another possibility is for a single fertilized egg to divide and create identical twins, with a second egg fertilized by a separate sperm to create a fraternal third baby. It's also possible for a single fertilized egg to divide three ways, resulting in three identical babies, although this is extremely rare.

Quadruplets (quads) and greater numbers of multiples most often result from four or more eggs fertilized by separate sperm. Naturally occurring quads or greater multiples is rare. The use of fertility drugs or assisted reproductive technology is almost always involved when there are four or more babies.

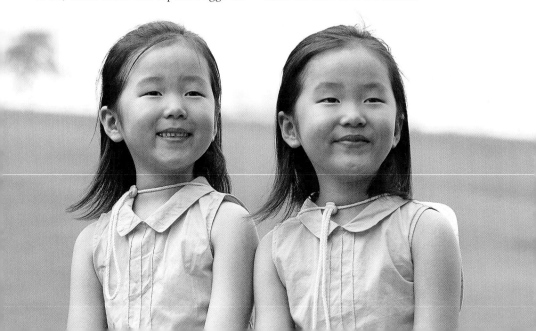

TWINS

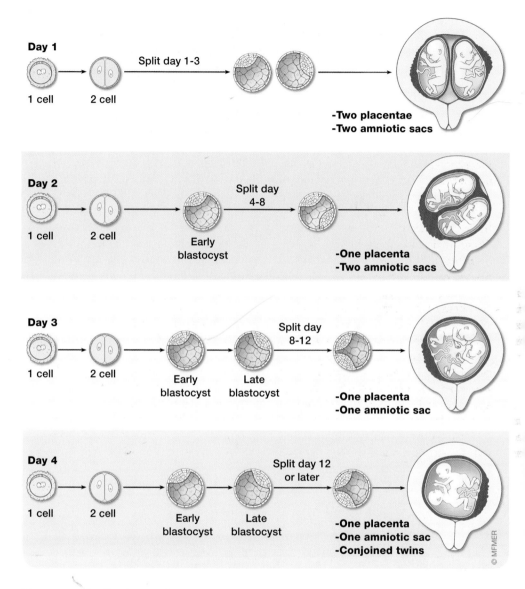

Day 1

1 cell → 2 cell — Split day 1-3 →

-Two placentae
-Two amniotic sacs

Day 2

1 cell → 2 cell → Early blastocyst — Split day 4-8 →

-One placenta
-Two amniotic sacs

Day 3

1 cell → 2 cell → Early blastocyst → Late blastocyst — Split day 8-12 →

-One placenta
-One amniotic sac

Day 4

1 cell → 2 cell → Early blastocyst → Late blastocyst — Split day 12 or later →

-One placenta
-One amniotic sac
-Conjoined twins

© MFMER

How soon a fertilized egg splits while in its blastocyst stage generally determines if identical twins will share a placenta and amniotic sac or have separate placentas and sacs.

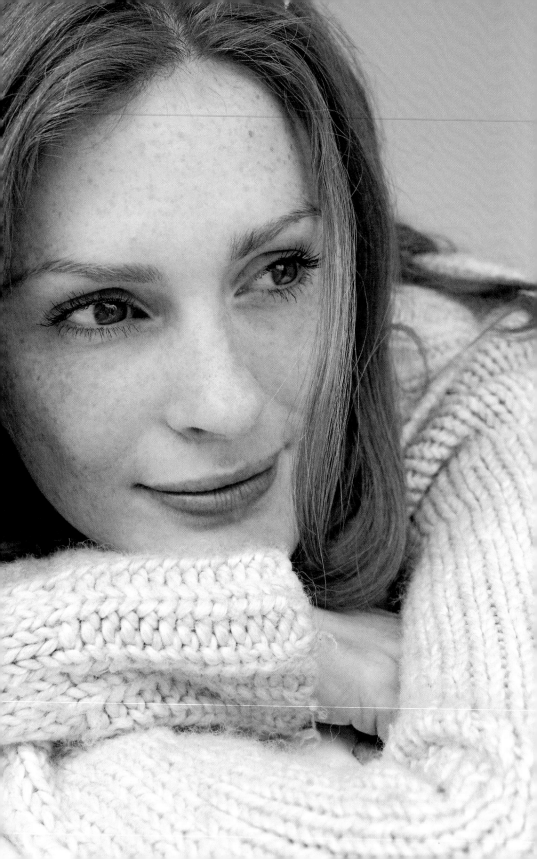

CHAPTER 6

Ovulation and fertility signs

The female body basically runs on a clock, and timing is important. Normal ovulation occurs once a month, and the lone egg that's produced literally vanishes about 24 hours after it's released. What that means is that there's a fairly narrow window of opportunity for sperm and egg to meet and to successfully mingle. So how do you know when the time is right to try to become pregnant?

What you need isn't so much pixie dust as a keen eye for detail. The signs and symptoms of ovulation can be subtle, but that doesn't mean they aren't there. Understanding these signs and symptoms and observing what happens to your own body can help you determine when you're most likely to be fertile, so that you can plan accordingly.

There are a number of ways you can keep track of where you are in your menstrual cycle, ranging from a glance at the calendar to using an ovulation predictor kit. But probably the best and least expensive way to figure out your fertility signs is to observe your body for a while.

After a few months, most women, though not all, are able to uncover definite patterns in the length of their cycles, the ups and downs of their resting body temperatures, and the changes that occur in mucus coming from the cervix. By following the clues revealed in your personal cycle, you'll be able to develop a pretty good estimate of when ovulation is likely to occur.

YOUR MENSTRUAL CYCLE

Before pregnancy was on your agenda, you probably didn't think much about your period, except maybe estimating when you would get it so that you could plan your activities or clothing choices accordingly and make sure you had tampons or other supplies on hand. Now that you're ready for a baby, though, getting your period takes on a whole new meaning. Biology may not be your thing, but it's worth getting a glimpse at the amazing amount of coordination and prep work your body goes through to become ready for pregnancy. Understanding the different phases can also help you use the tools discussed later in this chapter to determine when ovulation occurs for you.

For most women, the average menstrual cycle is right around 28 days. But it can be as short as 22 days or as long as 35 days and still be considered normal. There are three phases in a cycle — the follicular phase, the luteal phase and the ovulatory phase, which represents the transition between the other two.

The follicular phase: Prep time The follicular phase marks the first part of the menstrual cycle, a busy period when an egg is prepped and selected for possible fertilization and the lining of the uterus grows and proliferates, priming itself for potential pregnancy. This phase is also called the proliferative phase.

During this time, increases in follicle-stimulating hormone (FSH) from the pituitary gland signal a group of immature eggs to begin developing. For younger women, perhaps 15 to 20 eggs enter this phase in any given month, but typically only one egg ultimately matures enough to be ovulated. The immature eggs are contained in fluid-filled sacs called follicles.

Eventually, a single follicle becomes the dominant one, outcompeting the rest and growing in size until it attains a mature diameter of about an inch. At this point, the rest of the follicles gradually stop developing and dissipate.

At the same time, an increase in the hormone estrogen signals cells in the uterine lining to thicken, preparing the uterus for pregnancy. As estrogen levels continue to rise, there's often a noticeable increase in the amount and "stretchiness" of cervical mucus so that it resembles the white part of an uncooked chicken egg. The increase in mucus is for the benefit of incoming sperm, to facilitate their journey to the egg.

The length of the follicular phase varies from woman to woman and is the primary reason for differences in menstrual cycle length.

The ovulatory phase: Go time Partway through your cycle, switches are flipped and things change quickly. Estrogen peaks then drops. More FSH arrives and luteinizing hormone (LH) spikes dramatically in preparation for ovulation. Approximately 36 hours later, an egg bursts onto the scene, released by the dominant follicle. Ovulation has now occurred. The egg is a little like Cinderella at the ball, however, because its stay is short-lived.

The luteal phase: Resolution time Immediately after ovulation, the remainder of the follicle transforms into the corpus luteum, which begins to produce pre-pregnancy hormones, most importantly the hormone progesterone. Progesterone helps prepare the uterine lining for implantation by a fertilized egg. It also increases your basal body temperature by about 0.5 to 1 degree Fahrenheit (F). Sometimes this phase is called the secretory phase because the uterine lining releases (secretes) all kinds of molecules the embryo needs to develop.

If the egg is fertilized, the early embryo initiates the production of a substance called chorionic gonadotropin, which maintains production of progesterone. If pregnancy doesn't occur, estrogen and progesterone levels decrease late in the phase and basal body temperature drops back down to its usual level.

The length of the luteal phase is more constant than the follicular phase, averaging about 14 days every cycle.

YOUR FERTILITY WINDOW

The length of the fertility window in a woman's cycle depends on two variables:

▶ *The life span of the sperm inside the female reproductive tract.* Sperm can live as long as five days under the right conditions (plenty of cervical mucus). Technically, you could have sex on Monday but not become pregnant until the sperm finally meets the egg on Thursday or Friday.

▶ *The life span of the egg.* After it's released from the ovary, the egg lasts no more than 24 hours. You could still become pregnant the day after ovulation, but the odds tend to go down significantly after the first 12 hours.

What all this adds up to is a maximum of about six days wherein intercourse could lead to conception — the five days before ovulation and the 24-hour period after. Your goal is to find out where those six days fall in your menstrual cycle and determine what's the best opportunity for conception during those six days. Here are some ways you can do that.

Use a calendar A calendar can help you figure out the average length of your cycle and the approximate time around which ovulation typically occurs. If you don't already know your cycle length,

track your period for a few months — doing it for six to 12 months will give you greater accuracy.

Day one of your cycle is the first day of your period when you start bleeding, not just spotting. The last day of your cycle is the day before your next period starts. If you happen to have a smartphone, there are several apps available that can help you keep track. If not, a paper calendar will do just fine, and in some cases may even be simpler.

Once you have your average cycle length, you can get a general idea of when you're most likely to ovulate. Remember that the luteal phase — the time after ovulation when your body is determining if you're pregnant or not — is generally fixed at 14 days. Therefore, if your cycle is 30 days long, you'll likely ovulate on cycle day 16 (30 days - 14 days = day 16).

Using this example, your fertile window would fall between days 12 and 17. If you have sex about every other day during this time period, you're likely to have sperm ready and waiting when ovulation occurs.

If all this seems too confusing or like too much work, a group of researchers at Georgetown University developed a computer model that accounts for the various probabilities of conception on

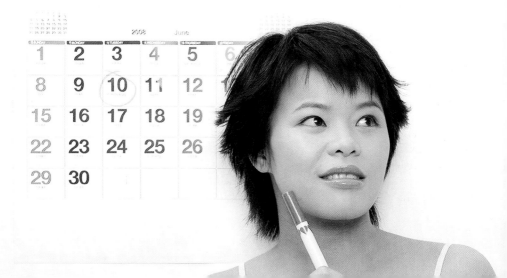

each cycle day. Based on this model, women who have regular cycles of 26 to 32 days will most likely be fertile sometime between days eight and 19.

Contrary to popular wisdom, ovulation at the exact midpoint — for example, day 14 of a 28-day cycle — isn't all that common and only happens in about a third of women. In most women, ovulation occurs in the four days before or after the midpoint. In addition, for many women, their cycles are less regular than they think. This means that your fertility window could come much earlier or even later than is typically described.

So if the calendar method doesn't seem to be helping, you might try looking for additional markers of fertility, such as temperature and cervical changes.

Monitor your temperature Another way to estimate your fertile window is by monitoring your body temperature. Right after ovulation, your basal body temperature — your temperature when you're fully at rest — increases slightly, by about 0.5 to 1 F. It then stays elevated until right

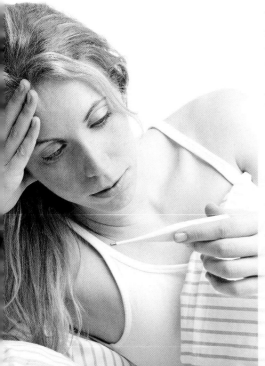

before your next period, when a drop in progesterone levels signals your body that pregnancy hasn't occurred and your temperature returns to its lower level.

The thing to remember here is that your temperature doesn't go up until you've ovulated, thus indicating the tail end of your fertile window. By the time you notice the change, the odds of conception may have decreased considerably. But by tracking your basal body temperature each day for a few months, you may be able to better predict the days before you ovulate. Here's what you need to do:

Take your basal body temperature every morning. You want to take your temperature right away in the morning before getting out of bed. Use a thermometer specifically designed to measure basal body temperature. Make sure you get at least six hours of uninterrupted sleep each night to ensure an accurate reading. Take your temperature before you do anything else, such as going to the bathroom or brushing your teeth. Once you start moving around, your body temperature tends to go up, masking any changes in your resting body temperature. If you're having trouble determining a pattern or a change in your temperature, you may consider taking your temperature vaginally. For the most accurate results, always take your temperature the same way.

Plot your readings on graph paper. Record your daily basal body temperature each day and look for a pattern to emerge. Typically, your basal body temperature will increase slightly when you ovulate. You can assume ovulation has occurred when the slightly higher temperature remains steady for at least three days in a row.

BASAL BODY TEMPERATURE CHART

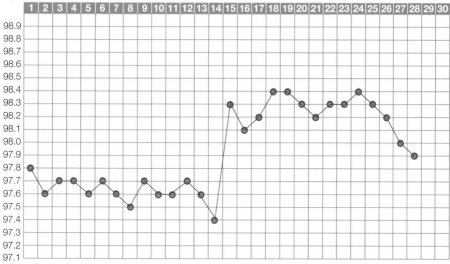

On a blank chart, each day record your basal body temperature. After a few months, you will begin to see a pattern. A slight but noticeable increase in temperature generally indicates that ovulation has just occurred.

© MFMER

Plan sexual intercourse accordingly. You're most fertile during the two to three days before your basal body temperature rises. This is the time to have sex.

Not all women experience a clear rise in temperature. In addition, a number of factors can affect basal body temperature, such as a fever, alcohol intake or not getting enough sleep. Though it's not necessarily the most reliable method for determining ovulation it's inexpensive and easy to do.

Watch for cervical changes Using your calendar and monitoring your basal body temperature can give you a rough estimate of when your fertile window is likely to occur. There are other clues to help you determine when you're most fertile. One of them is to learn to recognize the changing characteristics of your cervical mucus. Research indicates that changes in cervical mucus are highly pre-

dictive of ovulation and can offer a day-to-day estimate of potential fertility.

To do this, regularly check for mucus at the opening of your vagina and look for changes in quality and quantity. Cervical mucus changes with the different phases of the menstrual cycle.

Dry. For most women, the vagina typically feels dry for a few days right after menstruation. But if you generally have shorter cycles, you may notice some mucus shortly after your period, maybe even tinged with blood if you're still spotting.

Sticky. As your hormones ramp up for ovulation, your cervical mucus increases and you may notice some stickiness in your vagina or tacky vaginal discharge.

Wet and stringy. Just before ovulation, cervical mucus tends to become more abundant. It also looks somewhat clear and feels stretchy, wet and slippery — kind of like raw egg white. This type of fluid facilitates the passage of sperm through the cervix and helps the sperm reach full maturity. The last day that this type of fluid is present, the "peak" day, is considered your most fertile day. Ovulation usually occurs within a day or two of your peak day.

Thick and creamy. After ovulation, cervical mucus usually becomes thicker and less elastic and may eventually go away so that your vaginal area feels dry again.

To determine your usual pattern, check your cervical fluid a couple of times a day. Before you urinate is a good time to check. Wipe — front to back — with toilet tissue and record the color (yellow, white, clear or cloudy), consistency (thick, sticky or stretchy) and feel (dry, wet or slippery) of the secretions. Also, note any sensations of dryness, moistness or wetness in your vaginal area. Be careful not to confuse cervical fluid with semen or normal sexual lubrication, though.

You're most fertile when your vaginal area feels wet and your cervical fluid is slippery and stretchy, since this occurs right around ovulation. Days when you observe these sensations and secretions are the best days to have sex to get pregnant. Studies of women who tracked their cervical mucus changes found that the peak day of fertility almost always occurred within three or four days of the LH surge.

This method isn't for everyone. Not all women are able to detect changes in their vaginal discharge and some find monitoring and documenting these changes unappealing.

Putting it all together Rather than relying on just one method to determine your fertile window, you might consider using all three at once: charting your periods on the calendar, taking note of your basal body temperature and tracking your cervical mucus patterns. Being aware of all of these markers simultaneously is likely to give you a better big picture of your fertile window.

The calendar gives you the overall view, while cervical mucus changes signal that ovulation is near (and create ideal conditions for arriving sperm). A slight sustained increase in basal body temperature tells you that ovulation has occurred and may be your first indication that you're pregnant once you've missed your next period, since elevated temperatures can also accompany elevated levels of progesterone observed in early pregnancy.

PRODUCTS THAT CAN HELP

For some women, identifying patterns in their menstrual cycle is easier said than done. Irregular periods, no real noticeable shifts in body temperature and not being able to detect cervical fluid — or finding cervical fluid all the time — can make it difficult to track changes. This doesn't mean you can't conceive, it's just a little harder to tell when you're ovulating.

If this sounds like you, don't fret. Several products are available that can help you track the phases of your menstrual cycle. They can even let you know with the beep of a button when you're most likely to ovulate and give you color-coded indications of when your most fertile days are likely to be.

Ovulation predictor kits Over-the-counter ovulation kits (Clearblue, First Response, others) test your urine for the surge in luteinizing hormone (LH) that starts about 36 hours before ovulation.

You can buy ovulation kits at almost any pharmacy or discount store. The cost ranges between $20 and $70, depending on how many tests come in a kit.

Kits typically contain between five and 20 test sticks. Starting on the earliest possible ovulation date — generally day 10 or day 11 for a woman whose cycle ranges between 27 and 34 days — test your urine each day to see if LH is present. Hold the stick in your urine stream for a few seconds or place the stick in a urine sample you've collected in a sterile container. It's best to do this with the first time you urinate in the morning because all of the hormones your body made overnight are concentrated in a smaller amount of fluid since you weren't drinking while you were sleeping. Within a few minutes, an indicator appears on the stick — usually a color change of some sort — telling you whether LH is present or not. Follow the kit instructions carefully to get the best results.

Because the test measures hormone production over a number of hours, it usually detects the middle of an LH surge rather than its very start. Therefore, once the test indicates an LH surge, you know that ovulation will likely occur within the next 24 hours. At this point you can stop testing. This is also the best time to have sex.

Most home-based tests are pretty accurate at detecting the LH surge when it occurs. Studies comparing urinary LH tests with ultrasound visualization of ovulation found that LH levels correlated with ultrasound-confirmed ovulation almost every time. If you ovulate earlier or later than the midpoint in your cycle, it may take a few tries before you find the right time to start testing. Occasionally, ovulation may not occur or a false-positive result may happen, telling you LH is present when really it's not.

Fertility monitor Another option is to purchase a fertility monitor, a hand-held device that stores daily test results and shows you when your low, high and peak fertile days are. The most accurate monitors rely on urine tests to determine where you are in your cycle. One example currently available in the U.S. is the Clearblue Fertility Monitor.

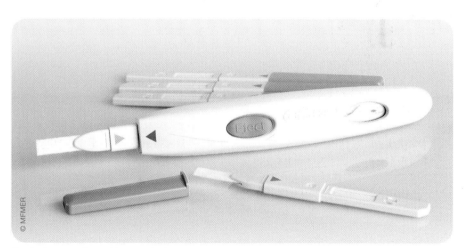

Ovulation predictor kits can help a woman predict when she's about to ovulate. After inserting a test strip in the device, you place the strip in your urine stream or a urine sample.

You start using this monitor on the first day of your period. Each day the monitor advises you whether or not to collect a urine sample right away when you wake up. It usually requests the first test on day six of your cycle and then tests daily for 10 days or more, depending on the length of your cycle and when it detects an LH surge (peak fertility).

Using a fertility monitor generally requires you to collect at least one cycle's worth of data before providing personalized feedback. After the first cycle, the monitor adjusts the initial test day based on what it "learned" from your last cycle.

Once you have a urine sample, you plug the test stick into the monitor. The monitor measures and stores the levels of estrogen and LH in the sample and tells you whether your fertility is low, high or at a peak range. When it detects an increase in estrogen, fertility is shown as high. Peak fertility is when the LH surge occurs. You can also get a printout of your monthly cycle data. As with other products, it's important to follow the instructions carefully to get the best results.

Evidence indicates that the Clearblue Fertility Monitor offers a fairly accurate portrayal of your fertile window. It can be expensive, however, starting around $180 for a starter kit and $40 for additional test sticks. For some women, this may be overkill. Many women find the low-tech

---

TESTS TO CONFIRM OVULATION

In some cases, your care provider may want to confirm that you are in fact ovulating and that the various phases in your cycle are occurring normally. There are a couple of ways to do this.

Progesterone blood levels One way is to measure the level of the hormone progesterone with a blood sample. The sample is taken about a week after you ovulate, the time you would expect to be in the middle of the luteal phase of your menstrual cycle. Levels of progesterone above a certain amount usually indicate that ovulation has occurred. Low levels may indicate that you haven't ovulated yet or that you have an abnormal luteal phase, an indication that the corpus luteum isn't functioning correctly. Your care provider may request more than one sample since levels can fluctuate.

Ultrasound Another method your care provider may use to confirm that ovulation has occurred is to perform a series of ultrasound exams, either abdominally or transvaginally. An initial scan may look for growing follicles, followed by a scan to identify the dominant follicle and then finally a scan to look for a collapsed follicle in the same location, indicating that the egg was released. Your care provider may correlate these results with blood or urine tests.

Ultrasound is one of the most accurate ways of detecting ovulation, but it's also expensive and inconvenient. If other methods seem to be working, you may not need this high-tech option.

methods described earlier work fine in determining when their fertile window is likely to occur.

Other devices Some monitors measure and store your daily basal body temperature and calculate your ovulation date and fertile periods based on temperature changes. However, as discussed earlier, temperature changes typically aren't the most reliable way to detect your fertility window.

Hormone changes may also be reflected in your saliva to a degree. Some ovulation tests and fertility monitors use samples of saliva to detect changes in estrogen that accompany a woman's fertility window. For example, some ovulation tests provide mini-microscopes you can use at home to observe samples of your saliva. When estrogen levels are high, special "ferning" patterns can be detected in dried saliva. When these patterns are present, your fertility is supposedly high. When absent, your fertility is considered low. Saliva-based fertility monitors collect and store information from saliva samples to help you determine high and low fertility days.

Not a lot of research has been done on temperature- and saliva-based monitors. What evidence is available indicates that these methods don't appear to be as accurate in detecting the fertile window as urine-based tests or combined methods.

DON'T BE AFRAID TO SEEK HELP

Your body can provide valuable information about when you're most likely to be fertile. But it can also be easy to get so caught up in tracking all of the various signs of fertility that you lose some of the

spontaneity and fun involved in making love. For some couples, ovulation testing is stressful.

Being aware of what's happening with your cycle is an important step toward conceiving. But if you become frustrated or if the methods described don't seem to be working for you, talk to your care provider or someone who's well-versed in natural family planning. He or she may be able to provide valuable information and advice.

And don't forget that if you're having frequent intercourse — every other day, on average — it's less important to clearly define your most fertile time.

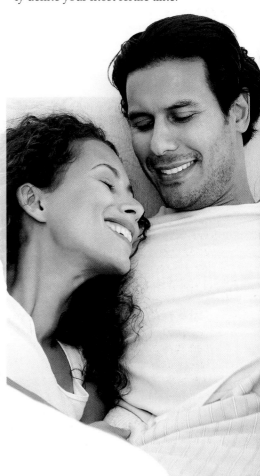

Amber's Story

My husband and I got pregnant the first month we tried. It really was that easy for us. We decided to start our family in September and were pregnant by October. We were shocked because so many people had told us that it usually takes a few months to happen. We wondered how we got so lucky.

We had our initial appointments and our first ultrasound and were given a July due date. Even though everything seemed to be going well, we kept our news to ourselves for the first 10 weeks. Then, when we felt we were safe, we started telling our family and friends. They were so excited for us!

About a week later, I started spotting. I didn't think much about it at first. I'd read that spotting for a couple of days is common. By the third day, however, I started to get nervous. That night, I went to the urgent care department where I learned that I had miscarried our baby.

The doctor called it a "missed miscarriage," meaning our baby was still there, but there was no heartbeat. I was given options on what to do next: I could wait for the baby to pass on its own, I could take oral medication that would cause me to go into labor (medical management), or I could undergo the dilation and curettage (D&C) procedure in which a doctor removes the fetal tissue from my uterus.

I chose D&C. I just didn't want to wait, knowing that my baby wasn't alive. The D&C was awful. I had to go to Labor and Delivery for the procedure — those words were even written above the door I went in. That just seemed cruel.

My husband and I were shellshocked. We weren't expecting anything bad to happen, and here we were facing the loss of our child. We were both crying when I had to go in for the procedure.

Christmas was difficult that year, but after the holidays we started trying again to have another baby. When we still hadn't conceived by May, we were referred to an endocrinologist, a doctor that specializes in hormone conditions. He discovered that I had Hashimoto's thyroiditis, a disorder that can affect fetal development.

I was put on a synthetic hormone and told to hold off on getting pregnant until my thyroid numbers returned to a normal range. After a couple of months, we were given the go-ahead to try again. Several months went by, and, still, we were unsuccessful. That's when we were sent to a reproductive endocrinologist, a doctor who specializes in fertility. She prescribed clomiphene (Clomid) a drug that stimulates ovulation. When Clomid didn't work, we moved on to hormone injections to stimulate follicle development and ovulation.

It was frustrating to have to go through these interventions — and frustrating not to be able to do something that came so easily the first time. But we were willing to do whatever it took to have a baby.

At long last, about a year and a half after our miscarriage, we discovered I was pregnant again. We had our first ultrasound at seven weeks. We'd been told we'd have a higher chance of twins and were excited about the possibility.

During the ultrasound, the tech said, "I see two sacs." We couldn't have been smiling any bigger. We were thrilled. But then the tech continued, "But I don't see any heartbeats."

In that second, we went from the highest of highs to lowest of lows. We couldn't believe it had happened again. The fact that it was twins made it seem even harder. We'd not only lost one baby, but two.

This time, my doctor recommended we take the medical management route, explaining that too many D&Cs can cause scarring, affecting my chances of getting pregnant in the future. I went home with the medication and took the prescribed 12 to 15 pills each day. For three weeks, I waited. But it turned out that I was in the tiny percentage of woman for which the medication doesn't work. I had to go in for a D&C after all.

By this point, I needed a break. At the same time, I couldn't help thinking that if I got pregnant and had a baby, I could make it "all better" — that I could somehow fix how I was feeling.

Less than two months later, I got pregnant. Our ultrasound looked great. After 10 weeks with no problems, they even set me up for an appointment in OB instead of reproductive endocrinology. The morning of my OB appointment, I started spotting. An ultrasound confirmed that we had miscarried again. That day, I had my third D&C. It had been less than five months since our last one.

There is no way to describe how devastated we were. I knew that a lot of people suffer multiple miscarriages, but

they also have children in between. I felt like having a baby was never going to happen for us. The experience sent me into a depression.

I decided I needed to talk to someone. I found a counselor who specializes in perinatal loss. She helped me process what we'd been through and get to a better place. She also prescribed an antidepressant to help me cope and sleep at night.

After a six-month break, I was ready to try again. We became pregnant immediately, but instead of feeling excited, we were filled with anxiety. Every little scare — spotting or a strange feeling — sent me to the doctor. An ultrasound at five weeks showed a yolk sac, but no heartbeat. We were warned that it might've just been too early, but that didn't make us worry any less. We left the appointment certain that we'd lost another baby. Waiting for our next ultrasound, a week away, was torture.

When that day finally came, the first thing the tech said was, "There's a heartbeat." We had never heard such beautiful words.

Ultrasounds at eight and 10 weeks were also successes. When we reached 12 weeks, it felt like a huge milestone. We had never made it that far before.

We delivered our healthy baby boy, Logan, more than three years after we started trying to have a family. Healthy and perfect in every way, we feel like he's our miracle baby. We look at him and thank God. It's almost unbelievable to us that he's ours.

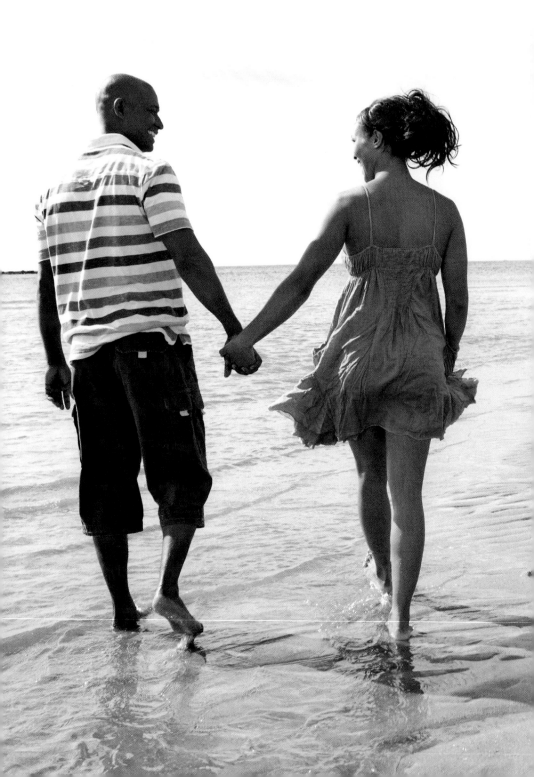

CHAPTER 7

Tips for increased success

Browse the Internet or flip through a health magazine, and it doesn't take long to notice that there's no shortage of advice on tips and tricks for getting pregnant — not to mention, plenty of opportunity to spend money on products that promise to help.

But do you really have to lie still or put your feet up on the wall for 30 minutes after having sexual intercourse to improve your chances of getting pregnant? And what about information that claims certain sexual practices can help you determine the sex of your baby? How do you know what's good information and what's not?

This chapter provides you with some general recommendations — based on existing evidence — to help you sort through all of the information out there on how to get pregnant faster. To a certain extent, you simply have to let nature take its course. However, you may be able to increase your chances of becoming pregnant by following some basic advice.

PLAN AHEAD

The best thing you can do to increase your chances of a successful pregnancy is to have a preconception visit with your care provider. Talking with your OB-GYN, family doctor or other care provider before you plan to become pregnant is a great way to begin your journey. He or she can assess your overall health and help you identify lifestyle changes that might improve your chances of a healthy pregnancy.

Preconception planning is especially helpful if you or your partner have any health issues. And keep in mind that preconception visits aren't only for women; they're just as beneficial and important for men.

For example, if you have a chronic condition such as high blood pressure or diabetes, a care provider can help you keep it under control so that you're in good health to begin your journey to pregnancy. Your provider can also review any medications you're taking and make appropriate recommendations including helping you choose prenatal vitamins to start taking right away.

A preconception visit can get you caught up on your immunizations, some of which are important to receive before you become pregnant to provide maximum protection for your baby. Depending on your age and family history and that of your partner, your care provider may discuss screening tests to identify potential genetic conditions. Sometimes, if the issues are complex, you may benefit from seeing a genetics counselor who can help you decide whether you should undergo testing, and if so, how to go about doing it.

Perhaps most importantly, your care provider can address any particular concerns that you or your partner may have regarding having a baby. By including your care provider early in the process, you'll not only be better prepared for the journey ahead but also have someone to turn to when additional questions or challenges arise.

Read Chapter 3 to get the whole scoop on preconception planning.

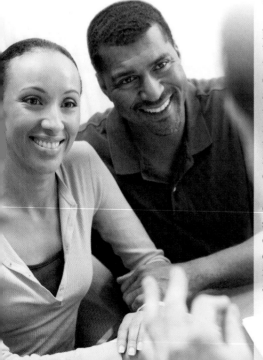

KNOW YOUR WINDOW

One thing that's evident from all of the data scientists have compiled on fertility is that there's a time frame in a woman's menstrual cycle when the odds of pregnancy are substantially higher — your fertile window. This window almost always occurs in the five days before ovulation and the 24-hour period after.

This calculation results from two factors: 1. Ejaculated sperm can live in the female reproductive system for up to five days. 2. Once ovulation occurs, the egg survives less than 24 hours. Theoretically, these six days provide the best odds for sperm and egg to meet.

In studies of healthy couples trying to conceive, pregnancy was most likely to occur when a couple had sex in the two to three days before ovulation. In a study published in the *New England Journal of Medicine*, investigators found that for couples who had intercourse only once during the six-day fertile window, the probability of conception was highest on the two days leading up to and including the day of ovulation.

Another report on a group of European couples broke down the probabilities by age group. For women between the ages of 19 and 26, the chances of becoming pregnant rose steadily from around 8 percent five days before ovulation to a peak of 53 percent two days before, and then decreased to 10 percent the day of ovulation. In the day or two following ovulation, the odds decreased even further to around 2 percent.

For women ages 35 to 39 years, the odds were lower but still followed the same pattern, rising from 6 percent five days before ovulation to a peak of 30 percent two days before ovulation, decreasing to 8 percent on the day of ovulation and lessening thereafter.

CONCEPTION VS. A SUCCESSFUL PREGNANCY

When scientists examine the odds of getting pregnant, they often measure the number of conceptions that occur. However, you should know that conceiving isn't the same as successfully delivering a baby. Out of all the conceptions that occur, about two-thirds result in babies being born. As you read earlier in the book, it's not uncommon for a miscarriage to occur before a woman knows she's pregnant.

Even in this chapter, the numbers described reflect conceptions, not live births. Conceptions are used primarily because it makes it easier to compare study results.

If you're looking into a fertility clinic or speaking with a care provider, it may help to keep this caveat in mind so that you can get a realistic picture of the numbers the clinic or individual may provide.

In other words, if you and your partner have sex within the two to three days leading up to ovulation, a good supply of sperm should be waiting to try to penetrate the egg when it's released from the ovary. The tricky part can be determining when ovulation occurs, but it's not impossible. You can learn more about recognizing the signs of ovulation in Chapter 6.

HAVE SEX OFTEN

You've probably heard and read about how frequently you should have sex to become pregnant. Generally, the more often, the better. For example, if you have sex every day throughout your cycle, your chances of conception are at their highest — somewhere around 37 percent, depending on your age. If you have sex every other day, your odds decrease a little but not by much — around 33 percent. At this rate, intercourse is bound to coincide with ovulation at some point. If you have sex just once a week, your odds in a given cycle drop to around 15 percent.

Having sex every day or even every other day may not be feasible, or even enjoyable, for many couples. However, the odds of conceiving are roughly equivalent whether you have sex every other day for the whole cycle or only a couple of times in the five days before ovulation.

If you're busy or you travel frequently and are away from your partner, it may be worth investing some time into determining your average fertile window so that you can maximize your efforts to become pregnant. If predicting your ovulation date proves difficult, rest assured that by having sex every other day starting soon after your period, your chances of conception are virtually the same as if you timed it.

Frequent sex and semen quality Perhaps you've heard that having sex too often might deplete the number and quality of sperm. It's true that closely spaced ejaculations can reduce the total sperm count, as well as the concentration of sperm and percentage of moving sperm. In theory, this might hinder chances of conception. Some studies report that one day of abstinence is enough to restore optimal semen quality while others say that four to seven days of abstinence is best.

Q. CAN YOU INFLUENCE THE SEX OF YOUR BABY?

A. What determines the sex of your baby is whether the sperm that ultimately fertilizes the egg is carrying an X or a Y chromosome. The egg already contains an X chromosome in its nucleus. If the lucky sperm brings another X chromosome, the baby will be a girl. If it brings a Y chromosome, the baby will be a boy.

An X chromosome contains roughly three times the genetic material that the Y chromosome does. A popular theory, therefore, is that Y chromosome-bearing sperm are lighter and able to swim faster than their X chromosome-bearing counterparts. Thus, if you have sex close to ovulation, the speedier sperm carrying Y chromosomes will reach the egg first and the result will be a boy.

On the flip side, X chromosome-bearing sperm are supposedly hardier and more likely to survive longer than the Y chromosome-bearing sperm. As a result, theory has it that if you have intercourse a few days before ovulation, chances are greater that the hardier X chromosome-bearing sperm will still be alive to penetrate the egg and the result will be a girl.

It seems to make sense, but many experts disagree, and available evidence on the timing of intercourse and the sex of children resulting from the sexual encounters have failed to confirm this theory. Some studies have even found the opposite — that more girls are born when sex is timed closely to ovulation.

Some high-tech procedures may increase the odds of having a child of one sex or another. One procedure known as sperm sorting uses a laboratory procedure called flow cytometry to separate male and female sperm by the amount of genetic material they contain, and then sperm of the desired sex can be used to fertilize eggs during intrauterine insemination or in vitro fertilization (IVF). However, this technique isn't foolproof, since there's some overlap between the amount of genetic material between the X- and Y-bearing sperm. There is always some contamination of male sperm in the female population and vice versa.

Another procedure called preimplantation genetic screening (PGS) is more accurate. PGS relies on genetic testing of the embryos to determine the sex. PGS requires couples to undergo IVF, since the embryos need to be sampled in the lab before they can be tested. This technique, sometimes referred to as "family balancing," is discussed on page 214.

If you're interested in having a child of a certain sex, you may want to ask your fertility provider if these techniques are available at his or her clinic and if there are restrictions to their use.

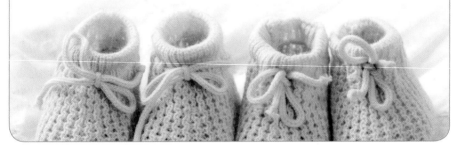

On the other hand, waiting too long can have detrimental effects, as well. Abstinence periods of 10 days or more can lead to a deterioration in semen quality.

Given that the highest pregnancy rates occur in couples that have sex every one to two days, it may be best not to give too much importance to allowing for periods of abstinence. Most experts don't recommend cutting back on intercourse for the sole purpose of improving sperm potency.

FORGET ABOUT POSITIONS AND ROUTINES

A lot of women wonder whether they should stay still or lie down after having sex. You may have heard this advice from others, or you may have noticed some leakage of semen upon standing following intercourse. You may even have had people advise you to put your legs up on the wall to prevent semen from leaking out.

These cautions really aren't necessary. The truth is that it only takes a few seconds for sperm to make their way into the cervical canal. Studies of small labeled particles placed in the vagina found that during the follicular phase of the menstrual cycle (prior to ovulation), the particles made it all the way into the fallopian tubes in as little as two minutes.

Semen itself is made up of lots of proteins and other substances in addition to sperm. Once outside of the male reproductive system, semen liquefies, making it easier for sperm to swim. What leakage may occur probably consists mostly of other substances with relatively few sperm still in it. So there's really no need to follow any special routine after sex to keep semen inside the vaginal tract.

Couples also wonder if certain positions during sex may improve the odds of conception or if it's important for the woman to have an orgasm during sexual intercourse if she wants to get pregnant.

The hormone oxytocin produced in a woman's body as a result of orgasm may help bring more sperm into the fallopian tubes, but no real link has been observed between female orgasm and fertility. Similarly, there's no scientific basis for the idea that certain positions during sex will enhance conception. By all means, though, feel free to get creative if you'd like!

AVOID LUBRICANTS

One piece of advice you may find helpful is to avoid using many of the sexual lubricants available in stores, such as K-Y jelly, Astroglide and Replens, to name just a few. When tested in a laboratory, these lubricants were found to either kill off sperm or impede their ability to swim. Some lubricants are sold as spermicide lubricants, intended to prevent pregnancy. So it pays to take a close look at the product label. Even home remedies such as olive oil and saliva have been shown to have damaging effects on sperm.

Whether lubricants actually impair fertility in real life is up for debate. But if you use lubricants during sex and you're having trouble getting pregnant, you might want to stop using them until you conceive.

Some manufacturers have created lubricants that are supposedly not toxic to sperm. Pre-Seed is an example. In lab testing, mineral oil and canola oil were found to be more sperm-friendly, as well. These products may be better options if you need to use a lubricant.

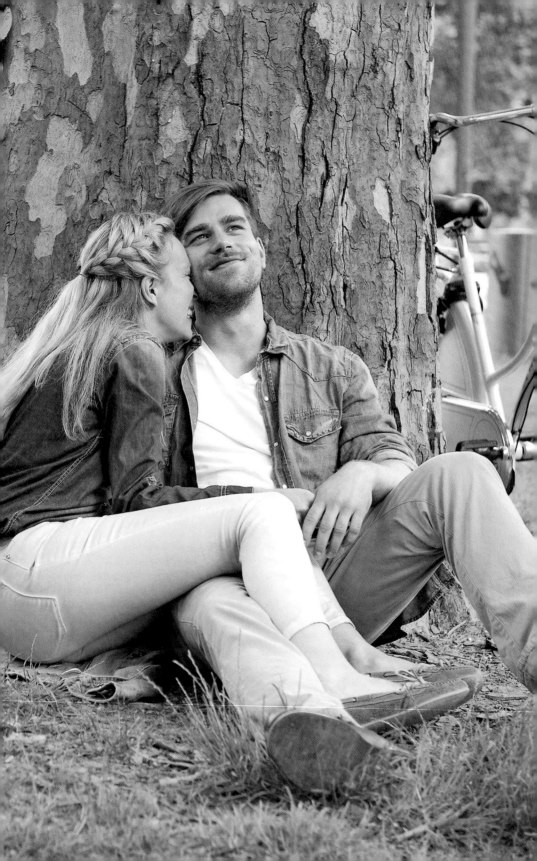

HAVE FUN

With all this talk of timing and percentages and varying odds, the idea of procreation can seem truly overwhelming. Having sex can become a chore rather than a pleasure and going through the motions can be less than fulfilling. Worst of all, the stress of trying to get pregnant can put a very real strain on your relationship.

As much as you can, try to set aside a few times a month when you're making love just for the sheer fun of it. Forget about having babies for a while, and make it a time to reconnect with each other and enjoy the love you share. That means a lot, too.

Try to take this approach beyond the bedroom. Meet for lunch, have coffee together, play a sport, get away for the weekend. If you focus too narrowly on just one specific aspect of your relationship — getting pregnant — you'll miss out on all the other fun parts.

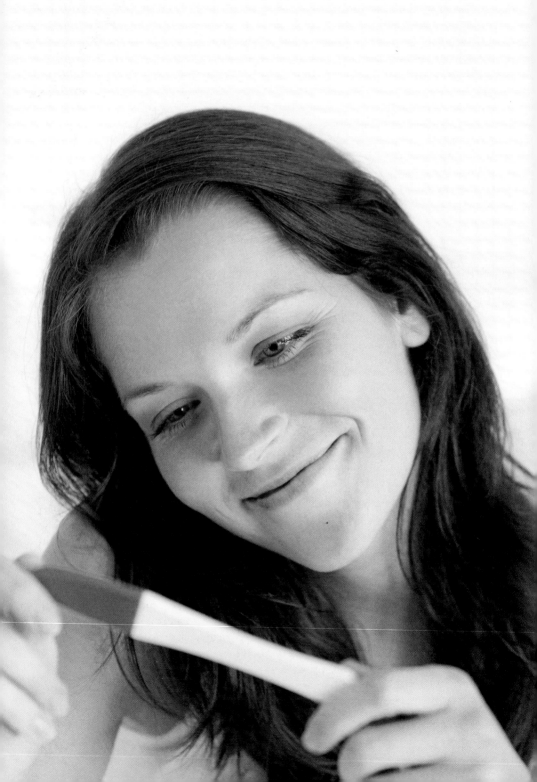

CHAPTER 8

Are you pregnant?

Maybe your period is a day or two late, or maybe it's just a gut feeling you have. You think you might be pregnant — and you must know, now! If you've been trying to conceive, you may wonder how you'll know if you're pregnant. A big clue, obviously, is if you miss your period. But it's possible you could experience subtle signs and symptoms even before then.

The only way to know for sure if you're pregnant is to take a pregnancy test. If you experience certain symptoms before you take the test, they could be clues to the test's results.

EARLY SIGNS AND SYMPTOMS

For some women, early signs and symptoms of pregnancy begin in the first few weeks after conception. Don't get too hung up on them, though. Some symptoms can indicate that you're getting sick or that your period is about to start. Likewise, you can be pregnant without experiencing any of these symptoms.

Tender, swollen breasts A woman's hormone levels rapidly change after conception. Your breasts may provide one of the first symptoms of pregnancy. As early as two weeks after conception, hormonal changes can make your breasts tender, tingly or sore. They may also feel warm, fuller and heavier.

Fatigue Fatigue also ranks high among early symptoms of pregnancy. During early pregnancy, levels of the hormone progesterone soar. High levels of progesterone can cause sleepiness.

Slight bleeding or cramping Sometimes a small amount of vaginal bleeding (spotting) is one of the first symptoms of pregnancy. The bleeding is different from a normal period and occurs earlier. Some women also experience abdominal cramping early in pregnancy that's similar to menstrual cramping.

Nausea with or without vomiting
Morning sickness, which can strike at any time of the day or night, is a classic symptom of pregnancy. For some women, the queasiness begins very early — two to three weeks after conception. Many pregnant women also have a heightened sense of smell, so various odors — such as foods cooking, perfume or cigarette smoke — may trigger waves of nausea.

Food aversions or cravings You might find yourself turning up your nose at certain foods, such as coffee or fried foods. Food cravings are common, too. Like most other symptoms of pregnancy, they can be chalked up to hormonal changes.

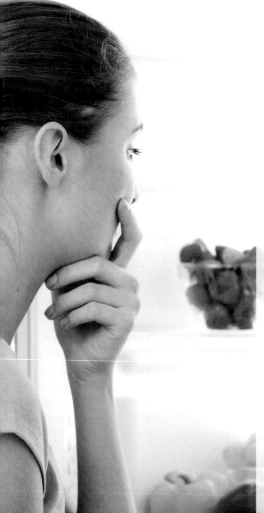

Increased urination You may find yourself urinating more often than normal. This is also related to a change in hormone levels.

Headaches and dizziness Increased blood circulation can trigger frequent, mild headaches. In addition, as your blood vessels dilate and your blood pressure drops, you may feel lightheaded or dizzy.

Mood swings The flood of hormones in your body in early pregnancy can make you unusually emotional and weepy. Mood swings are common.

Raised basal body temperature Your basal body temperature is your temperature when you first wake up in the morning after a full night's sleep. This temperature increases slightly soon after ovulation, and it remains at that level until your next period. If you've been charting your basal body temperature to determine when you ovulate, its continued elevation for more than two weeks may mean that you're pregnant.

It's important to remember that some of the symptoms just mentioned, such as tender breasts or cramping, also can happen right before your period. So, it's basically a guessing game — are you pregnant or aren't you? — until you take a pregnancy test.

HOME PREGNANCY TESTS

If watching for early signs and symptoms seems like a lot of work, relax. An easier way to find out if you're pregnant is to take a pregnancy test. Most women begin with a home pregnancy test. Home pregnancy test kits are user-friendly and they're widely available in stores. They work by detecting the level of human chorionic gonadotropin (HCG) in your urine, a hormone made by the pregnancy.

HCG is secreted into a woman's bloodstream and urine after a fertilized egg implants itself into the uterus, which typically happens within seven days after ovulation. This is the earliest that HCG can be detected with an ultrasensitive pregnancy test. During early pregnancy, HCG levels increase rapidly, doubling every two to three days.

Taking a home pregnancy test is fairly simple. To perform the test you hold a test stick in your urine stream while going to the bathroom. Or you dip the test stick into a cup of collected urine for a short period of time. The results window on the stick will show a control line (to indicate that the test is working) and the test result.

To make sure you get the best results when taking a home pregnancy test, keep these points in mind:

- The amount of HCG increases with time, so you may want to wait a week after a missed period to take the test. It will give you a more credible result. If you have an irregular menstrual cycle or you're uncertain when you had your last period, you may need to wait up to three weeks after the sexual encounter in which it's possible you may have become pregnant before taking a pregnancy test. If you can't wait that long, take a second test a week later to confirm the results.
- Test first thing in the morning, when your urine is the most concentrated.
- Check the expiration date on the package. You shouldn't use the kit after its expiration date because the chemicals in the kit may not work correctly after that date.

- Read and follow the directions supplied with the test. Perform the steps in the correct order.
- If a step needs to be timed, don't guess at the time. Use a clock.

Reading the results Women generally use home pregnancy test kits because the kits provide results quickly and they're convenient — you can perform the test at home at a time that works for both you and your partner. There are many brands of test kits available. All of them are performed in a similar manner, but how they display the results varies somewhat. Check the packaging that's included so you know what to look for.

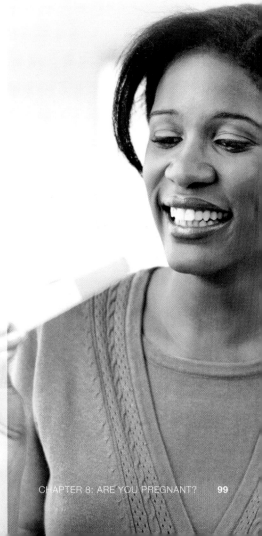

Q. WHEN SHOULD I TELL PEOPLE I'M PREGNANT?

A. There's no right or wrong answer, and it's up to you when to share your good news. Understandably, it can be very difficult to keep such a secret when you're so excited. You want to tell everybody! However, some couples prefer to wait until after the 13th week of pregnancy, when the rate of miscarriage goes way down. At that point, they feel they've gotten beyond the most dangerous stage of pregnancy. That doesn't mean, however, you have to wait that long if you just can't do it. Another option is a "limited release." Tell a few close friends or family members whom you know can keep a secret early on, and then wait until a bit later to share the news with everyone else.

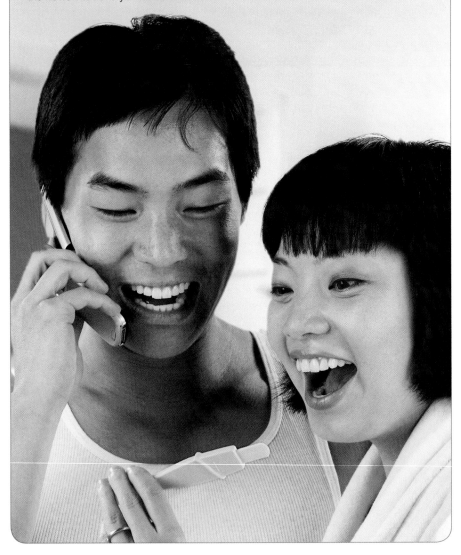

With some tests, you determine the results by noting the number of color bands, or lines, in the window. Some results show up as a plus (+) or negative (-) sign or a change in color. A few kits have a digital display that reads "yes" or "no" or "pregnant" or "not pregnant" on an LCD screen.

Test accuracy Although home pregnancy tests are very accurate, they may not be 99 percent accurate, as some manufacturers claim. A comparison of home pregnancy test kits found that some were 97 percent accurate on the first day of a missed period, while others were 54 to 67 percent accurate on the first day of a missed period. In general, positive test results are more likely to be true than are negative results.

The most common reason for a false-negative result — a result indicating you're not pregnant when you really are — is that the test was performed too soon after conception. This may be because ovulation and implantation occurred later than expected. If you think you may be pregnant, despite a negative test result, repeat the test in one week. If a second test a week later gives the same result, chances are good the result is accurate.

Another reason for a false-negative is that you drank a lot of fluid before taking the test and your urine was diluted. That's why it's recommended you perform the test first thing in the morning, when your urine is the most concentrated.

Follow-up blood test In some cases, a care provider may want to confirm the results of a home pregnancy test with a blood test that's more sensitive to HCG levels. Or you may not need one. Your care provider may schedule you for your first prenatal appointment without a blood test.

WHEN TO SEE A CARE PROVIDER

If the results of a home pregnancy test are positive, make an appointment to see your care provider. The sooner your pregnancy is confirmed, the sooner you can begin prenatal care. During your first appointment, your care provider will discuss symptoms that are common in pregnancy and that you can expect, and those that you should pay close attention to — that could be warnings of a problem.

Understandably, *a problem* are words you may not like to read about or hear from your care provider. And it's important that you not let yourself become consumed by worry or fear. Remember, the majority of pregnancies proceed normally. But it's also important that you be aware of symptoms that aren't normal, and that could signal something may not be right.

Bleeding A small amount of bleeding during pregnancy, often referred to as spotting, is common, especially during the first trimester. Spotting generally isn't a cause for alarm.

Early on, the spotting may be a result of what's called implantation bleeding — bleeding that occurs about a week after conception. Implantation bleeding may occur when the fertilized egg attaches to the lining of the uterus. This bleeding generally lasts for a short time and is usually much lighter and occurs earlier than a menstrual period.

Some women don't experience implantation bleeding and others don't notice it. It's also possible to mistake implantation bleeding for a period. If this happens, you might not realize that you're pregnant, which can lead to miscalculations when determining a baby's due date.

Implantation bleeding that's light and that stops on its own generally doesn't require treatment. If you experience heavier bleeding — you soak more than two pads or tampons in an hour for more than two hours — contact your care provider. Seek immediate care if your blood loss is accompanied by dizziness, lightheadedness, a racing heartbeat or severe pain.

Emergency symptoms In addition to heavy bleeding, contact or see your care provider right away if you experience these symptoms early in your pregnancy.

Nausea and vomiting. Nausea and vomiting with pregnancy is very common and it usually occurs within the first three months of pregnancy. This is nothing to worry about. However, if your symptoms are also accompanied by pain, fever, vertigo, diarrhea or headache, see your care provider. Also contact your care provider if you're unable to keep anything down. You may need intravenous (IV) hydration or prescription anti-nausea medication.

Urinary frequency. If you're urinating a lot, you may have an upper urinary tract infection (cystitis). Also contact your care provider if while urinating you experience pain or burning, blood or pus in the urine, a fever, or flank pain.

Pelvic pain. Mild pelvic pain is common as muscles and ligaments move and stretch and the uterus enlarges. However, if at any time you experience pelvic pain that's severe or that doesn't go away with time, rest or a change in position, contact your care provider.

Shortness of breath. Shortness of breath can accompany pregnancy but it's usually mild, comes on gradually, and isn't associated with other respiratory signs or symptoms, such as coughing or wheezing. If your shortness of breath is moderate to severe, accompanied by a fever or increased heart rate or symptoms such as coughing or wheezing, see your care provider. These could be indications of a pulmonary embolism or another cardiopulmonary condition.

Lightheadedness. When you've been standing for a period of time, especially in a warm environment, you may experience pregnancy-related lightheadedness. It should go away when you lie down or put your head in a head-down position. If it doesn't, contact your care provider.

Chest pain. Chest pain isn't a normal symptom in pregnancy. If you experience chest pain, you should see a care provider immediately. Keep in mind, though, that not all chest pain is heart related. Sometimes chest pain can result from heartburn (gastroesophageal reflux), which is more common with pregnancy.

Miscarriage and ectopic pregnancy
Two conditions that can develop early on and result in an unsuccessful pregnancy are miscarriage and ectopic pregnancy. The next chapter contains more information on these conditions, along with some coping strategies should they occur. Following are signs and symptoms to be aware of that could signal one of these conditions. Again, the purpose here is not to scare or frighten you — remember most pregnancies turn out well — but to help you better understand what warrants a quick response.

Miscarriage. Miscarriage is the spontaneous loss of a pregnancy before the 20th week. Most miscarriages occur because there was a problem with the egg or sperm or the way they came together to form the pregnancy. Contact your care provider if you experience any of these signs and symptoms:

▶ Vaginal bleeding of any kind (although spotting in early pregnancy is fairly common)

▶ Pain or cramping in your abdomen or lower back, which may range from mild to severe

▶ Passing of fluid or tissue from your vagina

Ectopic pregnancy. Normally, a fertilized egg attaches itself to the lining of the uterus. With an ectopic pregnancy, the fertilized egg implants somewhere outside the uterus, such as in a fallopian tube. An ectopic pregnancy can't proceed normally because the fertilized egg can't survive and the growing tissue might damage the mother's organs and structures.

Early on, the signs and symptoms might be the same as those of any pregnancy — a missed period, breast tenderness and nausea. Abdominal or pelvic pain and light vaginal bleeding are often the first warning signs of an ectopic pregnancy. If blood leaks from a fallopian tube, it's also possible to feel shoulder pain or an urge to have a bowel movement — depending on where the blood pools or which nerves are irritated. Heavy vaginal bleeding is unlikely, unless the ectopic pregnancy occurs in the cervix.

Seek immediate medical care if you experience severe abdominal or pelvic pain accompanied by vaginal bleeding, extreme lightheadedness or fainting.

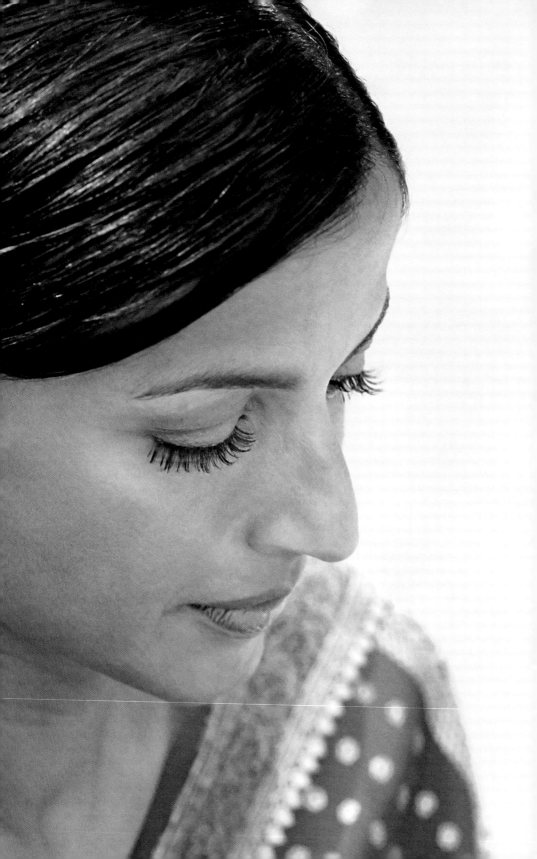

CHAPTER 9

Miscarriage and ectopic pregnancy

Sometimes pregnancy can be heart-breaking because it doesn't turn out as hoped. A loss occurs, and there's no new baby to hold in your arms. If this is your situation, it may be a time of grief, confusion and fear. Knowing why miscarriage and other forms of pregnancy loss occur won't stop the emotional pain, but it may help you and your partner understand why your provider recommends certain types of care, and what you can do to recover so that you can try again.

MISCARRIAGE

Miscarriage is the spontaneous loss of a pregnancy before the 20th week. About 15 to 20 percent of known pregnancies end in miscarriage. But the actual number is probably much higher because many miscarriages occur so early in pregnancy that a woman doesn't even know that she's pregnant. Studies suggest that about one-third of women trying to get pregnant have early miscarriages they aren't aware of.

With most miscarriages, the fetus begins to develop but then stops growing, often because of genetic problems. Miscarriage is a relatively common experience — but that doesn't make it any easier. A pregnancy that ends without a baby to hold in your arms can be difficult.

Signs and symptoms Signs and symptoms of miscarriage include:
 ▶ Vaginal spotting or bleeding
 ▶ Pain or cramping in your abdomen or lower back
 ▶ Fluid or tissue passing from your vagina
Keep in mind that spotting or bleeding in early pregnancy is fairly common. In most cases, women who experience light bleeding in the first trimester go on to have successful pregnancies. Sometimes even heavier bleeding doesn't result in miscarriage. However, you should alert your care provider if you have bleeding that soaks two pads or tampons an hour for two or more hours.

Rarely, women who miscarry develop an infection in their uterus. If you experience such an infection, called a septic miscarriage, you may also experience fever, chills, body aches, and vaginal discharge that's discolored (like pus) or has a foul odor. Call your care provider immediately if you experience these symptoms.

Sometimes, you may be asked to put the tissue that's passed from your vagina in a clean container and bring it to your doctor's office. It's unlikely that testing could define a cause for the miscarriage, but confirming the passage of placental tissue helps your doctor determine that your symptoms aren't related to a tubal (ectopic) pregnancy.

Causes Most miscarriages occur because the fetus isn't developing normally. Problems with the baby's genes or chromosomes typically result from errors that occur by chance as the embryo divides and grows — not due to problems inherited from the parents.

Some examples of abnormalities are:

▶ *Biochemical pregnancy.* In this situation the results of a pregnancy test are positive, but the pregnancy stops developing so early that nothing can be seen on an ultrasound test.

▶ *Early fetal demise, or missed abortion.* Here the embryo is present but has died before any symptoms of pregnancy loss have occurred. This situation may also be due to genetic abnormalities within the embryo.

▶ *Molar pregnancy.* A molar pregnancy, also called gestational trophoblastic disease, is less common. It's an abnormality of the placenta caused by a problem at the time of fertilization. In a molar pregnancy, the pregnancy tissue develops into a fast-growing mass of cysts in the uterus, which may or may not contain an embryo. If it does contain an embryo, the embryo will not reach maturity.

In a few cases, a mother's health may play a role. Uncontrolled diabetes, thyroid disease, infections, and hormonal, uterine or cervical problems can sometimes lead to a miscarriage. Other factors that increase a woman's risk of miscarriage include:

▶ *Age.* Women older than age 35 have a higher risk of miscarriage than do younger women. At age 35, you have about a 20 percent risk. At age 40, the risk is about 40 percent. And at age 45, it's about 80 percent. Paternal age also may play a role. Some studies indicate that the chance of miscarriage is higher if a woman's partner is age 35 or older, with the chance increasing as men age.

▶ *More than two previous miscarriages.* The risk of miscarriage is higher in

---

Q. CAN MISCARRIAGE BE PREVENTED?

A. There's no way to make sure that you won't have a miscarriage. But you can reduce your chances of having one by avoiding cigarettes, alcohol, too much caffeine and any injury to your belly. Having a fever or certain rare infections also puts you at risk of miscarriage, so you should talk to your doctor about how to avoid getting sick.

TYPES OF MISCARRIAGES

Depending on what he or she finds upon examination, your care provider may have a specific name for the type of miscarriage you experienced. Keep in mind that in this setting the terms *miscarriage* and *abortion* are often used interchangeably; they mean the spontaneous loss of a pregnancy. It can be confusing, and sometimes upsetting, when a couple hears their miscarriage referred to as an abortion.

▶ *Threatened abortion.* If you're bleeding but your cervix hasn't begun to dilate, you're experiencing a threatened abortion. After some rest, such pregnancies often proceed without any further problems.

▶ *Inevitable miscarriage.* If you're bleeding, your uterus is contracting and your cervix is dilated, a miscarriage is inevitable.

▶ *Incomplete miscarriage.* If you pass some of the fetal or placental material but some remains in your uterus, it's considered an incomplete miscarriage.

▶ *Missed abortion.* The placental and embryonic tissues remain in the uterus, but the embryo has died or was never formed.

▶ *Complete miscarriage.* If you've passed all of the pregnancy tissues, it's considered a complete miscarriage. This is common for miscarriages occurring before 12 weeks.

▶ *Septic abortion.* If you develop an infection in your uterus, it's known as a septic abortion. This requires immediate care.

women with a history of two or more previous miscarriages. After one miscarriage, your risk of miscarriage is the same as that of a woman who's never had a miscarriage.

▶ *Smoking, alcohol and illicit drugs.* Women who smoke or drink alcohol during pregnancy have a greater risk of miscarriage than do nonsmokers and women who avoid alcohol during pregnancy. Illicit drug use — particularly cocaine use — increases the risk of miscarriage.

▶ *Invasive prenatal tests.* Some invasive prenatal genetic tests, such as chorionic villus sampling and amniocentesis, carry a slight risk of miscarriage.

Getting medical attention If you're experiencing symptoms or you feel that you may have experienced a miscarriage,

contact your care provider. He or she will instruct you on who you need to see and when. In some circumstances, you may be instructed to go to a hospital emergency room.

Your doctor is likely to ask you a number of questions, including when you had your last menstrual period, when you began experiencing symptoms, and if you've had a miscarriage before. He or she may also perform one or more of the following tests:

▶ *Pelvic exam.* Your doctor will check to see the size of the uterus and if your cervix has begun to dilate.

▶ *Ultrasound.* This helps your doctor check for a fetal heartbeat and determine if the embryo is developing normally.

▶ *Blood tests.* If you've miscarried, measurements of the pregnancy hormone, human chorionic gonadotropin (HCG) can be useful in determining if you've completely passed all placental tissue. If it's not clear if a miscarriage has occurred, repeating the test 48 hours later may make things more clear.

- *Tissue tests.* If you've passed tissue, it can sometimes be sent to a laboratory to confirm that a miscarriage has occurred — and that your symptoms aren't related to another cause of pregnancy bleeding.

Treatment If you haven't miscarried but have symptoms of a threatened miscarriage, your doctor may recommend resting until the bleeding or pain subsides. You may be asked to avoid exercise and travel — especially to areas where it would be difficult to receive prompt medical care.

With the use of ultrasound, a doctor can often determine whether the embryo has died or was never formed — and that a miscarriage will definitely occur. In this situation, there are several options to consider. Before the use of ultrasound in early pregnancy, most women didn't know they were destined to have a miscarriage until it was already in process.

Expectant management. If you choose to let the miscarriage progress naturally, it usually happens within a couple of weeks after determining that the embryo has died, but it may take up to three to four weeks. This option is known as expectant management. At the time of the miscarriage, you may experience heavy bleeding and cramping, like a heavy period, which could last for several hours. You may also pass some tissue. Your care provider can advise you how to handle this tissue. Usually the heavy bleeding subsides within a few hours and light bleeding continues for up to several weeks. This can be an emotionally difficult time. If the miscarriage doesn't happen spontaneously, medical or surgical treatment may be necessary.

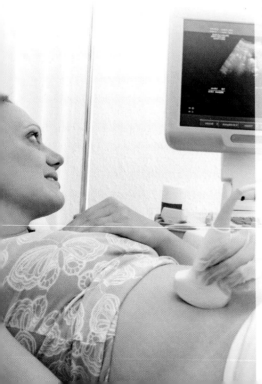

Medical treatment. If after a diagnosis of pregnancy loss you prefer to speed the process, medication may be used to cause your body to expel the pregnancy tissue and placenta. You can take the medication by mouth, but your care provider may recommend giving the medication vaginally to increase its effectiveness and minimize side effects, such as nausea, stomach pain and diarrhea. The miscarriage will likely happen at home. The specific timing may vary, and you may need more than one dose of the medication. For most women, treatment works within 24 hours.

Surgical treatment. Another option is a minor surgical procedure called suction dilation and curettage (D&C). During this procedure, the doctor dilates your cervix and gently suctions the tissue out

Q. IF I'VE HAD ONE MISCARRIAGE, WHAT ARE THE ODDS OF ANOTHER?

A. It's understandable to be worried about the possibility of another miscarriage, but fertility experts generally don't consider one miscarriage to be a sign that there's anything wrong with you or your partner. Miscarriage can be a one-time occurrence. Most women who miscarry go on to have a healthy pregnancy after miscarriage. Less than 5 percent of women have two consecutive miscarriages, and only 1 percent have three or more consecutive miscarriages.

of your uterus. Sometimes a long metal instrument with a loop on the end (curet) is used after the suction to scrape the uterine walls. Complications are rare, but they may include damage to the connective tissue of your cervix or the uterine wall. Sometimes additional surgical treatment is necessary to stop the bleeding. This option requires some type of anesthesia, and it typically takes place in an operating room or outpatient surgical facility.

Recovery Physical recovery from miscarriage generally takes a few hours to a couple of days. Expect your period to return within four to six weeks. Call your care provider if you experience heavy bleeding, fever, chills or severe pain. These signs and symptoms could indicate an infection. Avoid having sex or putting anything in your vagina — such as a tampon or douche — for two weeks after a miscarriage.

Emotional healing may take much longer than physical healing. Miscarriage can be a heart-wrenching loss that others around you may not fully understand. Your emotions may range from anger to despair. Give yourself time to grieve the loss of your pregnancy, and seek help from those who love you. Keeping the loss to yourself isn't necessary. Talk to

your care provider if you're feeling profound sadness or depression. Your care provider may advise you to wait a while before becoming pregnant again so that you can heal both physically and emotionally. Talk with him or her about when the best time would be for you to attempt pregnancy after a miscarriage.

RECURRENT PREGNANCY LOSS

Recurrent pregnancy loss is the loss of two or more pregnancies in the first trimester. As many as 1 couple in 20 experiences two pregnancy losses in a row. Up to 1 in 100 couples has three or more consecutive losses. Losses in the second trimester are less common.

Recurrent pregnancy loss can be emotionally traumatic, but it's important to remember that many women who experience three or more miscarriages still have a good prognosis for eventually having a successful pregnancy. In one study, 70 percent of women with recurrent pregnancy loss eventually had a successful pregnancy. In another study, 8 of 17 women with six or more unexplained miscarriages had successful pregnancy outcomes.

Causes Often, no reason for the miscarriages can be found — everything appears to be normal. Occasionally, a cause can be identified. Possible causes include:

Chromosomal alterations. One of the parents may have a chromosomal make-up that's altered, reducing the odds of getting the right combination of sperm and egg, leading to a higher rate of miscarriage. This problem can sometimes be addressed by doing in vitro fertilization and testing the embryos for the right chromosomes, or it can be addressed with donor sperm or donor egg procedures.

Problems with the uterus. If a woman has an unusually shaped uterus from the time of birth or from the presence of fibroids or scar tissue, it may lead to miscarriage. Surgery may be able to correct some problems with the uterus.

Problems with the cervix. Having a weakened cervix that can dilate without signs of labor also may be associated with an increased risk of miscarriage. Unlike most other forms of miscarriage, those associated with cervical problems tend to occur later, in the second trimester.

Blood-clotting problems. Some women are more likely to form blood clots that circulate through their blood. This can result in poor placental function and miscarriage. Testing can determine if a woman has anti-phospholipid antibody syndrome, a blood-clotting problem that can sometimes result in pregnancy loss. A variety of approaches may be used to reduce the risk of miscarriage.

Endocrine abnormalities. Poorly controlled diabetes increases the risk of miscarriage and increases the risk of birth defects. Women with diabetes whose blood sugar is under control before conception generally experience improved pregnancy outcomes. Women who have insulin resistance, such as obese women or those with polycystic ovary syndrome, have higher rates of miscarriage. Thyroid abnormalities and blood hormone prolactin may also be associated with miscarriage.

Sperm defects. Some evidence suggests that abnormal intactness (integrity) of sperm DNA may affect embryo development and possibly increase miscarriage risk. The data are still preliminary, and it's not known how often sperm defects may contribute to recurrent miscarriage.

Other factors have been suggested as causes of recurrent miscarriages. They include progesterone deficiency in early pregnancy, problems with implantation of the placenta and a variety of infections. However, there's no firm evidence that treating these problems affects the outcome of subsequent pregnancies. More than half the time, no cause for the pregnancy losses can be found.

Evaluation If you experience recurrent miscarriages, your care provider will likely want to do a complete evaluation. This may include your medical history, surgical history, genetic history and family history, as well as a physical exam. In addition, your care provider may:

▶ *Perform blood tests.* These include tests to check your immune system, blood-clotting system and hormone levels. They also include tests to check for certain medical conditions, such as thyroid disease or diabetes.
▶ *Do an imaging test of your uterus.* Different types of imaging tests may be performed to view the reproductive organs. A common test is a special type of ultrasound exam.

▶ *Look inside your uterus.* This involves having a thin tube with a camera and light on the end placed into your vagina and up into your uterus.

▶ *Perform chromosome tests.* This would involve both you and your partner. Before and after the testing, you talk with a person who specializes in genetic problems (genetic counselor).

Additional, more expensive tests generally aren't necessary. However, they may be done depending on your individual situation and if your care provider suspects a possible condition or abnormality.

Treatment If your care provider finds a possible cause that can be treated, he or she will likely want to treat it.

For example, problems in the uterus can sometimes be treated with surgery. Certain medical or hormone problems can sometimes be treated with medicines. If a cause can't be found, the next step is generally a discussion with your care provider about various options for increasing your chances of a successful pregnancy.

Dealing with a miscarriage can be very difficult, but don't give up hope. Even if you've had repeated miscarriages, you still have a good chance to have a successful pregnancy. This is true even if the causes of the past losses cannot be found. Future pregnancies may need early attention, so talk to your care provider about special care you may need.

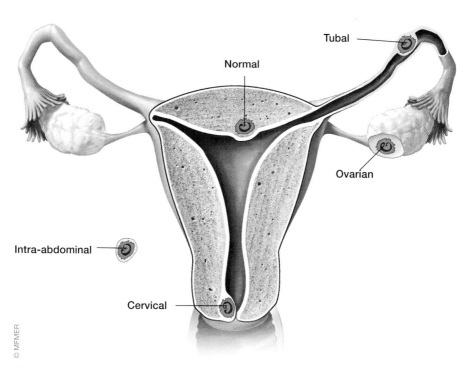

Normally, a fertilized egg attaches itself to the lining of the uterus. With an ectopic pregnancy, the egg implants somewhere outside the uterus. Often, an ectopic pregnancy occurs in one of the fallopian tubes. This is known as a tubal pregnancy. An ectopic pregnancy can also occur in the abdominal cavity, an ovary or the neck of the uterus (cervix).

ECTOPIC PREGNANCY

An ectopic pregnancy is one in which the fertilized egg attaches itself in a place other than inside the uterus. The vast majority of ectopic pregnancies occur in a fallopian tube (tubal pregnancy). They can also occur in the abdomen, ovary or cervix (see page 111). Because the fallopian tube is too narrow to hold a growing baby, ectopic pregnancies can't proceed normally. Eventually, the walls of the fallopian tube stretch and burst, putting a woman in danger of life-threatening blood loss.

There are strong associations between fallopian tube abnormalities and ectopic pregnancy. Factors known to increase the risk of tubal pregnancy include:

▶ An infection or inflammation of the tube that has caused it to become partly or entirely blocked
▶ Previous surgery in the pelvic area or on the fallopian tubes that has resulted in scar tissue around the tubes
▶ An unusually shaped fallopian tube or a fallopian tube that was damaged, possibly from a previous ectopic pregnancy or a previous surgery

The major risk factor for ectopic pregnancy is pelvic inflammatory disease (PID), which is an infection of the uterus, fallopian tubes or ovaries. The risk of ectopic pregnancy is also higher in women experiencing any of the following:

▶ A previous ectopic pregnancy
▶ Pregnancy after a tubal ligation
▶ Pregnancy while using an intrauterine device (IUD)
▶ Surgery on a fallopian tube
▶ Infertility problems or treatments
▶ Tobacco use

Signs and symptoms At first, an ectopic pregnancy may seem like a normal pregnancy. Early signs and symptoms are the same as those of any pregnancy — a missed period, breast tenderness, fatigue and nausea. Pain is generally the first sign of an ectopic pregnancy, but abnormal bleeding usually is present, too. You may feel sharp, stabbing pain in your pelvis or abdomen, generally on either the right or left side. Rarely the pain may occur in other places, such as the shoulder and neck. The pain may come and go. If you have severe pain, such as pain that wakes you from sleep or that persists despite rest, seek evaluation right away.

Other warning signs of ectopic pregnancy include gastrointestinal symptoms, dizziness and lightheadedness. If you experience any of these signs or symptoms, contact your care provider right away. There may be other possible causes for the signs and symptoms, but your care provider may first want to rule out an ectopic pregnancy.

Treatment If your care provider suspects an ectopic pregnancy, he or she will likely perform an abdominal and pelvic exam to locate the pain, tenderness or a mass. Unless your condition is obvious or you're clearly in an emergency situation, lab tests and ultrasound may be used to confirm the diagnosis.

An ectopic pregnancy must be treated to prevent rupture of the tube and other complications. Small ectopic pregnancies may be treated with the medication methotrexate, which is highly toxic to placental tissue and causes the embryo to stop developing. In many cases, however, surgery is required. A small incision is made in the lower abdomen and a long, thin instrument is inserted into the pelvic area to remove the mass. In some cases, the affected fallopian tube may need to be removed. Other times, the pregnancy tissue is removed but the tube remains in place.

HETEROTOPIC PREGNANCY

A heterotopic pregnancy is a rare situation in which a woman has one embryo growing in the uterus and one outside of the uterus (ectopic pregnancy) at the same time. Generally, the ectopic pregnancy is in a fallopian tube (tubal pregnancy), less often in the cervix or an ovary. Heterotopic pregnancy occurs most often in women undergoing assisted reproductive techniques. The goal is to try and remove the ectopic embryo while saving the uterine embryo. This is most often done with surgery or an injection of medication into the ectopic embryo that causes the embryo to stop developing.

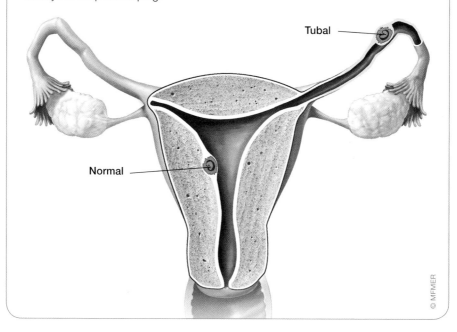

After treatment, your doctor will likely want to recheck your level of a pregnancy hormone called human chorionic gonadotropin (HCG) until it reaches zero. If the level remains high, it could indicate the ectopic tissue wasn't entirely removed, and you may need additional surgery or treatment with methotrexate. On rare occasions, a care provider may recommend no treatment except observation to see if an ectopic pregnancy will end on its own, through spontaneous expulsion or absorption, before any damage is done to the fallopian tube.

Future pregnancies If you've had one ectopic pregnancy, you're more likely to have another. However, successful pregnancy after an ectopic pregnancy may still be possible. Even if one tube was injured or removed, an egg may be fertilized in the other fallopian tube before entering the uterus. If both tubes were injured or removed, in vitro fertilization may be an option. In vitro fertilization involves retrieving mature eggs from a woman, fertilizing them with sperm in a laboratory and then implanting the fertilized eggs in the woman's uterus (see page 205).

If you've had an ectopic pregnancy, talk to your care provider before becoming pregnant again so that together you can work on the best strategy.

TRYING AGAIN

Pregnancy loss can be an extremely difficult experience. You may feel as if your hopes for the future have been taken from you. These feelings can occur even if the pregnancy was only a few weeks along. There's no set of rules about what you will or will not feel after a pregnancy loss. You may simply feel numb for a while. Allow yourself to have your feelings, and try to work through them. Grieving a pregnancy loss takes time.

Some couples think that they must try to conceive again right away in order to fix the problem or replace the hurt. Unfortunately, it's unlikely that a subsequent pregnancy will carry the same feelings of innocence and bliss. A pregnancy after a loss can be highly stressful because of anxiety and fear that something may go wrong.

Although a pregnancy loss can be extremely difficult, it doesn't mean you won't be able to have another baby. In most cases, your chances of having a normal, healthy pregnancy are still excellent. Your decision on whether and when to try again rests on the type of pregnancy you had, as well as your physical and emotional recovery. There's no perfect time to try to conceive again. In general, most care providers recommend waiting a few menstrual cycles before trying again.

Emotional recovery If you find yourself grieving deeply after a pregnancy loss, allow yourself the time to do so. Emotional recovery can, and usually does, take much longer than physical recovery.

Some people may wonder why you mourn for a child that you've never known. But in many ways you may have already bonded with the baby growing inside you. You and your partner may have already begun to imagine the days when you would hold your baby in your arms. The missed opportunity of watching your child grow and develop can be difficult to accept. Even if no embryo was ever present, you may still grieve when your dreams and expectations were to have a baby.

Keep in mind that you and your partner may deal with a pregnancy loss in different ways. It may not always be easy to recognize that the other person is hurting. You may wish to talk things out, and your partner may prefer to stay silent. In addition, one may feel the need to move on before the other is ready. Now more than ever you need to rely on each other for support. Try to listen and respond to each other while accepting the other person's feelings. You may wish to consider seeing a counselor or therapist for help in expressing your emotions and expectations in more neutral territory.

Physical recovery How long it takes to recover physically from a pregnancy loss often depends on the type of loss.

Miscarriage. Physically speaking, it often takes only a few days for a woman to recover from a miscarriage. It usually takes four to six weeks after a miscarriage before your period comes back. It's possible to conceive in those weeks between the miscarriage and your first menstrual cycle, but it's generally not recommended.

During this time, you may wish to use a barrier form of birth control, such as a

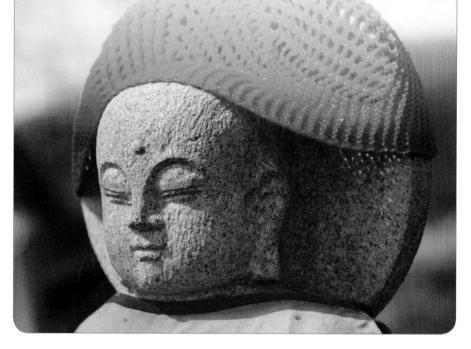
condom or diaphragm. If you and your partner feel ready to become pregnant again, there are several issues to consider. Before conceiving, talk to your care provider about your plans. He or she can help you come up with a strategy that will optimize your chances of a healthy pregnancy and delivery. If you had a single miscarriage, your chances of a subsequent healthy pregnancy are virtually the same as someone who has never had a miscarriage. Your care provider may suggest that you wait longer or have additional testing or monitoring if you've had recurrent miscarriages.

Ectopic pregnancy. Your chances of a successful pregnancy may be a bit lower after having had an ectopic pregnancy, but they're still good — between 60 and 80 percent if you have both fallopian tubes. The amount of time needed to heal will depend on how the pregnancy was treated. Talk to your care provider regarding how long you should wait before trying to conceive again.

Kristen and Chris' Story

Chris: After three and a half years of marriage, we decided it was time to start a family. It seemed like everyone around us was having children, and we were excited to join the adventure. We went off birth control and waited to see what would happen. And then we waited some more. Six, seven, eight months went by, and still, we weren't pregnant.

Kristen: I was starting to get frustrated. I couldn't understand why it wasn't working for us. Every month when I got my period, I was disappointed all over again. When we still weren't pregnant after a year, my doctor referred us to a fertility specialist.

There, we took test after test after test. We weren't sure what to expect when we went in to talk about our results, but we thought we'd be given recommendations for our next course of action. Instead, we were given some pretty tough news.

Chris: Based on our tests, the specialist told us that we had a 1 percent chance of getting pregnant on our own. That was a kick to the gut.

Then he immediately started talking about in vitro fertilization, and how it was our best option. It was a blur of information — an emotional bomb. I remember asking, "Are you telling me that we can't get pregnant on our own?"

He just kept saying, "Based on facts we have, you have a 1 percent chance."

I tried to be strong for Kristen, but it was heavy. The doctor was talking about freezing eggs, but we didn't even know if that was something we wanted to do. When we left that appointment, we both went to the bathrooms and cried.

Kristen: We learned that our problems conceiving came from both of us. I had polycystic ovary syndrome, which means that I had plenty of eggs, but they weren't maturing as they should. And Chris had irregular morphology, which means that his sperm was misshapen.

Despite these diagnoses, we decided we didn't want to try IVF. The cost was intimidating, and we were unsettled about the procedure. We knew IVF couldn't be our only option, so we sought a second opinion.

We felt more comfortable with our new doctor. We felt like she understood what we were going through. By this time, Chris had taken another test, and the doctor was encouraged by what she saw. These results were in the normal range, which opened some doors for us. It felt like there was hope.

I started taking clomiphene (Clomid), which stimulates ovulation. It took three months to find the right dose, but once we did, I got pregnant.

Chris: We were overjoyed. Seeing that positive pregnancy test was just incredible.

Anticipation mounted as the weeks went by leading to our first ultrasound. We spent the time talking and dreaming of our future with our baby. But then, when we went in for our first ultrasound at eight weeks, the ultrasound tech said, "I'm sorry, but I'm not seeing anything. There's nothing in the uterus."

We couldn't believe it. We have a strong Christian faith, and we knew God was with us, but my heart sank for my wife. There was nothing I could do to make this better.

Kristen: They performed a pregnancy test, and the numbers came back showing that I was pregnant. Yet, there was no baby in my uterus. We felt helpless.

It turns out there was a baby inside me, but it couldn't survive. They realized I was having an ectopic pregnancy, meaning that the egg had implanted in one of my fallopian tubes.

I was given a shot that would terminate my pregnancy. When that didn't work, I came back for another shot 10 days later. Still, it didn't work. A couple of days after the second shot, I experienced extreme pain in my stomach.

Chris: I rushed her to the hospital, and it was chaos. Every doctor on the floor was in our room, taking vitals, talking about her heart rate dropping, about internal bleeding. Her fallopian tube had collapsed.

They told me they needed to get her into emergency surgery. They were going to take her fallopian tube. Kristen was white as a ghost — losing that tube was the one thing she didn't want. We didn't know what this would mean for our future as a family, but it was the only option. Everyone could tell how devastating this was for us. Even the nurse was choking up. We weren't only mourning the loss of a child, but now this uncertainty: Would we ever have a baby?

Kristen: To our relief, the surgeon was able to check my other fallopian tube during surgery and it looked healthy. We were encouraged that there was hope. It took just a few months before I was both physically and emotionally ready to start trying for another baby.

I started taking Clomid again and was told that it was just as easy to conceive a baby with one fallopian tube as with two. But seven months went by, and I still hadn't become pregnant. Then we found out that I had a cyst on my ovary. This meant that I couldn't take the Clomid that month. I was so discouraged. Not only was I not pregnant, but now I couldn't even use the medicine that could help me get pregnant.

Chris: The doctor told us to take a break — to enjoy each other and not worry about getting pregnant for a month. We were actually at peace with it. That month, we stopped thinking about babies.

One night, we went to a wedding and there were kids everywhere. It was the day that our first baby was to be due. And I thought about how our child was supposed to be at that wedding, too. It was heavy. That night, I prayed, asking God why we didn't have a baby yet, telling him how much we wanted this. That is the night that our baby was conceived.

Kristen: It was such a miracle that the month we were told we wouldn't get pregnant is the month we did. I'd never been so happy. The pregnancy was flawless, incredible, amazing. And now we're enjoying our little girl.

PART 3

Common
Fertility Problems

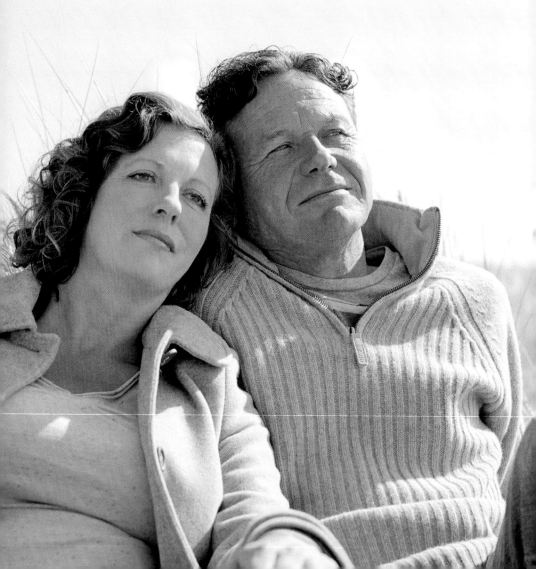

CHAPTER 10

Effect of age on pregnancy

If you put off having children too long, will it affect your ability to get pregnant? This is an important question many couples are asking. Women in particular are wondering how long they can wait before having a baby. Women, today, have more choices available to them in terms of their education and careers than in the past. Knowing that raising children requires time and effort, many women want to reach their educational, career, financial or other goals before committing to having a family. Most women also want to be in a stable relationship prior to having a baby.

The numbers reflect this trend. In general, women are now having their first child later than women did in the past. In 2011, the average age at which American women had their first baby was close to 26, as opposed to age 21 in the 1970s. In addition, the birthrate for women between the ages of 40 and 44 was the highest it's been in more than four decades.

As more women delay childbearing, the effects of age on fertility and pregnancy become more pressing. Most women are obviously aware that at a certain point in their lives, pregnancy is no longer possible. But exactly when does your potential for childbearing end? And what are your options as the years go by?

And what about men? If you're a man, does it matter how old you are if you want to have a baby?

As you'll see in this chapter, age does matter but in different ways for women and men.

FEMALE REPRODUCTIVE LIFE SPAN

To better understand the effect of age on a woman's fertility, it helps to look at the broader context of the female reproductive life span.

When a baby girl is born, she arrives with all the eggs she'll ever have — about 1 to 2 million of them. Even before birth, however, her total number of eggs has already been decreasing due to a natural process of growth and degeneration of the eggs (apoptosis). By the time she reaches puberty, the number of eggs available will be closer to 400,000. The process of egg depletion continues through adulthood. By age 37, about 25,000 eggs remain and by age 50, only about 1,000. Along the way, between 300 and 400 eggs actually make it to ovulation.

Eggs and the tiny sacs in which they develop (follicles) can mature in the ovaries largely independent of hormones, but only up to a certain point. To reach their final phase of development, the follicles require hormone stimulation. Production of these key hormones is directed by the hypothalamus, a central component of the brain, and the pituitary gland, a hormone-producing organ located at the base of the brain.

You're probably familiar with most of these important hormones by now — gonadotropin-releasing hormone (Gn-RH), follicle-stimulating hormone (FSH) and luteinizing hormone (LH). The hypothalamus releases Gn-RH, which prompts the pituitary to send out FSH and LH to the ovaries. FSH promotes growth of the follicles while LH regulates production of other hormones such as estrogen and progesterone. Estrogen and progesterone, in turn, play an important role in letting the brain know what's going on in the ovaries, so the production of Gn-RH and consequently FSH and LH can be regulated accordingly.

For successful ovulation to occur, eggs must be available and the signaling pathways between hypothalamus, pituitary and ovaries must be working smoothly (see page 135).

A cyclical pattern of hormone activity begins at puberty, resulting in the menstrual cycle women experience each month. In the first few years after puberty, cycles can be somewhat variable. But as you move into your 20s and 30s, cycles generally become fairly regular. These are the prime reproductive years for a woman.

As you move closer to your 40s, the typical decade before menopause, you start to lose eggs at a faster rate, so fewer eggs are available to compete for ovulation. And as the quantity of eggs diminishes, so does the quality of the ones remaining. The quantity and quality of your eggs is known as your ovarian reserve. Think of your ovarian reserve as a marker of you ovarian age. Changes in your ovarian reserve affect the feedback loops between the hypothalamus, pituitary and ovaries as your brain keeps trying to select the best egg possible from the ones remaining.

Toward your late 40s, hormone levels begin to shift: some increasing, others decreasing. Although you can still ovulate during this time, the follicular phase — before ovulation — tends to shorten by a few days, resulting in shorter menstrual cycles overall.

As you approach your 50s, you begin to skip cycles and ovulate less frequently. Eventually, you stop having periods altogether. Twelve months with no menstrual periods marks the official end of natural fertility and the start of menopause.

FEMALE FERTILITY AND AGE

So what does this mean for your chances of getting pregnant if you're in your mid-30s or older? For starters, keep in mind that although almost all women go through some variation of the phases described earlier, the ages at which these phases occur are by no means universal. In other words, there's no fixed age for the onset of what constitutes poor

NATURAL FERTILITY

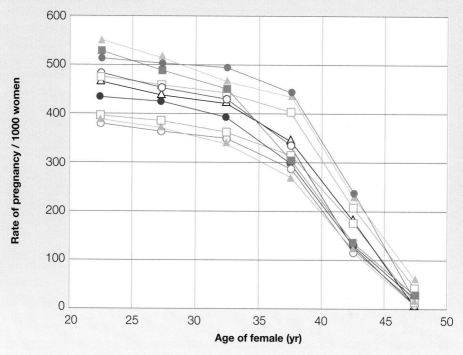

This graphic shows how fertility rates begin to decline fairly significantly after age 37. The 10 populations (in descending order beginning with the top entry on the left at ages 20 to 24) are Hutterites, marriages 1921–30; Geneva bourgeoisie, husbands born 1600–49; Canada, marriages 1700–30; Normandy, marriages 1760–90; Hutterites, marriages before 1921; Tunis, marriages of Europeans 1840–59; Normandy, marriages 1674–1742; Norway, marriages 1874–76; Iran, village marriages 1940–50; Geneva bourgeoisie, husbands born before 1600.

American Society for Reproductive Medicine Practice Committee. Optimizing natural fertility. *Fertility and Sterility*. 2008:90:S2. Used with permission.

reproductive potential. You're likely to be no less fertile the day after your 35th birthday than the day before. Everyone ages, but the effects occur gradually — on a continuum rather than at a particular cutoff point.

Women also vary. Some women have ovaries that act older than their age while other women don't begin to experience diminished ovarian reserve until their late 30s or even 40.

Clearly, women can get pregnant after the age of 35. Many of them do, some even in their early 40s. It's just that the further you move along the age continuum, the longer it may take to conceive. This is largely due to the decreasing quantity of eggs available and age-related changes to the hypothalamus-pituitary connection. At some point, the chances of getting pregnant naturally become pretty slim. And as the quality of the eggs diminishes, the risk of pregnancy complications and birth defects in the baby increases. Even with successful conception, the risk of miscarriage increases steadily with age.

Fertility over the years Studying natural fertility rates in contemporary American women can be a challenge because many women use some form of birth control at some point in their lives to prevent pregnancy. An alternative is to look at historical records of birthrates, when use of contraceptives was scarce and fertility tended to take its natural course.

Data from 10 different populations from the 16th through the 20th century show a fairly similar pattern over time (see graph on page 121). Between the ages of 20 and 35, birthrates remained fairly constant although with a slight, steady decline. After the age of 37 or so, rates declined sharply, becoming close to 0 between the ages of 45 and 50.

What about today? So what does fertility look like now? Today, the age-related decline in fertility may not be as great as what's reflected in historical records. Women today have fewer children (less stress on the body), better medical care during pregnancy and childbirth, and more effective treatment for conditions that might interfere with pregnancy. However, the general pattern still seems to hold true.

A large, well-designed study published in 2002 followed nearly 800 European women between the ages of 18 and 40 who weren't using hormonal contraceptives or taking medications that could affect fertility. The participants kept daily records of basal body temperature (to estimate time of ovulation), and recorded days on which intercourse or menstrual bleeding occurred. The participants were also broken down by age group: 19-26 years, 27-29 years, 30-34 years and 35-39 years.

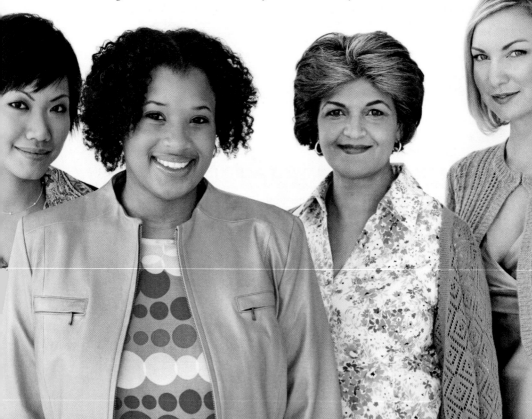

During the study, more than 400 pregnancies occurred, all resulting from one or more occasions of intercourse during the fertile window, which includes the 5 days leading up to ovulation and the day of ovulation itself, for a total of 6 days. The investigators found that neither the age of the woman or the man affected the duration of the fertile window. Older women didn't necessarily have shorter fertile windows compared to younger women. Also, the odds of becoming pregnant on a particular day followed a similar pattern for all age groups — chances of conception were highest two days before ovulation.

However, age did affect the overall probability of becoming pregnant during this window. Chances tended to decrease with increasing age. Within a single cycle, the average 19- to 26-year-old in the study had approximately a 50 percent chance of becoming pregnant on her peak fertile day, whereas the average 35- to 39-year-old had a roughly 30 percent chance of pregnancy on her peak fertile day.

This doesn't mean you have no chance of becoming pregnant if you're 37 or 38, just that your chances are lower when you compare them to a 23-year-old. Incidentally, women in their late 20s and early 30s had virtually indistinguishable rates of pregnancy.

Much of this depends on the timing of intercourse, too. If you're 37 and time intercourse so that it coincides with ovulation, your chances of pregnancy are higher than those of a 23-year-old who fails to have sex within the fertile window.

Interestingly, the investigators also noticed a substantial amount of variation within age groups. Among the women in the study aged 27 to 29, chances of pregnancy on the peak fertile day ranged from less than 10 percent all the way up to 80 percent. Scientists aren't sure of all the factors that account for such a huge variability among women of the same age (after accounting for the male partner's age and health), but it's likely a result of genetic and environmental factors.

All things being equal, however, it does become more difficult to get pregnant as you get older. An often-cited study examining fertility rates among women who received donor sperm because their male partners were infertile found that women who were older than age 35 had consistently lower conception rates and required more time to get pregnant.

The most recent national data on assisted reproductive technology success rates — using a woman's own fresh (not frozen) eggs — show substantially lower conception rates in women in their late 30s and early 40s compared with those younger than age 37. To give you an idea, live birthrates were around 42 percent for women under 35, 22 percent for women between 38 and 40, and 5 percent for women older than 42.

RELATED RISKS

Many women in their mid- to late 30s become concerned not just with getting pregnant but with the potential risks and complications that can occur in pregnancies that happen at a later age.

All pregnancies carry certain risks, no matter how old you are. At the same time, most pregnancies turn out just fine, including those among women older than age 35. But you should know chances for complications do increase with the mother's age, particularly once a woman reaches her 40s. The two biggies are pregnancy loss and chromosomal abnormalities (primarily Down syndrome). Other complications may occur, as well.

Q. IF I STILL HAVE REGULAR PERIODS, WHAT'S THE PROBLEM?

A. This is a good question and one that doesn't have a clear answer. After about age 37 or so, the average woman's fecundity — her ability to conceive in a single cycle — appears to take a sharp dive. Experts believe that this largely reflects a decrease in the quality of the eggs being released. There are several theories as to why this happens. Recall that a female is born with all the eggs she'll ever have. One idea is that the healthiest, highest quality eggs are selected for ovulation earlier in the reproductive life span, which translates into higher fecundity and lower miscarriage rates for younger women. Another theory is that the longer the eggs remain in the ovaries, the longer they have to be exposed to chemicals or radiation that may cause them to acquire genetic problems. Older eggs may also be more prone to problems with fertilization and abnormal embryo development, which can translate into higher rates of miscarriage when conception occurs.

Other factors, including environmental factors, also may play a role. Smoking, for example, is known to speed up the loss of follicles, leading to earlier menopause. In addition, as time goes by, women are at greater risk of developing disorders that may affect fertility, such as fibroids, endometriosis and pelvic infections.

The biological aging of your eggs doesn't always align neatly with your chronological age. This is reflected in the wide variation in fertility among women of the same age. Currently, there's no simple, direct way of determining the status of a woman's eggs. But there are several tests that can help doctors estimate your ovarian reserve (see Chapter 13). These results, in turn, may be helpful as you chart your next steps toward a family.

Pregnancy loss As you get older, staying pregnant becomes more difficult. An extensive survey of births to women in Denmark found that more than half the intended pregnancies in women older than age 42 resulted in loss of the pregnancy. At age 45 and older, more than 90 percent of pregnancies are lost.

Miscarriage — often occurring very early in the pregnancy and sometimes before you even know you're pregnant — accounts for the majority of losses. This is primarily because of a decrease in the quality of your eggs as time goes by, which can lead to irregularities in the way the cells divide and extra or missing chromosomes in some cells versus others. The female body will often identify a

fertilized egg with chromosomal abnormalities as not suitable for pregnancy and delivery. Hormonal shifts and changes in the way the uterus functions also may play a role in whether or not a pregnancy is sustained. Most miscarriages occur between six and 14 weeks of pregnancy.

The risk of ectopic pregnancy also increases with age, rising from a risk of 1.4 percent at age 21 to 6.9 percent at age 44 or older. An ectopic pregnancy is one in which the fertilized egg implants somewhere outside the uterus where it can't survive, often in a fallopian tube. As women get older, ectopic pregnancies become more frequent. This is probably due to risk factors that accumulate over a lifetime, such as possible exposure to more sexually transmitted infections, pelvic infection or inflammation, and fallopian tube problems.

Stillbirths — pregnancy loss after the 20th week of pregnancy — also occur more often in older women than in younger women. The reasons for this are unclear. The overall risk of stillbirth is small, though, even for women older than age 45. In the Danish study, the risk of stillbirth for a woman in her late 30s was less than half of a percent, and less than 1 percent for women older than age 45.

Chromosomal abnormalities Decreased egg quality also can lead to an increased risk of having a baby with a chromosomal defect. In a normal cycle, just before ovulation, hormones stimulate a waiting egg to finish the cell division process (meiosis) that was initiated years ago, before birth. But scientists speculate that the longer the time span between the initiation of the process and its completion — the older the egg, in other words — the more prone to errors the division process becomes. Cell division errors can result in extra or missing genetic material on one of the egg's chromosomes.

Most genetically abnormal eggs that are released from the ovaries and fertilized don't end with delivery of a baby, which is why rates of early miscarriage increase with age. But some altered eggs do survive, become fertilized and develop into full-term babies.

Down syndrome, one of the most common genetic abnormalities found in newborns, can result from just such a scenario. Because of division errors during the meiosis process, babies with Down syndrome typically carry a whole extra copy of chromosome 21 in addition to the standard two. Other chromosomal

MATERNAL AGE AND DOWN SYNDROME RISK

Maternal age (completed years)	Down syndrome risk at term:* 1 in _
20	1,477
21	1,461
22	1,441
23	1,415
24	1,382
25	1,340
26	1,287
27	1,221
28	1,141
29	1,047
30	939
31	821
32	696
33	572
34	456
35	353
36	267
37	199
38	148
39	111
40	85
41	67
42	54
43	45
44	39
45	35

*Based on Risk = $1/((1 + \exp{(7.330-4.211)}/(1 + \exp{(-0.282 \times (age-37.23))})))$ from Morris JK, et al. Journal of Medical Screening. 2002:9:2.

Rodeck, CH, et al. *Fetal Medicine: Basic Science and Clinical Practice.* 2nd ed. Philadelphia, Pa.: Churchill Livingstone Elsevier; © 2009. Used with permission.

abnormalities whose incidence increases with the mother's age are trisomy 18 (Edwards syndrome), trisomy 13 (Patau's syndrome) and sex chromosome defects, such as having an extra X chromosome (Klinefelter's syndrome) or missing an X chromosome (Turner's syndrome).

Compared with a younger woman, a woman in her late 30s or early 40s has a much higher risk of having a baby with a chromosomal abnormality. For example, the chances of a 29-year-old having a baby with Down syndrome are about 1 in 1,000. The chances of a 39-year-old are 10 times higher: about 1 in 100. This sounds dramatic, but keep in mind that the overall risk for the 39-year-old is 1 percent, which is still very low. Even for a 45-year-old woman, the overall risk is just under 3 percent (1 in 35). See the chart on page 125 for genetic risks based on the age of the mother.

Other complications High blood pressure and diabetes are common conditions that can complicate any pregnancy. As you get older, your risk of developing one or both of these conditions before becoming pregnant increases. In addition, the older you are the greater your risk of developing high blood pressure or diabetes during pregnancy. Generally, though, a mother in good health is more likely to have a good outcome than is a mother with a pre-existing health condition.

Becoming pregnant when you're older than age 40 can increase your risk of other complications, such as problems with the placenta and cesarean delivery. Congenital defects, low birth weight, preterm delivery and multiple births have been observed more frequently in older mothers, as well, but the size of the impact isn't always clear. In other words, some of these risks may technically increase as you get older, but the chances of it happening to you on an individual basis are much more variable.

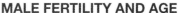

MALE FERTILITY AND AGE

Men age just as women do, but their reproductive timelines are different. In contrast to women, men don't run out of sperm like women run out of eggs at menopause. Under normal circumstances, men continue to produce sperm and male reproductive hormones throughout life. With age, however, male reproductive function gradually declines, which can affect a man's ability to father a child.

Research on aging and male fertility isn't as abundant as what's currently available on female reproductive aging, but a growing number of researchers are examining the subject. As with women, male reproductive aging occurs on a con-

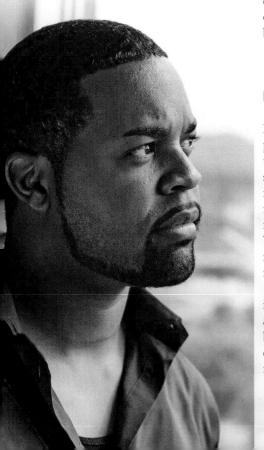

tinuum rather than at a specific cutoff point. So it's hard to pinpoint when age-related problems may begin. In addition, study results don't always agree on the impact a man's age can have on fertility and pregnancy rates. Scientists are still trying to tease out the nuances of male fertility throughout life, but here are some highlights from the research so far.

Effect on pregnancy rates Researchers who've compared semen quality between 30-year-old men and 50-year-old men have found that semen volume, the ability of sperm to move and the proportion of normal sperm all tend to decrease with age. But sperm quality doesn't always correlate well with the ability to achieve pregnancy, so it's an imperfect measure of male fertility.

Studies of how long it takes for a couple to get pregnant, particularly those that have accounted for the woman's age and other factors that might mask the true impact of the man's age, may offer a better reflection of a man's fertility over time. These studies indicate that it generally takes longer for men in their mid-30s and early 40s to achieve pregnancy than it does for younger men. A survey of British couples, after accounting for the woman's age and frequency of intercourse, reported that it took five times longer for men 45 years of age and older to achieve pregnancy than it did for men who were under age 25.

A large French study looking at women who were artificially inseminated with their husband's sperm found that the husband's age played a role in the likelihood of pregnancy, after adjusting for the effects of the wife's age. Among men younger than age 30, the pregnancy rate was 12.3 percent. After the age of 45, the pregnancy rate decreased to 9.3 percent a cycle (month).

Other studies have looked at couples receiving donor eggs from healthy, younger women — generally younger than age 35 — to see whether the father's age has any impact on fertilization and pregnancy rates. One such study, involving more than 1,000 males, observed an increase in pregnancy loss, decrease in live births and a decrease in healthy embryo development with men older than age 50.

Not all studies, though, have found that a man's age has a negative influence on pregnancy, and the factors involved in fertility are complex. Better-designed studies with larger groups of participants are needed. Age, whether that of the man or the woman, clearly isn't the only factor. But the general trend is that male fertility does tend to decline over time.

Health of aging sperm So, what happens to sperm as a man gets older that would lead to lower fertility rates? A popular line of investigation is the notion that sperm DNA become more vulnerable to damage and fragmentation with age. This may occur as a result of environmental factors, hormonal changes or other age-related events that occur as men get older. There's also some evidence that with age, the male testes have to work harder to perform quality control of sperm in line to be ejaculated. As a result, a greater number of ejaculated sperm with damaged DNA may slip by.

Oxidative stress also may contribute to sperm DNA damage over time. Oxidative stress occurs when excess free radicals, byproducts of your metabolism, begin to damage healthy cells. (See Chapter 4 for more information on combating oxidative stress.)

How damaged sperm DNA affects fertility is still unclear. Studies indicate that a woman's eggs have some capacity to repair a sperm's damaged DNA and make it viable. As a woman ages, however, her eggs' ability to rescue aging sperm may be decreased, so the age of each partner compounds the effects of the other. It also may be that current tests are unable to identify more subtle age-related DNA changes that may affect fertility.

RELATED RISKS

A number of studies also have shown that advanced male age may carry implications both for a successful pregnancy and for the health of the child.

The French study discussed earlier found that the age of the male partner had a substantial impact on the rate of miscarriages, almost doubling the risk after the age of 45. This increase isn't as strong as the impact of the woman's age (which more than doubled the rate of miscarriage), but it does play a role independent of the woman's age.

Studies also indicate a link between older fathers and later development of schizophrenia in the child. By examining the birth records of more than 600 people diagnosed with schizophrenia, researchers observed a remarkable association between the advancing age of the fathers and increased incidence of schizophrenia in the children of these men, independent of the mother's age. The relative risk of schizophrenia nearly doubled for children of men ages 45 to 49 and almost tripled for children of men older than 50, compared with children of men in their early 20s. Keep in mind, though, that the actual incidence of schizophrenia among children of men older than 50 is still pretty small, about 1 percent.

A connection also has been made between a father's advanced age and an increased risk of autism. Several studies have found that as the age of the father increases, so does the risk of autism spectrum disorders in his children.

Researchers hypothesize that age-related genetic mutations in the father's sperm may be responsible for the development of conditions such as schizophrenia and autism. However, other studies looking into these links have had mixed results, indicating there are likely other factors at play in addition to paternal age.

Statistics like these may sound frightening, but they shouldn't scare you away from having children. In general, if you're a man older than age 40, the possible increased risk of health problems to your children is still small in the grand scheme of things.

WHEN TO SEEK HELP

Fertility is a bit of a wild card. Genetics largely determine which women will still be fertile at age 40 and which won't. Knowing your mother's reproductive history may give you an idea of your fertility, but it's difficult to gauge and there are no guarantees. If time isn't on your side, you don't want to waste too much time trying to get pregnant on your own.

Keep in mind that most couples become pregnant within a year of trying. Sometimes it's just a matter of getting the timing right so that you're having sex as close to ovulation as possible. Chapter 6 contains a detailed discussion on how to identify the signs of ovulation and determine your fertile window. Adjusting your lifestyle also may help improve your fertility (see Chapters 1, 2 and 4).

If you're a woman older than age 35 and you and your partner have been trying to get pregnant for more than six months, it may be time to make an appointment with your care provider. This is according to recommendations from the American Congress of Obstetricians and Gynecologists and the American Society for Reproductive Medicine. Given that fertility tends to decline more rapidly as time goes by and considering the increasing risk of complications, it may benefit you and your partner to see what options are available to you. Your care provider also can help you decide whether you might want to try a little longer on your own to get pregnant or whether you and your partner should be evaluated for possible fertility complications.

If you're both younger than 35, don't be too concerned unless you've been trying regularly to conceive for at least a year. At that point, you may want to make an appointment with your primary care doctor or an OB-GYN.

Talk with your care provider sooner, though, if you're a woman and you have irregular or very painful periods, you've been diagnosed with endometriosis or pelvic inflammatory disease, you have a family history of early menopause, you've had ovarian surgery or cancer treatment, or you've had more than one miscarriage in the past. If you're a man, talk with your care provider if you have a history of testicular, prostate or sexual problems or treatment for cancer.

Then there's another issue. What if you would like to become pregnant and have a family in the future, but you don't think you're ready for a baby now? Discuss this with your primary care doctor or OB-GYN at one of your next appointments. One option may be fertility preservation, such as freezing your eggs (see Chapter 18). However, this approach isn't for everyone — it typically isn't covered by insurance and can be expensive.

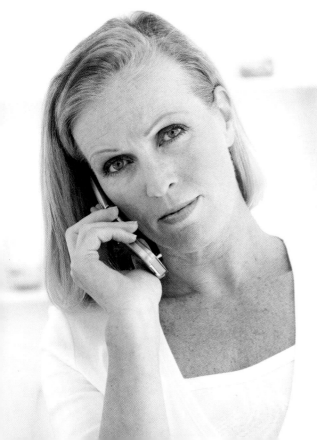

Jane's Story

I met my husband when I was 42 years old. It was a whirlwind romance, and I knew right away he was "the one" for me. We got engaged after just three months of dating, but waited a couple of years to get married.

When it came to getting to know each other and enjoying our time together, those years were valuable — but they also cost us a lot when it came to starting a family.

We learned that once a woman turns 44, it may not be best to use her own eggs to conceive a child, due to the increased risk of birth defects and other medical issues. This was devastating news to me. My husband had never had children before we met, and I had one child — a teenage son. I'd always hoped to have more kids, but it had taken a while to find my husband. We had been excited to start a family together.

After shedding many tears, talking with our doctor, and undergoing a lot of discussion, we decided to try to conceive a baby through an egg donor. This is when an egg is donated by another woman, fertilized with the father's sperm and transferred into the mother's uterus. It's an expensive process, but we decided it was worth it if it meant we could start a family.

There are different options when it comes to finding an egg donor — some perhaps less ethical than others. We chose to go through a medical facility that works with donated eggs. To start the process, we were asked to choose certain criteria — height, weight, hair type and eye color — for the egg donor.

Basically, I had to pick out "me" on paper: blonde, curly hair, 5 feet 6 inches, loves music and horseback riding.

At first, there were no donors available that fit our criteria. We worried there might never be. But then we got the call: They had three different candidates. I cried like a baby when we heard the news. We weren't able to see pictures of the donors, but we were provided with limited information such as blood type, results of a health screening (to ensure the donor is healthy), and physical characteristics such as height and weight.

Choosing our donor and beginning the transfer process was emotional. We hadn't been sure that we'd be able to have a family, and now we were so close. We were able to collect eggs, and 12 embryos were created in the lab, which was awesome. Doctors only planned to transfer two at a time, which meant I had several chances of conceiving a child.

I spent two months prepping for that first transfer, including getting progesterone shots, but it didn't work. We didn't become pregnant. We were disappointed, but we knew we needed to keep moving forward. By this time, I was 47 years old.

We had our next transfer approximately four months later. This time, our doctor thawed a third embryo because one hadn't grown properly. It takes about 10 days after a transfer before you know if you're pregnant. Those were 10 long days for us — but I was pregnant! Eight months later, we brought a beautiful daughter into this world.

We were thrilled and enjoyed every minute with our new baby. But we still had seven embryos left. So approximately 14 months later, we went through the entire process again and to our joy, I got pregnant again. Unfortunately, an early ultrasound showed that the baby wasn't developing as it should. Sadly, we miscarried that baby.

We tried again. But, unfortunately, it didn't work. I didn't become pregnant. By this point, I was 49 years old. If, 20 years earlier, someone would've told me I'd be trying to have a baby at 49, I never would've believed them. But we still had three embryos left. If we weren't going to use them for a final transfer, we had three choices: donate the embryos to another family, donate them to research or destroy them.

My husband and I talked at length about each of those options. We may have been using donated eggs, but we were also using my husband's sperm, and I felt strongly that they were my babies — my "frozen babies" is what I called them.

We went back in again, one last time, transferring all three embryos so that none were left behind. Eight months later we had another beautiful daughter.

I can't say that my pregnancies were without problems. While the first several months of my pregnancies were wonderful, we were warned that, because of my age, there was an increased risk of complications. I did end up with pre-eclampsia with both pregnancies, a pregnancy condition that causes high blood pressure and excess protein in the urine. Preeclampsia can be very serious, and, as a result, I did need to deliver my oldest daughter more than four weeks early and my second daughter five weeks early. We were fortunate, though, to have excellent medical care and everything ended up fine. There were no permanent effects to my health due to the preeclampsia.

Now, I'm just another busy mom running after two little girls. I know that I'm going to be called "grandma" sometimes, but I also know that I'm a better mother now, at age 50, than when I had my son at 31. I honestly believe that, for me, being an older parent is better than if I would've had these girls in my early 20s.

Sure, our life is crazy. And I'm often exhausted — in addition to the kids, I'm currently in graduate school and working full time — but it's a good exhaustion. (Just make sure you call before you come to visit, because the house is a mess!) Plus taking the egg donor route has caused financial burdens. We've spent many paychecks on that treatment and are still paying off some credit card debt.

But we know how lucky we are, and we wouldn't trade it for anything. I think about it on occasion — 20 years from now, what will I remember most? And that's having a family.

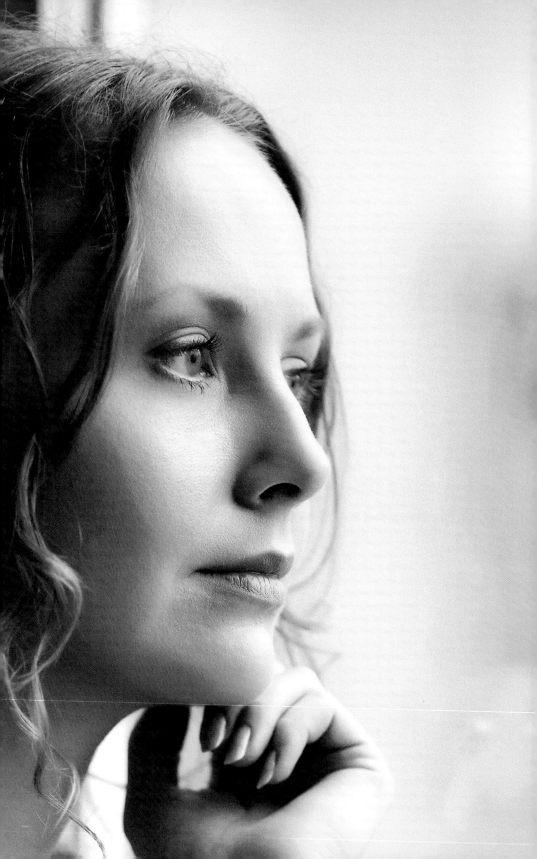

CHAPTER 11

Female problems: Common and unusual

Getting pregnant may sound easy at times, but if you've read through the previous chapters you can see that it involves complex processes of ovulation, sperm production and fertilization — factors that need to work together to get the pregnancy started. But things don't always go just right. For some couples trying to have a baby, the pieces fall shy of fitting together and pregnancy doesn't happen, despite months of trying.

If you're at this point, your care provider may start to talk about evaluation and treatment options for infertility. Don't be frightened by the term *infertility*, however. Infertility isn't the same thing as sterility. It doesn't mean you can never have a baby. It just means you haven't gotten pregnant within the usual time frame, and it's probably a good idea to see if there's a medical problem getting in the way. Timely treatment can prevent further delay in starting your family. And today there are more options than ever to help you conceive.

Sometimes, infertility is due to a problem involving only one partner, either the man or the woman. Other times, the cause may involve both partners, or it may never be fully explained. In any case, don't make the mistake of assuming the problem is with the woman. When a couple is having trouble getting pregnant, there's a 50-50 chance that at least part of the problem may lie with the male partner, according to the American Society for Reproductive Medicine.

For this reason, be sure to maintain your team effort as you plan your next steps. Talk with each other and see your care provider together. Tests for male infertility are much less invasive than are tests for female infertility and can easily be squared away before proceeding to a more complex female evaluation.

This chapter will help you understand potential problems from the female perspective. The next chapter discusses problems that may occur on the male side of the equation. Part 4 of this book guides you through finding the help you may need and different treatment options to consider.

OVULATION AND HORMONE ISSUES

Problems with ovulation and hormone regulation are some of the most common causes of infertility involving the female partner. If you have regular, predictable periods, you're likely ovulating. But if your periods are irregular or absent, or you don't typically experience any premenstrual symptoms — such as breast tenderness, cramps or moodiness — your body's ovulatory process may not be functioning quite the way it should.

Ovulation problems can be caused by flaws in the regulation of reproductive hormones by the hypothalamus or the pituitary gland, or by problems in the ovary itself. Here are some ovulation-disrupting conditions your care provider may check for.

Thyroid problems An overactive or underactive thyroid can affect the balance of hormones in your body, including the ones that regulate your menstrual cycles.

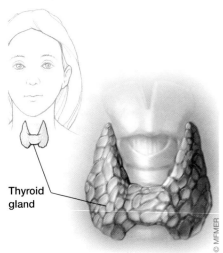

Thyroid gland

Both an underactive thyroid (hypothyroidism) and an overactive thyroid (hyperthyroidism) can affect fertility.

A small gland located at the base of your neck, your thyroid gland produces two main hormones, thyroxine (T-4) and triiodothyronine (T-3), that have a hand in every aspect of your metabolism. Directed by the hypothalamus and pituitary gland, your thyroid normally releases the right amount of hormones, which keeps your metabolism rate at the right pace — not too fast, not too slow.

If your thyroid starts to produce too much or too little of the hormones needed, your metabolism gets out of whack. Examples of factors that might affect your thyroid function include autoimmune diseases, such as Grave's disease or Hashimoto's disease, lumps in the thyroid gland and certain medications.

An underactive thyroid (hypothyroidism) can lead to irregular periods, as well as changes in the length of your menstrual cycles and the flow of your period. Several studies have found that even if your thyroid function is slightly off balance (subclinical hypothyroidism), it may affect your fertility. Also, hypothyroidism can interfere with the development of a fertilized egg, increasing the risk of miscarriage. Therefore, even if your thyroid tests are in the normal range, treatment may still be recommended if you're trying to get pregnant.

An overactive thyroid (hyperthyroidism) also has been linked to menstrual abnormalities and infertility. Having an overactive or an underactive thyroid can also affect a baby's development, so getting thyroid function right before pregnancy is doubly important.

Many care providers are becoming more vigilant about detecting and treating even subtle thyroid problems in women who seek help for infertility. If a thyroid problem is detected, your provider will likely treat it with medication and monitor your thyroid function more closely as you try to conceive and deliver a baby.

Elevated prolactin Some women have prolactin levels that are too high, which can affect the hormone regulation loop between the hypothalamus and the pituitary gland and lead to infertility.

Prolactin is a hormone produced by your pituitary gland. When you become pregnant, your pituitary gland produces higher levels of prolactin in preparation for breast-feeding. After birth, prolactin allows your breasts to produce milk.

In women who aren't pregnant or breast-feeding, too much prolactin can interfere with the communication between the hypothalamus, pituitary gland and the ovaries. In some cases, this leads to irregular ovulation, missed periods or the absence of menstruation altogether. Women with elevated prolactin levels may even produce breast milk when they haven't recently delivered a baby.

Pituitary tumors, even tiny ones that are usually benign, can cause an increase in the production of prolactin. An underactive thyroid, certain kidney problems, stress, exercise and certain medications also can increase prolactin levels. Sometimes, no cause can be found.

If you have irregular periods and you're having trouble getting pregnant, your care provider may request a blood test to check for high levels of prolactin. If the hormone is high, he or she may repeat the test to confirm the elevated value, and then recommend an MRI to check for an abnormal growth on your pituitary gland. Additional testing to check your thyroid and kidney functions may be advised.

Treatment usually involves medication to bring prolactin levels back to normal. Once your prolactin is normalized, you may have an easier time getting pregnant. Pituitary surgery is rarely required, unless a growth is very large and medication isn't helping.

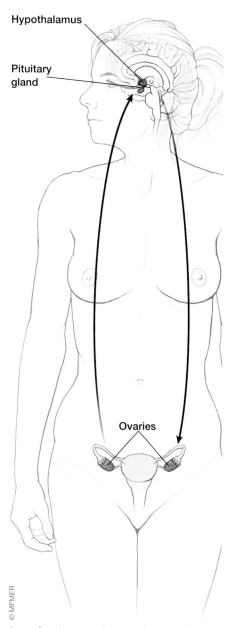

In a female, the hypothalamus, pituitary gland and ovaries compose what is known as the hypothalamic-pituitary-gonadal axis. Communication between these three organs is critical to the regulation of many of the body's systems, including the reproductive system.

Hypothalamic dysfunction Sometimes the communication loop between the hypothalamus, pituitary gland and ovaries doesn't kick off properly, leading to an imbalance in reproductive hormones and infrequent or absent ovulation.

Normally, your hypothalamus, a small but important region in your brain, releases gonadotropin-releasing hormone (Gn-RH), which prompts the pituitary to send out follicle-stimulating hormone (FSH) and luteinizing hormone (LH) to the ovaries. These hormones in turn regulate the growth of follicles in the ovaries and the production of estrogen and progesterone, all essential for releasing an egg for possible fertilization.

Extreme stress on the body — in the form of physical exercise, emotional stress or substantial, abrupt weight change — can suppress the hypothalamus's production of Gn-RH, with cascading effects on the pituitary gland and

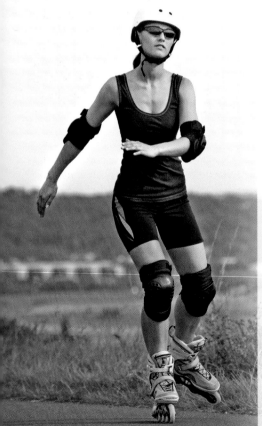

ovaries and the hormones they produce. The midcycle LH surge may not occur, follicles fail to develop normally and levels of estrogen typically decrease. As a result, ovulation may occur infrequently, if at all. Periods are usually light or absent. Over time, low estrogen levels can lead to reduced bone density and a higher risk of osteoporosis.

Gn-RH suppression is more common in professional athletes — ballerinas, runners and cyclists, for example — who strenuously work out for several hours every day. But women with eating disorders, such as anorexia or bulimia, may also experience this type of dysfunction. What they share in common is an energy deficit — they're losing more calories than they're taking in, which can affect the function of the hypothalamus. On the other hand, extreme emotional stress also can affect the hypothalamus.

Exactly how this happens, whether it's physical or emotional stress, is still unclear. It's possible that some women have a genetic profile that makes them more vulnerable to hypothalamic changes. It's also likely that each woman has a different set point for when — or if — hypothalamic dysfunction can occur. This is why some Olympic athletes still have periods like clockwork and other casual exercisers who take up jogging for the first time can experience menstrual irregularity.

Other factors may influence the hypothalamic-pituitary-ovarian axis. Diseases of any one of these three organs can affect the reproductive hormone loop between them. Chronic illnesses associated with nutritional deficiencies, such as untreated celiac disease, can be severe enough at times to affect hypothalamic Gn-RH production. Some women are born with a Gn-RH deficiency, in which case their periods may never start.

Eating enough calories to meet your body's needs, exercising less and reducing emotional stress may reverse the trend and allow spontaneous ovulation to occur again. Attitudes toward eating are often deeply ingrained, however. And many women find exercise to be their outlet for the stress of infertility. Some women find it helpful to see a dietitian or behavioral therapist to help them get back on track.

If the loop between the hypothalamus, pituitary gland and ovaries can't be jump-started with lifestyle changes, your care provider may recommend synthetic versions of FSH and LH to help restore ovulation. Estrogen supplementation also may benefit women with low estrogen levels, to prevent long-term consequences such as bone loss.

Polycystic ovary syndrome A common cause of infertility in women is polycystic ovary syndrome (PCOS). It affects between 5 and 10 percent of women. PCOS is marked by a collection of symptoms including:

▶ *Irregular ovulation.* Menstrual periods are typically more than 35 days apart, or you may have several skipped periods in a row.
▶ *Elevated androgen levels.* Androgens are primarily thought of as male hormones, but women also make androgens. Typically, most androgens are converted to estrogens within the body. In some women, higher than normal levels of androgens can result in acne or excess facial and body hair.
▶ *Cysts.* Often, but not always, ovaries may be enlarged and contain numerous small cysts located along the outer edge of each ovary. These cysts are actually small sacs containing immature eggs (follicles). The small egg sacs are crowded along the outer sur-

face of the ovary (cortex), often resembling a string of beads when the ovary is examined by ultrasound.

To diagnose PCOS, care providers look for at least two of these three characteristics. Blood tests can be done to check hormone levels, including androgens, and a pelvic ultrasound can show you and your care provider what your ovaries look like. Your care provider will also want to make sure that other causes of disrupted ovarian function — such as thyroid problems or elevated prolactin — are excluded before making a diagnosis of PCOS.

With PCOS, numerous immature follicles reside in the ovaries, waiting for the right signals to get the ovulation process started. Although it's not entirely clear why, communication within the ovaries required for egg development may be irregular or absent. Because of this, ovulation can occur erratically or, in some cases, not at all. When ovulation doesn't occur, progesterone isn't produced by the ovaries, and the menstrual cycle is thrown off balance. It's not clear what causes PCOS, but genetics may play a role since the condition is more likely to occur in families. In many women, insulin resistance may contribute to the development of PCOS.

Although not part of the criteria for diagnosing PCOS, more than half the women with PCOS have a body mass index (BMI) that's considered obese. High cholesterol, high blood pressure and diabetes also are common in women with PCOS. These factors increase long-term risk of heart disease, so discovering that you have PCOS can help you focus on your long-term health in addition to your fertility goals.

Weight loss through diet and exercise can improve your body's use of insulin and normalize hormone levels. Studies have shown that losing as little as 5 to 10 percent of your body weight can improve ovarian function and increase your ability to conceive within six months of weight loss. You can learn more about lifestyle changes to improve fertility in Chapters 1 and 2.

Your care provider also may prescribe medication to help increase your body's sensitivity to insulin, which may improve ovulation and reduce your risk of developing diabetes. In addition, your provider may recommend medication to specifically induce ovulation to increase your chances of conception.

Rarely, a surgical therapy called ovarian drilling may lower androgen levels and restore ovulation. This laparoscopic technique makes small holes in the surface of the ovary and alters hormone production by the ovary. For the procedure, a surgeon inserts a slender viewing instrument (laparoscope) through a small incision near your navel and inserts surgical instruments through one or two other small incisions in your lower abdomen. However, for most women, a combination of lifestyle changes and medication is a better option than is surgery.

Another option for getting pregnant if you have PCOS is in vitro fertilization (IVF), where eggs are removed from the ovaries and fertilized in a lab. IVF can substantially increase your chances of becoming pregnant in any given cycle, but it's more costly. Read Chapter 14 for more on fertility medications and surgical treatments. Chapter 15 describes IVF and other options for reproductive assistance.

Primary ovarian insufficiency About 1 percent of women younger than age 40 experiences what's known as primary ovarian insufficiency (POI), a condition where the ovaries stop working as they should years before the typical onset of menopause. An older term for this problem is premature ovarian failure.

In some cases, the problem is that a woman's egg supply is lower than normal from the time of birth, and the available eggs run out sooner than for the average woman. In other cases, a woman may have undergone treatment for cancer or other serious medical illnesses that resulted in permanent egg loss as a side effect. Although the effects of these therapies vary from woman to woman, they can damage, sometimes irreparably, the genetic material in the ovarian follicles. Some women recover ovarian function, others don't.

Autoimmune diseases, including those affecting the thyroid and adrenal glands, are another known cause of POI. In other cases, the condition is associated with a genetic disorder, such as Turner's syndrome, a condition in which a woman has only one X chromosome instead of the usual two, or a problem with a gene that can result in fragile X syndrome, a major cause of intellectual disability. Most of the time, there's no clear-cut reason why the ovaries are failing.

No matter what the cause, though, the ovaries don't release eggs regularly, and they don't produce the normal amounts of estrogen. Infertility is a common result.

Similar to women going through menopause, women with POI have symptoms typical of estrogen deficiency, including irregular or skipped periods, night sweats, hot flashes, vaginal dryness, and decreased sexual desire. Women with POI may have irregular or occasional periods for years and may even become pregnant, although the chance of this is low.

Unfortunately, there's no treatment proved to restore fertility in women with this condition. Although some women do conceive naturally in spite of POI, the chances of becoming pregnant using your own eggs, with or without medical help, are low — somewhere between 5 and 10 percent.

An alternative option is to use eggs from another woman (donor eggs). The eggs can be fertilized with your partner's sperm in a lab and then placed in your uterus. During this process, you take medication that allows your uterus to support a pregnancy. Once the pregnancy is established, you stop taking the medication and the pregnancy proceeds naturally to the delivery.

In addition to addressing infertility concerns, your provider is likely to recommend therapies to treat symptoms of estrogen deficiency. The treatment, which typically includes estrogen and progesterone replacement and calcium and vitamin D supplementation, can make you more comfortable and help prevent long-term complications, such as osteoporosis. Usually, you take hormone replacement until around age 50, the average age for natural menopause.

It's possible, though not always feasible, to preserve your eggs before receiving chemotherapy or radiation therapy. If you're getting ready to undergo cancer treatment and want to learn more about options for fertility preservation, turn to Chapter 18.

Luteal phase defect A normal menstrual cycle is marked by three distinct phases. In the initial follicular phase, several follicles start to mature but one beats out its competitors and is prepared to be released from the ovary. Ovulation follows, marking the transition to the luteal phase, where the now eggless follicle transforms into the corpus luteum and begins to produce high levels of progesterone. Progesterone is a hormone designed to help prepare the lining of your uterus (endometrium) for potential implantation by a fertilized egg. Once the embryo is implanted, the corpus luteum continues to produce progesterone until about the eighth week of pregnancy. At that time, the placenta — a structure that attaches the amniotic sac holding the baby to the mother's uterus — is established enough to produce the hormone on its own.

Luteal phase defect (deficiency) is the term for a condition where not enough progesterone is being produced during the luteal phase to develop the endometrium properly and to sustain embryo implantation and growth. Theoretically, this can prevent a pregnancy from progressing.

Although luteal phase defect has been associated with conditions involving infertility — such as eating disorders, excessive exercise, obesity, PCOS, thyroid problems and other infertility-related disorders — scientists have also noted that progesterone levels vary from cycle to cycle in healthy, normally menstruating women. As a result, there's some disagreement as to whether luteal phase defect is a true cause of infertility. Also, for luteal phase defect to be an obstacle to fertility, it needs to occur consistently, month after month.

Diagnosing luteal phase defect can be problematic, as well. Although care providers have used several tests to try to identify deficiencies in the luteal phase — such as measuring progesterone levels and examining samples of endometrial tissue — none of the tests can reliably distinguish a fertile woman from an infertile one.

If your care provider thinks you may have luteal phase deficiency, he or she will most likely try to identify and treat any underlying problem that might be causing it, such as a thyroid disorder, hypothalamic dysfunction or hyperprolactinemia. Once the problem is addressed, the luteal phase defect should be resolved, too. If none of these disorders are present, your provider may recommend medications, such as progesterone supplements or agents to recruit multiple eggs, to promote endometrial development and support implantation and early pregnancy.

STRUCTURAL AND ANATOMICAL ISSUES

In addition to an optimal hormonal environment, fertilization and pregnancy rely on a number of key logistical operations to be successful — transportation of egg and sperm to the right meeting place, preparation of the uterus for pregnancy, and the right shape and space for it all to take place.

For these logistics to run smoothly, your fallopian tubes, cervix and uterus need to provide accessible, hospitable environments for normal processes to be carried out. Abnormalities in the structure of your reproductive organs can impede these logistics and present fertility problems.

Some women are born with structural abnormalities that present challenges to fertility. Other problems develop later. A pelvic infection, surgery or a previous ectopic pregnancy, for example, can damage healthy organs, leading to scarring and tissue changes that impede the processes of fertilization and implantation.

Following are some of the more common structural and anatomical problems that can lead to infertility. Although treatment isn't necessary in every case, various methods are available to help overcome these obstacles and optimize your ability to get pregnant.

Fallopian tube damage or blockage

Your fallopian tubes (oviducts) are a pair of hollow tubes that serve as conduits for eggs to travel from your ovaries to your uterus. One of the main functions of the fallopian tube is to receive the egg upon its release from the ovary and channel it toward the uterus. The tube is lined with delicate finger-like projections that help it perform this task. It's in a fallopian tube where the sperm usually meets the egg and fertilization occurs. The fallopian tube also provides the egg and fertilized embryo with the nutrients they need.

When fallopian tubes become damaged or blocked, they can keep sperm and egg from meeting or close off the passage of the fertilized egg into the uterus, preventing implantation. Potential causes of fallopian tube damage or blockage include:

Inflammation. Infection of the pelvic area (pelvic inflammatory disease) can inflame the fallopian tubes and destroy the microscopic hairs (cilia) that line the tubes and help sweep the egg toward the uterus. Inflammation can also lead to scarring of the tube and obstruct the tube's passageway between an ovary and the uterus.

Sexually transmitted infections such as chlamydia and gonorrhea are common causes of pelvic infection and fallopian tube damage. You don't always have to feel or see the symptoms for damage to occur. Chlamydia, in particular, seems to increase the risk of infertility. As you might imagine, the more severe the infection, the greater the damage. Seeking prompt care when you experience significant pelvic pain, especially if you have a fever, can help prevent fertility complications.

Q. WHAT'S A HYDROSALPINX?

A. In some women, an old pelvic infection or scars from a previous surgery can block a fallopian tube near its opening to the ovary, causing the tube to fill with fluid and enlarge. A tube in this condition is called a hydrosalpinx, derived from the words *water* (hydro) and *fallopian tube* (salpinx).

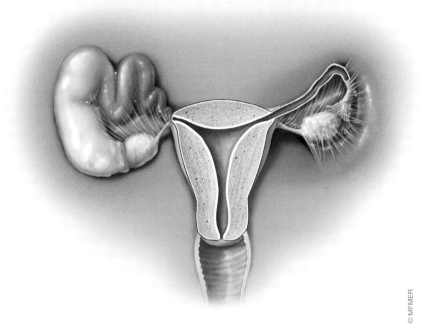

© MFMER

If you have a hydrosalpinx, getting pregnant can be difficult because there's no pathway for egg and sperm to meet and for the embryo to travel to the uterus — similar to any other type of tube blockage.

Some women with a hydrosalpinx experience frequent pain in their lower belly and sometimes a vaginal discharge. But some women don't feel anything at all. To check for a hydrosalpinx, your care provider may request an X-ray or ultrasound or perform surgery.

Rarely can a hydrosalpinx be corrected with surgery. If there's too much damage, your care provider may recommend another way to get pregnant, such as in vitro fertilization (IVF). With IVF, an egg is fertilized in a laboratory with your partner's sperm and then placed in your uterus where it can grow.

Depending on how damaged the tube is, fluid from a hydrosalpinx can leak back into the uterus and cause problems with an IVF pregnancy. Because of this, your provider may recommend removing the damaged tube or placing a clip on it, similar to what's done with a tubal ligation, before starting IVF treatment.

Previous abdominal or pelvic surgery. Scar tissue left over from a previous operation on your abdomen or pelvic area or inside your uterus can distort the fallopian tubes and lead to fertilization or implantation problems.

Previous tubal pregnancy. Sometimes a fertilized egg will attach itself to the inside of a fallopian tube rather than to the uterus, resulting in a tubal (ectopic) pregnancy (see the illustration on page 111). This type of pregnancy can't proceed normally and requires prompt treatment before it becomes life-threatening. A tubal pregnancy can also cause permanent damage to the tube, which may interfere with fertility later on.

Severe endometriosis. Endometriosis is a condition where the type of cells that line your uterus in preparation for pregnancy begin to grow in other places. Over time, endometriosis can form scar tissue that blocks the fallopian tubes and inhibits the transportation of eggs and sperm.

Your care provider can perform tests to see if your fallopian tubes are blocked, especially if you have a history of any of these conditions. If they are blocked, your provider may recommend surgery to open up the tubes and improve your chances of becoming pregnant.

Endometriosis A fairly common obstacle to fertility is a condition called endometriosis. This is an often painful disorder in which tissue that normally lines the inside of your uterus (endometrium) implants itself outside your uterus. These endometrial implants may be found on your ovaries, fallopian tubes, the outer surface of the uterus and the tissues between these organs.

In endometriosis, displaced endometrial tissue continues to act as it normally would — it thickens, breaks down and bleeds with each menstrual cycle. Because this displaced tissue has no way to exit your body, it becomes trapped. Surrounding tissue can become irritated, eventually developing scar tissue and adhesions — abnormal tissue that binds organs together. In severe cases, the endometrial tissue may invade other organs, creating blood-filled cysts and massive adhesions.

Endometriosis can cause pain — sometimes severe — especially during your period. However, the amount of pain doesn't necessarily correlate with the severity of the condition. Some women with mild endometriosis have severe pain, while others with advanced endometriosis may have little pain or even no pain at all.

Varying stages of endometriosis can be found in up to half the women seeking help for infertility. In its severe stages, endometriosis can alter the structure of your pelvic organs in a way that prevents the release of eggs from the ovaries or prevents the fallopian tubes from picking up eggs that have been released. It can also keep sperm from entering the fallopian tubes.

However, the link between mild endometriosis and infertility isn't as clear. Some studies report that women with minimal endometriosis conceive at a monthly rate that's about five times lower than healthy women. Experts speculate that endometriosis may have subtle effects on your pelvic environment, perhaps through inflammation or hormonal changes that make conception more difficult.

If you have painful periods and other tests haven't identified any possible causes of infertility, your care provider may recommend a laparoscopic procedure to look for endometriosis. If endometriosis is present, your provider can

Q. I'VE BEEN TOLD I HAVE A 'TIPPED UTERUS.' COULD THIS MAKE IT MORE DIFFICULT FOR ME TO GET PREGNANT?

A. No. A tipped uterus, also known as a tilted or retroverted uterus, isn't associated with any known fertility problems. Just like a person's nose can be tipped up or tipped back, so can some uteri. Most uteri tip forward at the cervix. One that tips backward is generally considered a normal anatomical variation. The position of your uterus can also vary for other reasons. Depending on how full your bladder is or what position your body is in, your uterus may appear to be tipping backward at one time and forward at another.

remove the patches of endometrial tissue right then and there. Surgery can help with pain and may provide a slight boost to fertility. Surgery to identify endometriosis generally isn't done if you don't have pelvic pain or other suggestive symptoms because there are other, less invasive ways to increase your chances of pregnancy.

If surgery doesn't help you achieve conception, your provider may recommend medications to enhance your fertility or some type of assisted reproductive technology, such as IVF, to help you become pregnant.

Congenital abnormalities About 3 percent of women are born with structural abnormalities of the uterus, fallopian tubes or upper part of the vagina. Some of these variations can hinder efforts to become pregnant.

When a baby girl is taking shape in her mother's uterus, two ducts, called müllerian ducts, fuse together to form a single uterus with a hollow cavity and two fallopian tubes, one on each side of the uterus. Occasionally, the formation of these organs doesn't proceed as it should, resulting in structural abnormalities known as müllerian anomalies or defects. There are two common types of anomalies: one where some of the reproductive organs are absent (müllerian agenesis) and another where the organs fuse incorrectly (fusion disorders). Imaging techniques, such as X-rays in combination with dye (hysterosalpingogram), ultrasound or MRI, can help diagnose these types of anomalies.

Müllerian agenesis. Rarely, the uterus, fallopian tubes, cervix and upper vagina don't develop correctly, or at all. This is called müllerian agenesis. In women with this condition, the ovaries, breasts, clitoris and vulva develop normally but the vaginal opening is small or just a dimple. There may be small, undefined remnants of a uterus. Most girls don't even know they have müllerian agenesis until they fail to get a period. Healthy sexual relationships are entirely possible with help.

If you have müllerian agenesis, using dilators to steadily enlarge the vagina so that you can have intercourse is often the normal route of treatment. Rarely, surgery may be needed to enlarge the vagina or create a vaginal canal. Since your ovaries are working fine, you're still producing eggs, which means you can have a baby but not in the normal way. You'll need to use in vitro fertilization and have a gestational carrier carry the baby for

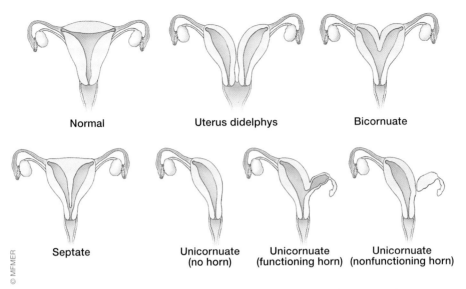

Normal   Uterus didelphys   Bicornuate

Septate   Unicornuate (no horn)   Unicornuate (functioning horn)   Unicornuate (nonfunctioning horn)

© MFMER

Fusion disorders occur when the müllerian ducts fail to join together correctly.

you because a uterus can't be created. Girls born to women with müllerian agenesis typically have normal reproductive tracts, even if their mothers don't.

Fusion disorders. A number of anomalies can result when the uterus, cervix and upper vagina don't develop properly. Menstruation and sexual function are often normal, but depending on the nature of the defect, conception may be more difficult and the risk of miscarriage higher.

These anomalies are often discovered during an evaluation for infertility or another gynecologic or obstetric disorder. Sometimes, they're first discovered when you have a pregnancy-related ultrasound. Some fusion disorders need surgical correction to allow for pregnancy, others don't. Many women are able to have babies with few, if any, problems.

Commonly described types of fusion disorders include:

Uterus didelphys. Sometimes, the two müllerian ducts fail to fuse at all, creating two sets of reproductive structures — usually two separate uteri and cervices, although sometimes duplication of the vaginal canal and other structures may occur, as well. This is sometimes called a double uterus. Despite the presence of duplicate structures, women with a uterus didelphys typically have normal menstrual cycles and successful pregnancies and deliveries and don't require treatment. Women may even alternate pregnancies between the uteri — having one pregnancy in the right uterus and the next in the left. But if complications occur — such as painful periods, recurrent miscarriages or preterm delivery — or if the vagina is divided and causing difficulty with intercourse or vaginal delivery, your care provider may recommend reconstructive surgery to repair the affected structures.

Bicornuate uterus. Sometimes, the müllerian ducts become only partially fused, leading to various degrees of separation between the two upper portions (horns) of the uterus. Sometimes people refer to this as a "heart-shaped" uterus since each horn sticks out a little. The separation can be complete, partial or minimal. A bicornuate uterus may or may not interfere with pregnancy. Most women have similar pregnancy rates to women with normal uteri. If complications arise, surgery can unite the two sides to create a better environment for pregnancy.

Septate uterus. In a septate uterus, the two tubes come together but the central area doesn't dissolve normally, so there is a single uterus. This central area or septum is not normal muscle and is more fibrous like scar tissue. The septum may extend only part of the way into the uterus, or it may extend all the way through. This defect happens when the final fusion between the two müllerian ducts fails to resorb into the body during fetal development. Having a septum does appear to increase the risk of miscarriage. Therefore, surgical removal of the fibrous band, usually through a minimally invasive procedure called a hysteroscopy, can make it easier to carry a pregnancy.

Unicornuate uterus. This occurs when one of the müllerian ducts doesn't develop completely, leaving a one-horned appearance to the uterus or a very small (rudimentary) horn on one side. There may or may not be an open connection between the two horns. Frequently, the rudimentary horn isn't functional and no treatment may be necessary. In this situation, fertility isn't really affected.

In some cases, the small horn may contain functional albeit abnormal endometrial tissue. Because this can lead to complications — such as chronic pain or ectopic pregnancy — your care provider may recommend surgical removal of the rudimentary horn. Because the kidney and uterus develop in tandem, women with a unicornuate uterus are more likely to have a missing kidney or an abnormal kidney on the same side as the missing or rudimentary horn.

Arcuate uterus. An arcuate uterus is marked by a small indentation at the top of the uterus. It usually doesn't cause any difficulties with conception or pregnancy and doesn't require any type of treatment. Most women probably never know they have it. There's even some controversy as to whether this is a true defect or just a variation of a normal uterus.

Because these situations can vary from one woman to the next, it's important to talk with your care provider and take your own history into account so that you can evaluate the risks and benefits of different approaches to treating any infertility related to müllerian anomalies. For women with variations that are associated with an increased risk of early delivery, avoiding fertility procedures that carry an increased risk of multiple pregnancies is important. When you become pregnant, your care provider may advise extra monitoring as your pregnancy progresses and to be aware of the risk of preterm delivery. But overall, most women have successful pregnancies and deliveries even when corrective surgery is needed.

Uterine growths For some women, growths inside the uterus such as fibroids or polyps can sometimes, though not very often, interfere with conception or implantation of a fertilized egg. Both types of growth are usually benign, although in rare cases either can be confused with cancer. Having uterine fibroids or polyps shouldn't keep you from trying to have a baby. But if it appears that they're making it difficult for you to get pregnant, your care provider may recommend their removal.

Uterine fibroids. These common growths develop from the smooth muscular tissue of the uterus (myometrium). A single cell divides repeatedly, eventually creating a firm, rubbery mass distinct from nearby tissue. Fibroids often occur in multiples and grow at different rates.

Fibroids come in a variety of sizes and positions. Most women with fibroids get pregnant and deliver without difficulty. Sometimes, though, fibroids can grow to occupy critical uterine real estate, making it more difficult to get pregnant. Problematic fibroids include those that grow inside the uterine cavity (submucosal fibroids) or large fibroids within the uterine wall that protrude into the cavity, distorting the shape of the uterus. Fibroids can also increase the risk of miscarriage and are associated with other pregnancy complications.

Fibroids are common. However, if you're having fertility problems and you have fibroids, you can't automatically jump to the conclusion that the fibroids are the problem. If after a thorough evaluation of you and your partner, it's determined that fibroids are distorting your uterine cavity or causing your symptoms, they can be removed through surgery, depending on their size and number. Other treatments designed to destroy or shrink uterine fibroids that don't require surgery also exist. However, not all fibroid surgeries improve your chances of pregnancy and each fibroid treatment

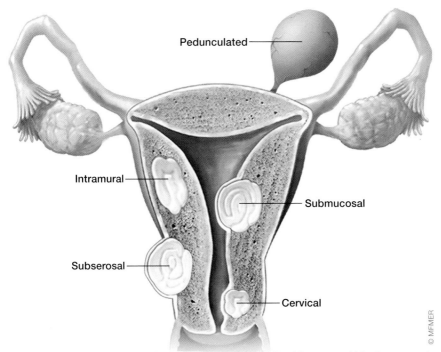

Pedunculated

Intramural

Submucosal

Subserosal

Cervical

© MFMER

There are different types of uterine fibroids. Intramural fibroids grow within the muscular uterine wall. Submucosal fibroids bulge into the uterine cavity. Subserosal fibroids project to the outside of the uterus. Some subserosal or submucosal fibroids are pedunculated — they hang from a stalk inside or outside the uterus. Cervical fibroids grow in the wall of the cervix (neck of the uterus).

has its own effect on fertility. So it's worth a detailed conversation about fibroid treatments and fertility with your care provider before proceeding with treatment.

Uterine polyps. Overgrowth of cells in the lining of the uterus can lead to the formation of uterine polyps, also known as endometrial polyps. These polyps are usually noncancerous (benign), although rarely some can be mistaken for cancer or eventually turn into cancer (precancerous polyps).

The sizes of uterine polyps range from a few millimeters — basically no larger than a sesame seed — to several centimeters — about the size of a golf ball. They may attach to the uterine wall by a large base or a thin stalk.

Very large polyps pushing out on the uterus may obstruct sperm travel and implantation, similar to fibroids. Polyps may also cause inflammation or produce biochemical effects that hinder implantation and embryo development.

Polyps may show up during testing for infertility. Small polyps without symptoms usually don't need to be treated, unless you're at risk of uterine cancer, and they may shrink on their own. If no other causes of infertility are found, removal of larger polyps might allow you to become pregnant.

Uterine polyps may also increase the risk of miscarriage in women who undergo in vitro fertilization (IVF). If you're considering IVF treatment and you have uterine polyps, your provider may recommend removing the polyps before transferring an embryo to your uterus.

Cervical narrowing or blockage

Cervical problems also can affect fertility. Normally, the cervix serves as a passageway for sperm to reach the egg. It also produces mucus during the mid-part of your menstrual cycle, making it easier for sperm to swim through the vagina and cervix and up toward the fallopian tubes.

Some women are born with cervical abnormalities that obstruct the passage of sperm or that make the production of cervical mucus difficult. An infection or surgery also can damage the shape and function of the cervix.

Congenital cervical abnormalities. Rarely, a girl is born with no cervix or an underdeveloped cervix. This results from failure of the müllerian ducts to come together and form properly during fetal development (see page 143 on müllerian agenesis). An absent or underdeveloped cervix can make it very difficult to conceive naturally. In rare cases, surgery may help repair an underdeveloped cervix, but it's also possible to plan a pregnancy using intrauterine insemination to bypass the cervix and place the sperm in the uterus as close to the egg as possible. The baby can then be delivered via cesarean section.

Cervical narrowing. Some women are born with a very narrow passageway through the cervix (cervical stenosis). More commonly, though, this condition results from scarring after a biopsy, surgery or radiation therapy of the cervix. Infections of the upper genital tract also can change the structure of the cervix.

In addition to blocking the passage of sperm and causing infertility, cervical stenosis can cause menstrual abnormalities, such as light or scant periods, painful periods, and abnormal bleeding. At a care provider's office, it's generally easy to tell if you have cervical stenosis because the narrow opening won't allow for the use of instruments used in Pap tests and other gynecologic tests.

A narrowed cervix can be gradually widened by gently inserting progressively larger dilators — small, lubricated metal rods. This can be done in your care provider's office. The first dilator used is usually very thin, and then thicker ones are used as your cervix widens. Sometimes, a tube (cervical stent) may be temporarily left in place to keep the cervix open. To achieve the best results, the procedure may need to be repeated.

Pregnancy is possible after dilatation, although the risks of miscarriage and premature delivery are increased. Your care provider will want to monitor your pregnancy closely to check for cervical incompetence or other factors that might lead to premature labor.

UNEXPLAINED INFERTILITY

For about 30 percent of couples seeking help for infertility, the cause of the infertility remains unexplained. For these couples, tests for possible fertility problems come back normal or the problems discovered are too minor to be considered the cause of infertility on their own. Eggs are available, ovulation is going fine, the fallopian tubes are open, the uterus is normal, and sperm are swimming.

It can be frustrating to go through all of the testing only to discover there's no apparent reason for why you can't seem to get pregnant. In some cases, it can be tempting to want something to be wrong just so that it can be fixed and dealt with.

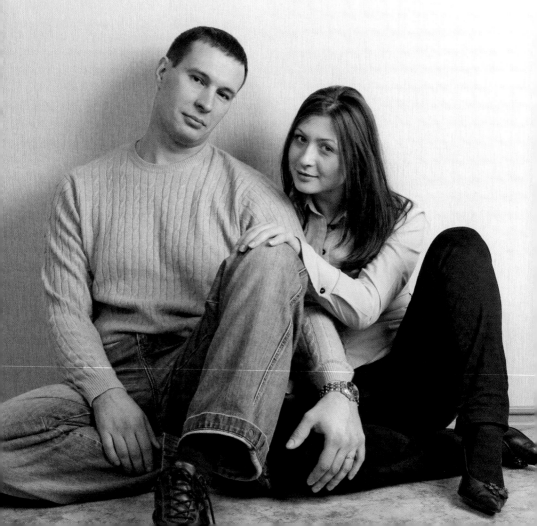

Twenty or 30 years ago, doctors would keep performing tests to see if they could find an answer. They might check the mucus in your cervix shortly after you've had sex to see if the sperm were swimming well, test for antibodies to sperm and even check to see if the sperm would fertilize a hamster egg. However, none of these tests proved very useful, and they're rarely performed today.

The good news is that you've covered all of your bases and nothing major is wrong. It may be that subtle abnormalities in how the sperm and egg get together or the way in which the embryo is implanted are preventing pregnancy from happening. Many cases are probably a combination of both female and male factors. It's also possible that current tests aren't sophisticated enough to detect what's causing the problem.

If you think about it, unexplained infertility has been around for generations, but only recently has been viewed as a problem. In your great-grandmother's day, when there weren't good birth control methods and couples often married at a young age, not getting pregnant quickly was a good thing. You'd rather have time to establish your relationship than get pregnant on your wedding night or in the first few months of life as a couple. Now that women can take birth control pills until they're ready to get pregnant, our expectations are different.

If both you and your partner are young — particularly when the female partner is younger than age 32 — your care provider may recommend trying to conceive naturally for a bit longer. This is because 1 to 4 percent of couples with unexplained fertility become pregnant each month. Lifestyle changes may be of benefit, as well.

In any case, you still have options. Many of the same treatments used for specific disorders are applicable to unexplained infertility. Medications can help stimulate ovulation, or intrauterine insemination can bypass any problems that may be occurring with sperm transport. The next few chapters will help you understand the processes of evaluation and treatment.

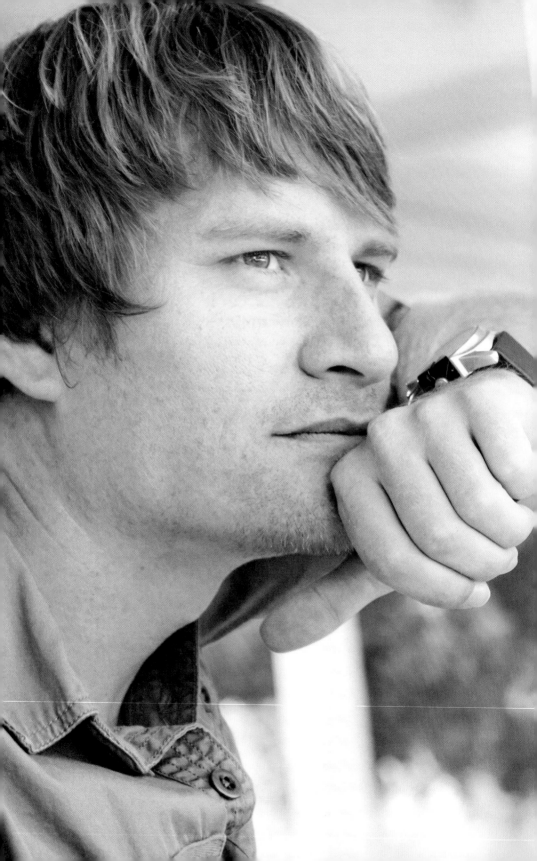

CHAPTER 12

Male problems: Common and unusual

Male infertility is a common problem. It affects an estimated 35 to 75 percent of infertile couples. Because of this high rate for couples having difficulty achieving pregnancy, it's recommended that both the male and the female partner undergo fertility evaluations.

At first glance it may seem that male infertility is pretty straightforward — it's all about the sperm, right? Male fertility does, in fact, depend on a healthy production of sperm and unobstructed delivery of the sperm to the female vagina. The production of sperm, however, is a complex process. It requires normal functioning of the testicles (testes) as well as the hypothalamus and pituitary glands — organs in your brain that produce hormones that trigger sperm production. Once sperm are produced in the testicles, they spend months there maturing before delicate tubes transport them to be mixed with other seminal fluids and be ejaculated out of the penis.

Problems with any of these systems can affect sperm quantity or quality or both, and possibly reduce a couple's fertility. Also, abnormalities in sperm shape (morphology) or movement (motility) can affect male fertility.

An evaluation for possible male infertility begins with a thorough history, and often a physical examination as well as a simple semen test, called a semen analysis. Because a semen analysis is relatively simple and noninvasive, it's an excellent initial test that provides a large amount of information. Results of the analysis will determine if further testing is necessary, including blood or imaging tests or other procedures.

A wide range of factors may contribute to male infertility, and sometimes the cause of the infertility remains unknown. A man may have an abnormal semen analysis, and doctors may not be able to find a reason why (idiopathic male infertility). Or the results of the physical examination, laboratory tests and semen analysis may all come back normal, but a man may still experience infertility (unexplained male infertility).

Knowing this, it may be tempting to skip all of the diagnostic testing and go straight to using assisted reproductive technology (ART) to get pregnant faster. But a thorough male evaluation is important. An evaluation may uncover a condition that's treatable. It can also identify serious health problems. In addition, testing and treatment can help increase the chances of success with ART, possibly preventing unnecessary procedures.

Also keep in mind that male fertility evaluations are performed within the context of the female partner's health and age. For example, recommendations regarding treatment of various male conditions may vary if the female partner is older than age 35, to reduce unnecessary delays.

There are numerous causes of male infertility. In this chapter, we briefly discuss some of the more common findings

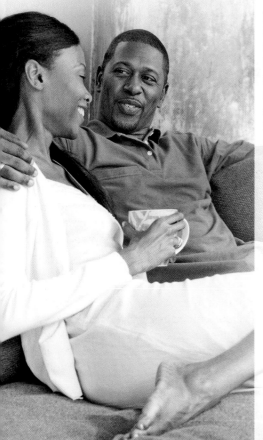

associated with infertility and the role of various diagnostic tests. Treating male infertility, as with female infertility, is an emerging science. As you work with your care provider, talk with your partner about the process and the steps you're willing to take as a couple to pursue pregnancy.

SPERM MATTERS

Currently, the best way to evaluate sperm is through a semen analysis (read about what to expect in this test in Chapter 13). Because semen production is based on a number of different factors — including how many days you've abstained before ejaculation — and can vary from day to day, more than one sample may be obtained to achieve greater accuracy.

In general, to assure accurate results, you should abstain from ejaculating for at least 48 to 72 hours prior to a semen test. Although a semen analysis is the best measure currently available of a man's fertility potential, it's not a perfect test. Many men with abnormal findings on a semen analysis continue to be fertile, while those with normal results may experience infertility. In analyzing this "overlap" of results, studies have shown that sperm movement (motility) is likely the most important factor in predicting the ability to achieve a pregnancy.

Information gained from a semen analysis includes:

▶ *Semen volume.* For most men, the typical amount of semen collected measures about one-half to one full teaspoon. Small amounts of semen most often indicate that some of the sample was lost during ejaculation, although it may also signal a problem with ejaculation, including a possible obstruction blocking the semen. Right after ejaculation, semen is usually thick. But after about 10 to 30 minutes at room temperature, it should naturally liquefy. If it doesn't, it may be too thick for sperm to move freely.

▶ *Sperm number.* Total sperm count refers to the number of sperm within the whole ejaculate sample. Sperm concentration is the number of sperm per unit volume of semen. Normal sperm concentrations range from 15 million to greater than 200 million sperm per milliliter of semen. Your sperm count is considered low (oligospermia) if you have fewer than 15 million sperm per milliliter. Higher total sperm counts increase your chance of getting your partner pregnant up to a certain level (about 40 to 55 million). Beyond this amount, increasing numbers aren't likely to have a significant impact. Some men have no sperm in their semen at all (azoospermia).

▶ *Sperm movement (motility).* Because sperm must travel to reach the female egg, motility is very important to achieving pregnancy. The sample is considered abnormal if fewer than 40 percent of the sperm are motile.

▶ *Sperm shape (morphology).* A semen analysis also studies the size, shape and appearance of the sperm in the sample. Defects of the head, body and tail are noted, as well as immature sperm forms. There are different methods to assess morphology, therefore, this number may vary significantly between laboratories.

Additional factors that may be evaluated include semen acidity (pH), semen sugar content (fructose) and the number of white blood cells (leukocytes) in semen. Other tests including DNA fragmentation, reactive oxygen species, antisperm antibodies, sperm viability testing, sperm-cervical mucus interaction, zona-free hamster egg tests and computer-aided sperm analysis are less common and may be used in select cases to assist in making treatment decisions.

What causes a low sperm count? A persistently low sperm count can result from a number of health issues and medical treatments. These may include anatomical or structural problems with the male reproductive organs — due to tumors, infection, surgery and cancer treatments — hormone imbalances, problems with ejaculation, or genetic abnormalities. Many of these problems are discussed below in greater detail.

A reduced sperm count affects your fertility in that there are fewer sperm coming near the egg when you have intercourse with your partner. It's true that all it takes is one sperm, but starting off with fewer sperm than normal can reduce your chances of getting even one of them to the right place at the right time so that it can do its job. In addition, a low sperm count is frequently associated with poor-quality sperm, ones that don't move well or are abnormally shaped. These sperm are less apt to travel well and penetrate the egg.

When there's no sperm In some men, no sperm are found in a semen analysis. This may occur because of an obstruction in the male reproductive tract that prevents sperm from being ejaculated (obstructive azoospermia) or because of a problem with the production of sperm in the testicles (nonobstructive azoospermia).

An obstruction may result when there's been damage to some part of the male reproductive tract. For example, severe or repeated infections of the male reproductive tract can cause inflammatory damage that obstructs sperm storage or transport. Previous surgery — including a vasectomy, a male birth control procedure — can block the normal progress of sperm through the reproductive tract. Blockage may also result from a birth defect of the reproductive tract. Men with certain variants of cystic fibrosis are often born without the tubes that transport sperm from the testicles to the ejaculatory ducts in the penis (vas deferens) so that sperm never make their way out of the testes. For some men, this blockage is the first evidence they have of an abnormal cystic fibrosis gene.

Failure of the testicles to produce sperm at all can result from congenital conditions, such as an undescended testicle or a genetic abnormality, or damage to the testicles because of infection, trauma or cancer treatment. Using high-dose testosterone or other anabolic steroids also can suppress sperm production from the testicles.

Men who have an obstruction that's causing azoospermia typically have normal-sized testicles and are producing normal amounts of reproductive hormones. Men with nonobstructive azoospermia often have hormone imbalances and smaller testicular volume.

Another reason for lack of sperm in your ejaculate may be a condition called retrograde ejaculation. It occurs when the bladder neck fails to tighten properly during orgasm, and semen flows backward and enters the bladder rather than going out the penis (see page 162). If the volume of your ejaculate is very low and

LEUKOCYTOSPERMIA: IS IT A PROBLEM?

A number of studies have found a link between male infertility and abnormally high levels of white blood cells (leukocytes) in semen, a condition called leukocytospermia. However, other reports haven't confirmed this, and the mechanisms by which leukocytospermia might damage sperm or impede fertility are still unclear. It's also not clear how to treat leukocytospermia.

White blood cells are normally recruited by your immune system to help fight infection. They're also found in low levels in sperm and may be important in maintaining normal sperm function. If the levels of white blood cells become too high, this may lead to decreased fertility, sperm damage or early loss of pregnancy.

An elevated white blood cell level may result for various reasons, including an infection or inflammation, environmental exposures, tobacco or marijuana use, or heavy alcohol consumption.

For several reasons, an elevated white blood cell count generally doesn't affect the treatment of infertility. The majority of men who have a high level of white blood cells in their semen don't show other signs of infection. Many of the current tests used to evaluate semen don't correctly differentiate between true white blood cells and other types of cells that appear similar, resulting in higher reported values than are actually present. In addition, the treatment of leukocytospermia with antibiotics has had mixed results. If your test results show a high white blood cell count, talk to your care provider about your options.

no sperm can be found in it, your care provider may want to perform additional tests to check for retrograde ejaculation.

STRUCTURAL AND ANATOMICAL ISSUES

There are a number of problems related to the way a man's reproductive organs are structured that can contribute to infertility. Many of these problems can be repaired, often through surgery, in ways that can optimize the chances of conception.

Varicoceles Varicoceles are enlarged veins that can develop within the pouch of skin that holds your testicles (scrotum). They're similar to varicose veins that can develop in your leg. Varicoceles occur in approximately 15 to 25 percent of the male population and among 35 to 60 percent of infertile men.

Normally, the testicular veins, which transport oxygen-depleted blood away from the testicle, form a web of blood vessels around the testicular arteries, which bring fresh blood to the testicle. This arrangement of veins over arteries in combination with the testicles being located outside of the abdomen produces a cooling mechanism that helps to maintain an appropriate temperature for optimal sperm production and survival.

Problems within the testicular veins, however, can lead to excessive dilation, resulting in a backup of flow. This may cause the temperature in the testicles to rise, possibly affecting sperm count, shape (morphology), movement (motility), testosterone production and fertilizing potential of the sperm. Varicoceles may also lead to progressive destruction of the testicle and cause it to shrink,

which may further contribute to a decreased sperm count.

Most of the time, varicoceles don't cause infertility or any symptoms, although some men may notice swelling around the testicle or dull, aching testicular pain, which worsens following prolonged periods of standing. Varicoceles usually develop on the left side. The larger the veins get, the more noticeable they become. Sometimes, they may feel like a bag of worms. Your care provider can usually diagnose them during a physical examination.

Varicoceles are the most common reversible cause of male infertility. They're generally treated with surgery. Among men with varicoceles that can be felt on exam, studies have demonstrated improvements in sperm count, morphology, motility and fertilizing capacity with treatment. Some studies show increased spontaneous pregnancy rates and better assisted reproductive technology (ART) outcomes, including in vitro fertilization.

Undescended testicles Sometimes, during fetal development, one or occasionally both testicles fail to descend from the abdomen to their proper position in the scrotum. This is more common among premature infants, and most of the time it resolves on its own within the first few months after birth.

If a testicle fails to descend to its normal spot, or if surgical repair is delayed, this can lead to low sperm counts, poor sperm quality and decreased fertility. Men born with an undescended testicle also are at increased risk of testicular cancer.

An undescended testicle is usually corrected with surgery. The surgeon carefully manipulates the testicle into the scrotum and stitches it into place. This procedure is most often performed in infants, but it may be performed later.

Men with a history of two undescended testicles experience higher rates of semen abnormalities and reduced pregnancy rates, while those with only one undescended testicle have similar paternity rates compared to men without a history of undescended testicles. Among men undergoing ART, a prior history of undescended testicle doesn't appear to reduce success rates.

Sperm duct abnormalities The tubes that transport sperm around the male reproductive tract can be abnormally formed at birth, or they may be damaged by illness or injury. Sometimes they're intentionally or accidentally closed during surgery, as in the case of a vasectomy or during inguinal hernia repair. The result is that sperm may be completely or partially blocked during ejaculation, leading to infertility. An obstruction in the reproductive tract may occur at any location, the most common locations are at the ejaculatory ducts, vasa deferentia, and epididymides.

Ejaculatory ducts. In the case of ejaculatory duct obstructions there's a blockage in the prostate gland, near the junction of the seminal vesicles and vasa deferentia (see page 69). The blockage may have been present since birth or may have resulted from recurrent infection or inflammation, stones, trauma or a prior surgical procedure. Treatment may include surgery to remove the blockage. Another option is ART.

urine sample for laboratory analysis. The presence or number of sperm may be a sign of retrograde ejaculation (see page 161).

▌ *Genetic tests.* If the number of sperm is extremely low or sperm are absent, genetic causes could be involved. A blood test can reveal whether there are missing or extra chromosomes or subtle changes in the Y chromosome that may be contributing to infertility (see page 163). Genetic testing may also be ordered to diagnose various congenital or inherited syndromes, such as Klinefelter syndrome or cystic fibrosis.

▌ *Testicular biopsy.* This test involves removing tissue samples from the testicle by way of a surgical procedure or with a small needle. The results can often tell if sperm production is normal. A testicular biopsy may also be used to retrieve sperm for treatment with ART.

▌ *Anti-sperm antibody tests.* These tests check for immune molecules (antibodies) that attack sperm. However, how anti-sperm antibodies affect fertility is controversial.

▌ *Specialized sperm function tests.* A number of tests may be performed to check how well your sperm survive after ejaculation, how well they can penetrate an egg, and whether there's any problem attaching to the egg. These tests may be done if your semen analysis is normal and your partner's tests have also come back normal. While there are several specialized sperm function tests available, many are primarily for research purposes and their practical relevance isn't always clear.

Vasa deferentia. Blockages in the vas deferens are most commonly the result of prior vasectomy procedures, but they can result for other reasons, including injury from prior scrotal surgery or inguinal hernia repair. The vasa deferentia may also be abnormal due to conditions such as cystic fibrosis or another genetic disorder. Treatment options may include a vasectomy reversal or ART, depending on the underlying condition.

Epididymides. Some men experience dysfunction or obstruction of the ducts surrounding the testicles (epididymides). Even though the testicles are producing sperm normally, sperm can't pass through one or both of the epididymides. An infection resulting in chronic inflammation of an epididymis or testicle can lead to scarring and obstruction of the ducts. Prompt treatment may reduce the chance of this kind of scarring.

Similar to other obstructions, surgery may or may not fix the problem. If surgery isn't an option, the next best way to achieve pregnancy is often with reproductive technology. Sperm is taken directly from a testicle or an epididymis by aspiration and placed in one of the following locations:

▌ Your partner's uterus (intrauterine insemination)

▌ Close proximity to your partner's egg in the laboratory (in vitro fertilization)

▌ Directly into your partner's egg in a laboratory (intracytoplasmic sperm injection, or ICSI)

With all blockages and abnormalities, the decision of whether to have surgery is dependent, in part, on your partner's age. If the female partner is beyond a certain age, a fertility specialist may recommend ART over surgery, particularly given that it often takes several months for sperm counts to return following surgery, such as vasectomy reversal.

Hypospadias Hypospadias is a condition in which the opening of the tube that drains urine from the bladder (urethra) is on the underside of the penis instead of on the tip. In mild cases, the opening is near the tip of the penis. In more-severe cases, the opening is in the middle or near the base of the penis. The condition is usually diagnosed and treated in infancy. If it persists into adulthood, it may contribute to infertility due to the abnormal placement of semen at the time of ejaculation.

This relatively uncommon cause of infertility may be easily overcome by way of corrective surgery or assisted reproductive technologies, such as intrauterine insemination.

Tumors Men who are infertile and have abnormal semen analyses are at increased risk of testicular cancer. Inversely, men with a prior history of testicular cancer are at an increased risk of infertility due to testicular abnormalities and the effects of treatments. Infertile men may also be at an increased risk of colorectal cancer, melanoma or prostate cancer, although further studies are required to confirm these associations.

In addition to having direct effects on the testicles, tumors can disrupt normal functioning of the hypothalamus and the pituitary gland, parts of the brain that stimulate the production of reproductive hormones in the testicles.

Removal or treatment of a brain tumor may bring a return of normal fertility. On the other hand, cancer treatment — including surgery, chemotherapy and radiation — can lead to infertility (see Chapter 18). Effects of treatment may be temporary, but in some cases infertility is permanent.

HORMONE IMBALANCES

Similar to the way a woman's reproductive system works, a man's reproductive system depends on carefully balanced communication between the hormones produced by the hypothalamus, the pituitary gland and the testicles.

The hypothalamus produces gonadotropin-releasing hormone (Gn-RH), which signals the pituitary gland to make follicle-stimulating hormone (FSH) and luteinizing hormone (LH). Luteinizing hormone then signals the testicles to produce testosterone. Testosterone helps initiate the production of sperm during puberty and helps maintain sperm production throughout adulthood. FSH also stimulates the testicles to make sperm, and it contributes to sperm production through other, indirect ways. Hormones produced by the testicles and other organs, in turn, travel to the hypothalamus and pituitary gland where they help regulate the release of more or less Gn-RH.

Problems with any of these communication loops can disrupt the normal calibration of hormones and lead to a decrease in sperm and testosterone production. Hormone problems that affect the testicles directly are referred to as primary hypogonadism. Problems of the hypothalamus and pituitary glands are called secondary hypogonadism.

Either type of hypogonadism may be caused by an inherited (congenital) trait or something that happens later in life (acquired), such as an injury or infection. Hypogonadism doesn't always cause symptoms. When it does, symptoms may include fatigue, decreased energy, impaired erectile function, impaired desire for sex (libido), difficulty in gaining muscle mass and lack of personal drive. In many cases, men with hypogonadism already have a feeing they could be infertile because of their symptoms.

Primary hypogonadism Common causes of primary hypogonadism include:

▶ *Klinefelter syndrome.* This inherited condition results from an abnormality of the sex chromosomes X and Y. Normally, a man has one X and one Y chromosome. Someone with Klinefelter syndrome carries one or more extra X chromosomes. The extra X chromosome causes abnormal development of the testicles, which in turn results in abnormal sperm development and decreased testosterone.

▶ *Undescended testicles.* Before birth, the testicles develop inside the abdomen and normally move down into their permanent place in the scrotum. Sometimes one or both of the testicles may not be descended at birth. A history of undescended testicles is associated with decreased fertility, regardless of when the problem is corrected. However, early repair, especially before ages 1 to 2 years, may help preserve testicular function.

▶ *Mumps orchitis.* If a mumps infection involves the testicles as well as the salivary glands (mumps orchitis), it may result in long-term testicular damage and decreased fertility. Vaccination for the mumps virus virtually eliminates the risk of this complication.

▶ *Hemochromatosis.* This condition, which is marked by too much iron in the blood, can cause testicular failure or pituitary gland dysfunction affecting testosterone production.

▶ *Chronic infection or illness.* A number of chronic conditions, including liver and kidney failure, can have a damaging effect on the testicles and on hormone production. In addition, chronic infections of the testicle or epididymis may damage or scar the testicle or the tubes that transport sperm (vasa deferentia). Other inflammatory conditions such as sarcoidosis and histiocytosis may impair hormone production in the hypothalamus and pituitary gland. Infections such as HIV/AIDS and tuberculosis may affect hormone production as well as the reproductive organs themselves.

▶ *Exposures.* A number of environmental chemicals, including pollution, pesticides, and polychlorinated biphenyls (PCBs), may impair semen quality. Other factors that can impair fertility include heavy metals, radiation,

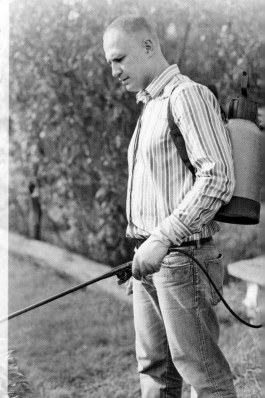

solvents, heat and cellular phone radiation. It's important to recognize that many of the studies that have identified these associations are very limited and require further research to confirm findings.

▶ *Medications.* Several medications are associated with impaired semen analyses and infertility. These medications may impair fertility either through direct action on the testicle itself or through alteration of hormones. The medications include certain blood pressure drugs, psychotherapeutics, antibiotics and hormonal agents. Testosterone or other performance-enhancing substances also may have a negative effect on fertility, which may persist for several years following discontinuation. If you're currently on any medications, review them with your care provider to see if they may be contributing to infertility. Don't make changes to your current medications without first discussing this with your care provider.

▶ *Injury to the testicles.* Because they're situated outside the abdomen, the testicles are prone to injury. Damage to normally developed testicles can result in hypogonadism. Damage or loss of one testicle doesn't significantly change testosterone production or reduce your ability to achieve pregnancy except if reduced fertility is already present.

▶ *Primary germ cell abnormalities.* Occasionally, an illness can lead to abnormal production of sperm, including cases where sperm cells don't develop normally (Sertoli-cell-only syndrome) or where sperm stop growing at certain stages (maturational arrest). Many men with these conditions may still father children with the help of assisted reproductive technology.

▶ *Cancer treatment.* Chemotherapy or radiation therapy for the treatment of cancer can interfere with testosterone and sperm production. The effects of both treatments may be temporary or permanent, depending on the medi-

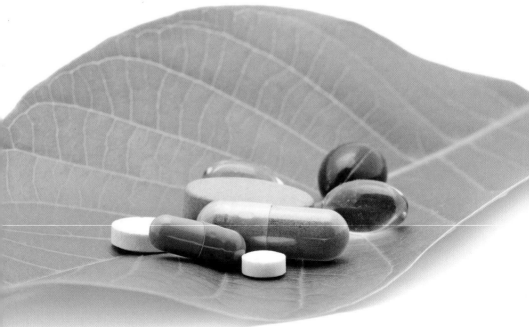

cations used and the duration of the treatment. Although many men regain their fertility within a few months after treatment ends, all men wishing to preserve their fertility should discuss storing sperm prior to beginning therapy (see Chapter 18).

Secondary hypogonadism With secondary hypogonadism, the testicles are normal but they function improperly due to a problem with the pituitary gland or hypothalamus. A number of conditions can cause secondary hypogonadism. In addition to infections, inflammation and medications discussed in the previous section, causes of secondary hypogonadism include:

▶ *Kallmann syndrome.* Abnormal development of the hypothalamus can cause hypogonadism. This rare inherited abnormality is also associated with impaired development of the ability to smell (anosmia). It's often successfully treated.

▶ *Pituitary disorders.* An abnormality in the pituitary gland can impair the release of hormones from the pituitary gland to the testicles, affecting normal testosterone and sperm production. Treatment of a brain tumor, such as surgery or radiation therapy, may also impair pituitary function and cause hypogonadism.

▶ *Obesity.* No matter what your age, being significantly overweight — having a body mass index (BMI) greater than 30 — is associated with decreased testosterone levels, reduced sperm concentrations and decreased success rates with ART. Weight loss and exercise improve testosterone production and likely improve fertility.

Because of testicular damage that often occurs with primary hypogonadism, in many cases there's no effective way to restore fertility. However, in the majority of cases, sperm can be identified and retrieved through various surgical techniques. If some sperm are available, intracytoplasmic sperm injection (ICSI) may be a possibility. Another option may be to seek sperm from a donor to be used to fertilize one of your partner's eggs. These treatments are discussed in Chapters 15 and 16.

In the case of secondary hypogonadism, your care provider may recommend various therapies, including weight loss or hormone supplementation, to help restore sperm production. Men with low testosterone levels who want to maintain their fertility shouldn't be treated with testosterone alone because it will worsen their fertility.

EJACULATION ISSUES

Conception and pregnancy can sometimes be hindered by problems with the way sperm exit the penis. In some cases, semen may be going the wrong way (retrograde ejaculation). In other cases, sperm and semen production are fine, but the timing of ejaculation or the lack of an erection present a problem.

Retrograde ejaculation and anejaculation Retrograde ejaculation occurs when semen enters the bladder instead of emerging through the penis during orgasm. With anejaculation, no sperm exit the genital tract. You still reach orgasm, but you may ejaculate very little or no semen.

During a male orgasm, sperm are released from each of the epididymides. Tubes called the vasa deferentia transport the sperm to the prostate gland, where they mix with other fluids to produce liquid semen (ejaculate). The muscle at the opening of the bladder (bladder neck) tightens to prevent the ejaculate from entering the bladder as it passes into the tube inside the penis (urethra). This is the same muscle that holds urine in your bladder until you urinate.

With retrograde ejaculation, sperm travel backward into the bladder rather than being ejected out through the penis. With anejaculation, sperm are never released into the urethra.

Several conditions can cause problems with the muscle that closes the bladder during ejaculation. These include:

▶ Prostate or bladder neck surgery
▶ Side effect of certain medications used to treat high blood pressure, prostate enlargement and mood disorders
▶ Nerve damage caused by a medical condition, such as diabetes or multiple sclerosis, or by surgery involving the nerves responsible for ejaculation
▶ Disease of the urethra, such as narrowing (stricture)

If your semen volume is low and no or few sperm are present, your care provider may examine your urine for the presence of semen after you have an orgasm. If sperm are found in your urine, you may have retrograde ejaculation.

If the problem is associated with nerve damage, your care provider may recommend medications that help keep the bladder neck muscle closed during ejaculation. Medications to treat retrograde ejaculation include certain antidepressants, antihistamines and decongestants.

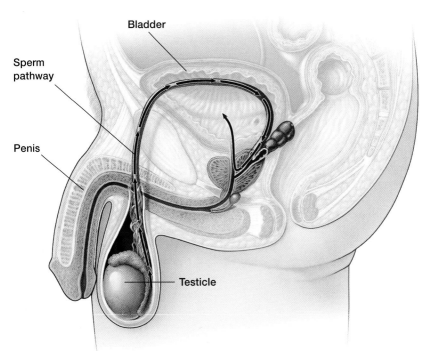

Bladder

Sperm pathway

Penis

Testicle

© MFMER

Retrograde ejaculation occurs when semen is redirected into the bladder instead of being ejaculated out of the penis. Although you still reach sexual climax, you ejaculate very little or no semen (dry orgasm).

If medication isn't helpful, you may need to consider assisted reproductive technology (ART). Sperm can be recovered from the bladder, processed in the laboratory, and used to inseminate your partner or her eggs.

Erectile dysfunction Male sexual arousal is a complex process that involves the brain, hormones, emotions, nerves, muscles and blood vessels. Erectile dysfunction, the inability to achieve or maintain an erection firm enough for sexual intercourse, can result from a problem with any of these. Likewise, stress and mental health problems can cause or worsen erectile dysfunction. Sometimes a combination of physical and psychological issues causes erectile dysfunction. For instance, a minor physical problem that slows your sexual response may cause anxiety about maintaining an erection. The resulting anxiety can lead to or worsen erectile dysfunction.

Erectile dysfunction can also result from a number of physical conditions, particularly those that impair blood flow to the nerves in the penis or damage the nerves. Examples include vascular disease, high blood pressure, diabetes, multiple sclerosis, and previous surgery or other treatments affecting the pelvic area. Use of certain medications, as well as tobacco and alcohol, also can contribute to erectile dysfunction. So can psychological issues such as depression, anxiety and stress.

Medications — either oral or injected — can successfully treat erectile dysfunction in many men and may lead to pregnancy. Often, in cases of erectile dysfunction resulting from anxiety or stressful situations, medications are used temporarily to regain confidence in being able to achieve and maintain a satisfactory erection. Medications alone often improve symptoms in most men. However, for those men who don't respond to medications or who are concerned about drug interactions, alternative therapies are available. Often, a counselor or a therapist can be of help in finding ways to reduce associated stress or anxiety.

CHROMOSOME DEFECTS

Your genes are involved in your body's most basic level of functioning. Genes code for proteins that help your cells operate normally. If something goes awry at the genetic level, it can throw off normal body functions in big or small ways.

Problems with fertility and the normal workings of the male reproductive system can result from larger changes at the chromosomal level, such as what occurs with cystic fibrosis (see page 154), Klinefelter syndrome (see page 159), Kallman syndrome (see page 161) and other inherited conditions. These genetic anomalies may result from extra chromosomal material or swapping of genes between chromosomes that corrupt the genetic message. These types of genetic mutations often cause other problems in addition to infertility.

With recent advances in genetic research, scientists are observing that even very small changes in gene arrangement can cause complications. One example of this is the deletion of small parts of several genes along the Y chromosome — the chromosome only men have that contains many of the genes critical for sperm production and testicular development. These deletions, called Y-chromosome microdeletions, are small enough to be missed on a conventional genetic test but can now be captured with newer, more sophisticated techniques.

As it turns out, Y-chromosome micro-deletions are much more common in men with very low or no sperm in the ejaculate. These deletions may explain many male infertility cases previously designated as having an unknown cause. As research progresses, investigators are hoping to obtain a more complete picture of the genetic changes involved in infertility, as well as the influences of a man's individual environment, metabolism and ethnic background, among other factors.

Currently, genetic causes of infertility can't be fixed to achieve natural conception. But it may be possible to retrieve enough sperm to attempt ART. Before doing so, however, you and your partner may want to talk to a genetics counselor, since these conditions may be passed on to your children. A genetics counselor can help you understand what the odds are and how best to proceed. It's possible to screen embryos for certain genetic conditions before the eggs are placed in the uterus to prevent a disorder from being passed on (preimplantation genetic diagnosis).

timed as best you can to coincide with your partner's ovulation. Among couples where low sperm count is a factor, about 30 percent of them conceive naturally over a period of two to three years.

However, if you have a severe condition or your partner is of an older age, you may want to pursue reproductive assistance. You can read more about the treatments in Chapter 15.

WHAT HAPPENS NEXT?

When a problem is discovered, such as a hormone imbalance or an obstructed tube, it's often possible to treat the problem and restore your fertility.

It's not uncommon, though, to go through all the testing and come away without an answer — an identifiable cause for your fertility problems. This can be frustrating, but it's not the end of the road. If your sperm count isn't terribly low and your partner is young and healthy, your care provider may recommend that you have frequent intercourse

EVALUATING INFERTILITY
A summary of the evaluation process

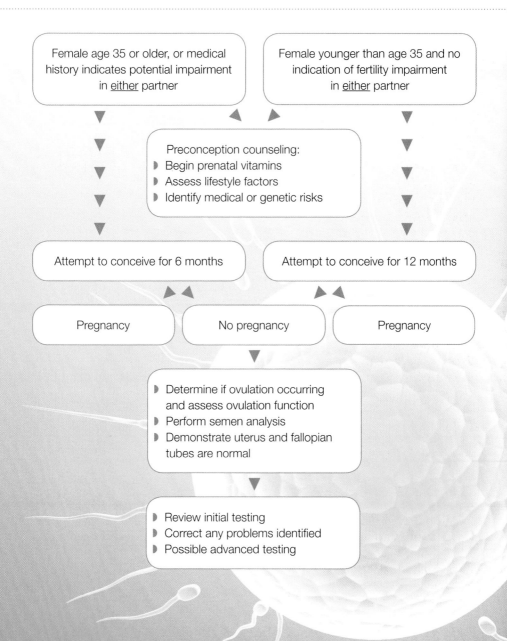

Female age 35 or older, or medical history indicates potential impairment in <u>either</u> partner

Female younger than age 35 and no indication of fertility impairment in <u>either</u> partner

Preconception counseling:
▶ Begin prenatal vitamins
▶ Assess lifestyle factors
▶ Identify medical or genetic risks

Attempt to conceive for 6 months

Attempt to conceive for 12 months

Pregnancy

No pregnancy

Pregnancy

▶ Determine if ovulation occurring and assess ovulation function
▶ Perform semen analysis
▶ Demonstrate uterus and fallopian tubes are normal

▶ Review initial testing
▶ Correct any problems identified
▶ Possible advanced testing

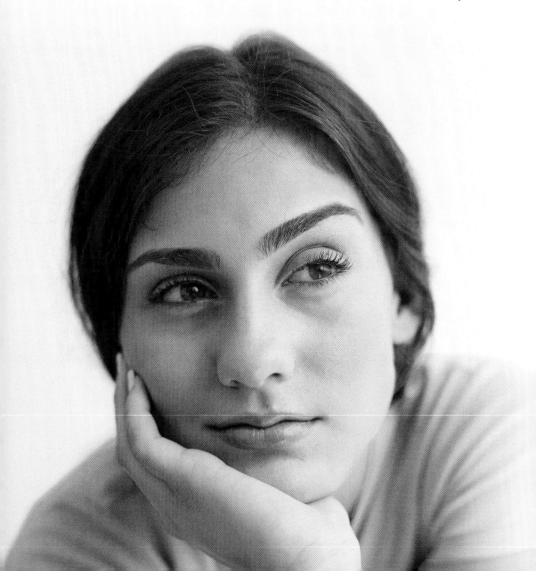

PART 4

When You Need Some Help

CHAPTER 13

Seeing a doctor

If you've been trying to have a baby for a while without any success, you may be frustrated. Angry. Anxious. Embarrassed. Sad. Scared that it just might never happen. All of these emotions are normal. If you're bickering and fighting with your partner, that's perfectly normal, too.

But your emotions and actions may be an indication it's time to seek some help. There's absolutely no shame in seeing a doctor to help determine what's keeping you from having a baby. Seeing a doctor doesn't mean you're a failure. It doesn't mean you can't have a baby "the natural way." And it doesn't mean you're surrendering to a future of hormone injections and in vitro fertilization.

Just the opposite: Seeing a doctor can help identify if you or your partner has any of the common fertility problems described in Part 3 of this book — some of which can be easily rectified. Working with a fertility expert may relieve some of the stress you're feeling and help you stay optimistic and hopeful about your chances of having a baby.

In this chapter, you'll learn when to seek help, what to expect at your first appointment and what diagnostic tests you might need to undergo. If you decide to see a specialist, it's important that you and your partner approach the process as a team and schedule a joint visit. (Remember, you're in this together!)

It's also essential that both of you are honest and candid every step of the way. Your doctor won't judge any of the information you share during your appointments. Instead, he or she will search your personal history for possible clues in your struggle to become pregnant so that you and your partner can move forward in your plans to start or expand your family.

WHEN TO SEE A DOCTOR

By definition, infertility means not being able to get pregnant despite having appropriately timed, unprotected sex for at least a year. If this describes your situation, it's time to talk to a doctor. In some cases, you shouldn't be quite so patient. It's probably a good idea to see a doctor after six months if:

◗ You're a woman older than age 35
◗ You aren't having menstrual periods (amenorrhea), your periods are more than 35 days apart (oligomenorrhea), or they're very light
◗ You or your partner has undergone chemotherapy or radiation treatments
◗ You or your partner has a history of fertility problems with another partner
◗ You know or suspect that you have uterine problems, tubal problems, pelvic infection or endometriosis
◗ Your partner has a history of testicle trauma or surgery, adult mumps, or sexual dysfunction

Just remember to schedule a joint appointment — not just an evaluation for the person you think may have a fertility problem. Women often assume it's best to start with a female evaluation and then bring in their partner once they've been "cleared." This isn't a good tactic. It can lead to months of tests that all come back normal, only to discover that the real problem is related to sperm quality. And that's a lot of wasted time!

If your partner is reluctant to seek medical help for infertility, talk to him about why he doesn't want to go. Understandably, he may be scared of what the doctor will discover. He may worry that his manliness is being scrutinized. He may be concerned that the troubles you're having are his fault. He may be uncomfortable masturbating into a container and submitting his sperm for judging. (Who wouldn't be?) These feelings are normal and common. Let him know that. But also help him understand that it doesn't make sense for you to go through infertility testing without him.

When it comes to infertility, knowledge really is power. Most infertility problems can be successfully treated. But, first, doctors have to understand what the problem is, if, in fact, there is one. Try to discuss these issues with your partner and focus your attention on your dreams of building a family. Be steadfast in your belief that your goal of having a baby is worth some uncomfortable moments. Encourage your partner to do some research or talk to his primary care doctor. Also, try to give him some time and space to process his emotions. People often become anxious when seeing a doctor about a sensitive issue.

Who should you see? When couples decide to seek professional help for fertility problems, they traditionally turn to the woman's gynecologist or primary care provider as their starting point. That's a reasonable place to begin. Many obstetrician-gynecologists (OB-GYNs) and primary care providers can perform some of the initial diagnostic tests used to determine why you're having difficulty becoming pregnant. Besides, you may have a long-standing, trusted relationship with this person, so it's a comfortable setting to talk about your situation.

However, you may eventually need to see a doctor who specializes in treating disorders that prevent couples from conceiving. Reproductive endocrinologists, commonly referred to as fertility specialists, are OB-GYNs who have received additional training in the diagnosis and treatment of infertility and related disorders. Fertility specialists generally receive an additional three years of training beyond the four-year residency required to become a general OB-GYN. This specialized training typically includes experience in ultrasound imaging and ovulation induction, in vitro fertilization, microsurgery, laparoscopic and hysteroscopic surgery, as well as clinical or laboratory research.

Reproductive endocrinologists are specialists in both male and female infertility and disorders affecting both reproductive systems. If it turns out that you need surgery, medication or complicated procedures to help you have a baby, a reproductive endocrinologist can guide you through the entire process.

Reproductive endocrinologists often work at specialized fertility clinics or within large medical centers where they have the equipment and resources to perform high-tech procedures. Urologists who specialize in fertility care also may be part of the team.

If you're considering assisted reproductive techniques, it may best to seek out a reproductive endocrinologist, if there's one available in your area.

HOW TO CHOOSE A FERTILITY DOCTOR OR CLINIC

Whether you start with a list of recommended doctors, talk to close friends and family members, or search the Internet for specialists in your area, it's important that you do your research before picking an infertility clinic. You'll probably find some information about the staff and the clinic on the clinic's website, but you may have additional topics you want to discuss on your first visit. Here are some questions you might want to ask:

▶ What's your training?
▶ Did you complete a fellowship in reproductive endocrinology?
▶ Are you board-certified in this subspecialty?
▶ How long have you been in practice?
▶ What percentage of your patients are fertility patients?
▶ How do you typically work with patients? What's your philosophy?
▶ What treatments do you offer?
▶ What do treatments cost?
▶ Which insurance plans do you accept?
▶ What's your success rate?

It's tempting to focus a lot of attention on success rates published by the Centers for Disease Control and Prevention and other organizations in order to find the "best" clinic. But it's important to interpret success rates with caution and to discuss the clinic's or doctor's reported rates in the context of the practice's philosophy and approach.

Success rates aren't a direct reflection of the training, experience and quality of services at a particular clinic. Some clinics accept more couples with complex infertility problems than do others, which can lower success rates. On the flip side, some clinics offer high-tech procedures to couples that might have become pregnant with less technologically advanced procedures, which will generally increase success rates. So it's important to assess fertility clinics with a critical eye. Try to identify success rates among couples that are similar to you.

Beware that some people who call themselves fertility specialists have not received additional training. The Society for Reproductive Endocrinology and Infertility can help you find a certified doctor (see page 274).

WHAT TO EXPECT

Determining why a couple is having difficulty becoming pregnant isn't always easy. And often, there isn't an obvious reason. Expect that the process could take several appointments and, potentially, a range of different diagnostic tests. The first visit is usually focused on a complete medical history and possibly a physical examination of one or both partners. It's a good opportunity for you and your partner to get to know your fertility doctor and vice versa.

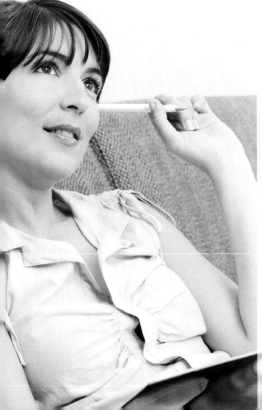

This is also a good time to get things off your chest, perhaps questions or concerns that have been nagging you. Write down a list of questions you want to ask your doctor, so you don't forget some of them during your appointment. If you're nervous or you get wrapped up on a particular topic, it's easy to forget about something you wanted to address. You may also want to bring along a notepad and pen, so you can take notes as your doctor talks, rather than trying to recall important details later.

Medical history You and your partner should anticipate that your doctor will likely have a long list of questions about your medical history and lifestyle. Plan ahead, so you can provide complete and accurate answers to these questions.

Consider bringing a copy of your medical records if either of you has had reproductive problems or prior reproductive tests and a list of any medications, vitamins and other supplements you're taking. It also may be worthwhile to chart your menstrual cycles and associated symptoms for a few months. Use a calendar or notebook to write down when your period starts and stops. Make note of the days when you have sex and any symptoms you're having. These details can be important pieces of information.

Be ready to answer the following questions:

Personal history. Have you or your partner ever had any major surgeries, serious illnesses, infections or previous hospitalizations — especially related to your abdomen, pelvis or reproductive organs? Do you have allergies? Do you have any chronic conditions? Have you ever had an abnormal Pap test? What medications do you take? Are your vaccinations up to date?

Family history. Do you have a family history of genetic disorders or birth defects? Have other people in your family struggled with infertility? What is the racial and ethnic background of each of your families?

Menstrual history. At what age did you have your very first period? When was your last period? How long are your typical periods? On average, how many days pass between the beginning of one menstrual cycle and the beginning of your next menstrual cycle? What is the bleeding pattern like? Do you experience other symptoms with your periods, such as cramping, abdominal bloating or breast tenderness? Have you ever tried using ovulation predictor kits or checking your basal body temperature?

Male partner history. Do you have any serious medical illnesses or take any medications? Did your testicles descend normally in infancy? Have you ever had hernia surgery? At what age did you experience puberty? Have you ever fathered a pregnancy with another partner? Have any of your family members had fertility problems? Do you have sexual dysfunction?

Sexual history. How long have you been trying to become pregnant? Do you know when is the best time to have intercourse when you're trying to get pregnant? How often do you have intercourse? Do you have pain with intercourse? Do you use lubricant with sexual intercourse? What types of birth control have you used? How many sexual partners have you had? Have you ever been pregnant before? If so, what was the outcome of that pregnancy? Have you ever been exposed to a sexually transmitted infection? Have you ever had

an abortion? Have you ever been a victim of sexual abuse? Do you have little interest in sex? Do you have trouble achieving orgasm?

Lifestyle habits. Do you smoke? Did you smoke in the past? Do you drink alcohol? How much do you drink? Do you use recreational drugs or steroids? How much do you exercise? Have you recently changed your diet? Have you recently gained or lost a lot of weight? What is your stress level?

Work conditions. What's your occupation? Are you exposed to any toxic chemicals in the workplace? Do you work a night shift?

No doubt, some of these questions may make you squirm. Do your best to put aside any embarrassment or nervousness you may feel and answer the questions with candor and honesty. Remember that your doctor isn't judging your responses. Truthful answers to all of these questions can provide clues as to what may be stopping you from having a baby. If you and your partner haven't discussed some of these topics before, you may want to have a heart-to-heart before you step foot in the doctor's office.

Physical exam For your first infertility evaluation, you and your partner may undergo a physical exam. An exam can give your doctor an idea of your general health and help identify common fertility problems. If you see a gynecologist for an infertility evaluation, an appointment may be made for your partner to see a urologist. The exam will likely start with the basics: determining your weight and height and checking blood pressure and pulse. You may undergo a basic head-to-toe evaluation or the exam may focus on just a few things.

For women, the appointment may include a pelvic examination. Your doctor will be looking for obvious abnormalities and signs of infection in the vagina or cervix, as well as any tenderness in the pelvis or abdomen. He or she will also check the size, shape and position of your uterus.

Men may undergo a thorough examination of the testicles, scrotum and penis. The doctor will be checking for any tenderness, swelling or signs of infection. He or she may also perform a digital rectal exam. In this exam, the doctor inserts a gloved finger into the rectum to determine if the prostate is enlarged, swollen or inflamed.

Each part of the physical examination can help your doctor identify or rule out possible causes of your infertility. But this is just the first step in the process. Your doctor probably won't be able to give you any definitive answers at the end of the first appointment.

Fertility tests What happens after that first visit partly depends on the information your doctor gathered during your medical history and physical exam. In general, though, a series of fertility tests is often the next step.

These tests should be conducted in a systematic, efficient and cost-effective manner. First off, your doctor wants to identify all of the relevant factors that may be at the root of your infertility. He or she isn't necessarily looking for a single culprit. In fact, it's not uncommon for couples to have more than one factor contributing to their infertility problems. So it's generally best to take a broad approach. But at the same time, your doctor should be keeping your best interests and your partner's in mind. There's no need for expensive, high-tech procedures if a few basic tests will do.

A basic infertility evaluation includes tests aimed at the most important causes of infertility — ovulatory dysfunction and ovarian reserve, semen abnormalities, and fallopian tube and uterine abnormalities. In short: eggs, sperm, tubes and uterus.

Depending on the exact tests your doctor chooses, a basic fertility evaluation may take one or two menstrual cycles, because some tests need to occur on a particular day of your cycle. Additional tests may be needed, depending on the results of the first batch of tests.

TESTS FOR WOMEN

Women are responsible for three parts of the fertility equation: eggs, tubes and uterus. Basic infertility testing in women is focused on these factors.

It's likely that your doctor will request some form of testing to confirm that you're ovulating on a regular basis, as well as an exam of your uterus and fallopian tubes to look for abnormalities. Another type of testing related to your egg supply — called ovarian reserve — is recommended for women older than age 35, as well as younger women with certain conditions or in certain situations. Your doctor may suggest additional tests, depending on your individual circumstances and personal medical history.

Ovulation tests As you learned in Chapter 5, ovulation is one of the most important events in the making of a baby. During ovulation, an egg is released from its follicle within one of your ovaries. This often happens about midway through your menstrual cycle, although the exact timing may vary. After ovulation, the egg is swept into one of the fallopian tubes, where a sperm can fertilize it.

A variety of problems can prevent or disrupt this monthly process, including thyroid or pituitary disorders, polycystic ovary syndrome, stress, or a tumor or structural blockage. So it's important to know if you're ovulating normally.

Your menstrual history may be the only assessment of ovulation that you need. It's not uncommon for women to miss a period now and then — traveling, strenuous exercise, illness and high stress can cause an occasional skipped period. However, if your menstrual history is very abnormal, that's generally a good indication that you're not releasing an egg each month.

Your doctor may look to other methods to confirm that you're ovulating regularly. Some women track their basal body temperature to check for slight rises in temperature that occur following ovulation. Some women use an over-the-counter ovulation prediction kit, which detects a surge in luteinizing hormone (LH) in urine. LH is the key hormone that triggers ovulation, so detecting a surge of this hormone at the right time of the month helps confirm that ovulation is occurring normally.

If it's unclear if you're ovulating, your doctor may order a blood test to measure levels of the hormone progesterone. Heightened progesterone levels provide reliable, objective evidence that ovulation has recently occurred. The timing of this test is important, though. If you don't have regular menstrual cycles, it can be difficult to time the test correctly in order to see the rise in progesterone levels.

In rare cases, a transvaginal ultrasound exam may be used to confirm ovulation. During this exam, your doctor or a medical technician inserts a wand-like device (transducer) into your vagina while you lie on your back on an exam table. The transducer emits sound waves that generate images of your pelvic organs, including your ovaries. A transvaginal ultrasound can measure and monitor the wall of an ovarian follicle as it matures and ruptures, releasing an egg. The procedure isn't painful, but you may need multiple ultrasound exams to determine when ovulation has occurred.

Ovarian reserve tests All women are born with a fixed number of eggs. At some point — usually in your early 50s — the eggs run out and menopause begins. However, years earlier, the number and quality of the remaining eggs begins to diminish. *Ovarian reserve* is a term used to describe the number and quality of the immature egg cells (oocytes) in the ovaries. There's no perfect test to count the number of eggs present. But there are ways to determine if you have a reasonable supply compared to other women your age. This helps estimate your fertility potential and the likelihood that you can successfully have a baby.

Decreased or diminished ovarian reserve is a normal part of the aging process. It can also occur because of ovarian surgery, chemotherapy or radiation treatments, genetic abnormalities, and, possibly, smoking. There are several tests to measure ovarian reserve, some of which are performed on specific days of your menstrual cycle. Those most commonly used include:

Follicle-stimulating hormone (FSH) test and estradiol. These blood tests are the most common tests for ovarian reserve. They're drawn on day three of your menstrual cycle. As mentioned earlier, FSH is the key hormone that causes immature eggs in the ovaries to begin maturing. It's produced in the pituitary gland, located at the base of your brain.

A high level of FSH indicates that your body is working extra hard to get the eggs in your ovaries to develop, which means that the number and quality of eggs is diminishing. FSH levels continue to increase as your egg supply decreases and you begin menopause.

Estradiol is the ovarian hormone made by the developing follicle, the fluid-filled sac where the developing egg grows. Estradiol stimulates the growth of the uterine lining to prepare the uterus for pregnancy. It also signals the brain that the FSH is working. By analyzing both hormones, doctors sometimes uncover problems they wouldn't see by looking at FSH alone. Testing takes place the first few days of the menstrual cycle.

Anti-müllerian hormone (AMH). This hormone is produced by small ovarian follicles. Each available follicle contributes a small amount of AMH. Thus, high amounts are associated with a good ovarian reserve, while low levels of AMH indicate a declining egg supply. AMH can be measured with a blood test at any time during the menstrual cycle.

Antral follicle count (AFC). Antral follicles are small follicles that appear on your ovaries at the beginning of your menstrual cycle. The number of antral follicles reflects the underlying egg supply left in the ovaries. Antral follicles can be counted during a transvaginal ultrasound. This is typically during the early part of your menstrual cycle. This test doesn't provide any information about the quality of the remaining eggs — just the quantity.

Ovarian reserve tests are often used in combination. Together, the tests can provide a good gauge of your remaining eggs and help determine the treatments that will be best for you.

Uterine and fallopian tube tests It doesn't matter how many good eggs you have and how regularly you release them if the sperm can't get to them or the embryo can't find a safe place in the uterus to grow and implant. That's why it's important to identify problems or obstructions in your uterus and fallopian tubes. Common fallopian tube and uterine problems include tubal blockage or damage, polyps, adhesions, uterine fibroids, and abnormalities such as a uterine septum. According to one study, damage to the fallopian tubes accounts for 14 percent of fertility problems. Problems with the uterus or cervix are less common but important to be aware of.

There are several imaging tests that can check the shape of your uterus and make sure your fallopian tubes are open (patent):

Hysterosalpingography (HSG). This special X-ray procedure is frequently performed. Its use dates back more than 100 years, but it's still the standard for confirming that the uterine cavity is normal and the fallopian tubes are unblocked.

HSG begins similar to a pelvic exam. You'll be asked to undress from the waist down and put on a gown. Then you'll lie on a table under a real-time X-ray imaging machine called a fluoroscope. Your doctor or a radiologist will insert a speculum — a plastic or metal-hinged instrument shaped like a duck's bill — to open your vaginal walls. Then he or she will clean your cervix with a swab and place a catheter into the cervix, before removing the speculum.

The catheter is used to fill the uterus with a small amount of liquid or dye. As the dye spreads through the reproductive tract and fills up your uterine cavity and fallopian tubes, your doctor will be able to see any blockages or abnormalities on

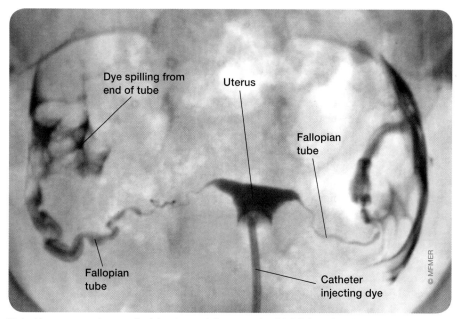

Labels on image:
Dye spilling from end of tube
Uterus
Fallopian tube
Fallopian tube
Catheter injecting dye
© MFMER

This X-ray procedure called hysterosalpingography highlights the female reproductive tract and can identify blockages or abnormalities. *Note:* The lower part of the uterus is obscured in this image by a balloon at the end of catheter.

the X-ray monitor. If a particular area isn't filling, there may be a polyp or other structure blocking the liquid from moving into that area.

The procedure typically takes about 15 to 30 minutes, although the time you're exposed to X-rays is almost always less than one to two minutes. It may cause some discomfort or mild cramps. It's also common to have mild spotting for a few days afterward.

An HSG provides the most detail of the fallopian tubes. Most of the time the inside of the uterus is seen, too. Because the most commonly used type of catheter has a balloon at the end of its tip, sometimes the balloon can limit the view.

Sonohysterography. Also known as saline sonography, this is an ultrasound exam that also includes the injection of fluid through the cervix into the uterus.

The fluid expands the uterus so that you can see inside instead of just seeing it as a thin stripe on a traditional ultrasound. This type of imaging can detect problems in the uterus, such as an abnormally shaped uterus, scarring inside the uterus, or abnormal growths inside the uterus such as fibroids or polyps. It's sometimes used instead of HSG, but it provides less information about the fallopian tubes. This may be the best test if, based on your history and exam, you're more likely to have a uterine problem than a fallopian tube problem.

For this procedure, a traditional transvaginal ultrasound exam is done first. Then, fluid is injected into the uterus and the transvaginal ultrasound is repeated.

The process is similar to HSG or a pelvic exam. You'll be asked to undress from the waist down and put on a gown. You'll lie on an examination table for the first transvaginal ultrasound. Then, your doctor will use a speculum to open your vaginal walls. He or she will pass a swab through the speculum to clean your cervix and then place a catheter into the cervix, before removing the speculum. Finally, the transvaginal ultrasound transducer is placed in the vagina again, and a sterile salt water is slowly passed through the catheter as the ultrasound resumes. The whole procedure takes about 10 or 15 minutes. Like HSG, you may feel cramping because of the injected fluid. You may also have spotting after the procedure.

Hysteroscopy. In this procedure, your doctor inserts a slender surgical telescope with a small camera (hysteroscope) into your vagina and through the cervix to view the inside of your uterus. It's the gold standard for evaluating inner uterine problems, but it's more expensive and invasive than an ultrasound-based test. It also doesn't examine the outer uterine walls or the ovaries. Therefore, it's usually scheduled only if other tests aren't sufficient or your doctor suspects a particular problem in the uterus.

Laparoscopy. Laparoscopy was once a key component of an infertility evaluation. A surgeon would perform laparoscopic surgery to look at the reproductive organs to see if they appeared normal. Today this procedure, which is invasive and expensive, is rarely used. However, laparoscopy may be performed if your doctor knows (or suspects) that you have endometriosis, pelvic adhesions, an ovarian cyst, blocked fallopian tubes or similar conditions, and he or she needs to get a closer look inside your reproductive organs.

If you undergo laparoscopy, you'll receive general anesthesia before the procedure begins. A surgeon will insert a needle through your bellybutton and fill your abdomen with carbon dioxide gas. The gas pushes the abdominal wall away from your internal organs to make it safe for the laparoscope to enter. The laparoscope, a slender tube with a camera at its tip, is inserted through an incision in your bellybutton. During the procedure, the surgeon views and takes images of the uterus, fallopian tubes and ovaries. Often, a few other small incisions are made so that other instruments can be inserted to help the surgeon see better or fix a problem.

After the procedure, it's common to have a tender navel area and bruised abdomen. Some women also experience nausea from the anesthesia or discomfort in the shoulders, chest and abdomen from the carbon dioxide gas. There's also a risk of a bladder infection or skin irritation. In rare cases, other complications are possible. Women are usually encouraged to take it easy for a few days after the procedure.

Hormone tests Sometimes, infertility can stem from a problem with your endocrine system, the body system that regulates the production and release of hormones. Your doctor may request a blood test to check the following hormone levels:

Thyroid-stimulating hormone (TSH). If you have an underactive thyroid gland, the gland isn't producing enough of certain important hormones (hypothyroidism). For women, sometimes there's a link between hypothyroidism and infertility and having a healthy pregnancy. Low levels of thyroid hormone can interfere with the release of an egg from your ovary (ovulation), which impairs fertility. In addition, some of the underlying causes of hypothyroidism — such as certain autoimmune or pituitary disorders — may impair fertility. Other signs and symptoms of hypothyroidism may include fatigue and an enlarged thyroid gland.

There's also increasing evidence that what is a normal level of thyroid function for most people may not be optimal for women trying to become pregnant or women who have experienced repeated miscarriages. This problem, called subclinical hypothyroidsm, is often treated in women trying to become pregnant and then discontinued once the baby is born.

Prolactin. This milk-producing hormone is secreted by the pituitary gland in your brain. If your body produces a high level of prolactin, it causes a decrease in estrogen that interferes with ovulation. This is good for women who are breastfeeding (lactating), but it's not good if you're trying to get pregnant.

Prolactin overproduction may be caused by a noncancerous tumor (adenoma) of the pituitary gland. It can also result from certain medications, other types of pituitary tumors or an underactive thyroid. Women with high levels of prolactin may also notice milky breast discharge or painful intercourse due to vaginal dryness.

Some doctors routinely test for these hormones as part of a basic fertility evaluation. If your doctor orders these tests, it doesn't necessarily mean that he or she suspects a problem.

TESTS FOR MEN

As you read earlier, for pregnancy to happen, the male partner must produce healthy sperm. At least one of his testicles must be functioning correctly, and he must produce testosterone and other hormones to trigger and maintain sperm production. Next, enough sperm need to be carried into the semen, and the sperm must be shaped correctly and able to move quickly. If the movement (motility) or shape (morphology) is abnormal, the sperm may not be able to reach or penetrate the egg.

The goal of fertility testing in men is to confirm that all of these things are happening properly. A basic infertility evaluation for men generally includes a complete medical history and physical exam and a semen analysis. Additional tests may be ordered, based on the results of these initial tests.

Semen analysis Semen analysis is the cornerstone of infertility testing for men. Couples are asked to avoid sex for a few days before a scheduled semen analysis, because intercourse can diminish the

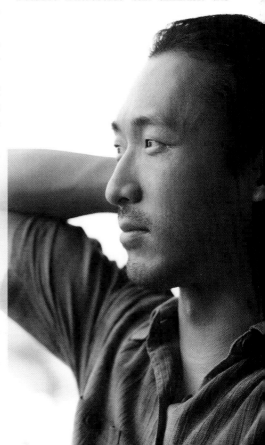

sperm count and interfere with the reliability of the test.

A semen sample is generally collected by masturbating and ejaculating into a special sterile container at the doctor's office. This is done in a private room or bathroom, with or without the other partner present, whatever is most comfortable for both of you. Videos or magazines may be available as aids.

If you live close to the doctor's office or lab, the sample may be collected at home and delivered shortly after collection. Your doctor also may give you the option of collecting the sample during intercourse, using a special condom that doesn't contain an additive that kills sperm.

Regardless of the collection method used, the lab will analyze the sample and check for the following:

▶ Semen volume
▶ Sperm count
▶ Sperm shape (see page 59)
▶ Sperm movement (motility)
▶ Acidity and sugar content
▶ Signs of problems, such as infections

Having an abnormal sperm test doesn't automatically mean there's a problem. Men produce millions of sperm each day, and not every sperm will be perfect. Also, there's a variation in sperm production from day to day, week to week and month to month. So having to undergo a second test isn't uncommon. When a semen analysis reveals an abnormality, another sample is often taken and analyzed to determine if the problem is consistent, and if it is, how significant it is.

Other tests Depending on the results of the semen analysis and what your doctor learned during the medical history, additional tests may be performed.

Scrotal ultrasound. This exam can help your doctor see obstructions or other problems in the testicles and supporting structures, including swollen veins around the testes (varicoceles). After applying a gel to the scrotal sac to help transmit sound waves, your doctor or a medical technician moves the ultrasound transducer over the scrotum to create images and look for abnormalities.

Hormone testing. Just as hormones play a key role in female fertility, they're also important to male fertility. Hormones produced by the pituitary gland and testicles affect male sexual development and sperm production. Abnormalities in other hormonal organs also may contribute to infertility. Your doctor may recommend blood tests to check levels of testosterone, follicle-stimulating hormone (FSH), luteinizing hormone (LH), prolactin and thyroid function.

KEEPING A POSITIVE OUTLOOK

Understandably, fertility testing can be stressful, and it's certainly not enjoyable. As you head down this path, it's important to view the process in the right frame of mind. All of the testing that you and your partner undergo provides more pieces to the puzzle. As your doctor puts these pieces together and begins to see the bigger picture, he or she can help you decide the next steps you should take.

For some couples, testing reveals a clear reason why conception isn't happening. In other cases, the evaluation process ends without a lot of concrete answers. This can be frustrating, but it doesn't mean all is lost. If you find yourself in this category, take heart. The good news is that no significant obstacles to pregnancy have been identified, and there are still several steps you can take.

TESTS YOU DON'T NEED

The field of medicine is constantly changing and advancing. What was standard procedure yesterday is often no longer today. Some tests that were long regarded as essential components of an infertility evaluation are now deemed to be outdated and unnecessary. If your doctor recommends these tests, inquire as to why they're needed. You shouldn't be paying for something you don't need.

Postcoital testing For this test, couples are instructed to have sex just before coming to the doctor's office. The doctor then examines the quality and quantity of cervical mucus production and the number of sperm swimming.

This test has been discontinued for many reasons: First, it's difficult to interpret because there are no standard measurements. Second, researchers and doctors have discovered that abnormalities in cervical mucus are rarely the real cause of infertility but rather a side effect of infertility problems that can be detected through other tests. Finally, as you may imagine, postcoital testing is inconvenient and embarrassing for many women and stressful for the couple.

Endometrial biopsy A biopsy of the lining of the uterus (endometrium) was a routine part of infertility testing for decades. The biopsy was used to confirm that ovulation had occurred and to evaluate whether the lining was in sync with how far along it should be to support a pregnancy. Today, the idea that the uterus can "lag behind" and cause infertility has been debunked. In fact, researchers have found that many women who have no trouble getting pregnant have an endometrial lining that would be considered out of sync.

An endometrial biopsy may still be appropriate when problems with the endometrial lining are strongly suspected, such as when you have irregular bleeding or infrequent periods. But doctors are much more hesitant to recommend this invasive, expensive, uncomfortable test for all women.

Routine laparoscopy As mentioned earlier, laparoscopy may be appropriate to investigate a specific problem, but it's no longer recommended simply to take a look around and make sure that everything looks OK.

Sperm antibodies For many years tests were done to check for antibodies to sperm in cervical mucus, blood or even sperm. These tests were intended to look for special proteins (antibodies) that attack a man's sperm — similar to an allergic reaction. Current thinking is that because there isn't an effective treatment for sperm antibodies, testing for them generally isn't necessary.

If your doctor recommends tests you're not familiar with or you don't understand why they're being done, research them and ask questions — especially if the tests are expensive or supposedly could be a quick fix to your problems. As the old saying goes, if something sounds too good to be true, it probably is.

Lisa and Scott's Story

Lisa: After we got married, we decided to stop taking birth control. When it came to getting pregnant, we said, "If it happens, it happens." But I have to admit we were hoping it would "happen" right away. Scott worked at a college and had his summers off. If we got pregnant soon after our summer wedding, it would've been perfect timing.

Unfortunately, it didn't happen right away. In fact, it took us nine months to finally get pregnant. And then, one day before our five-week mark, I miscarried.

This was a tough loss for us, but we coped by diving right back in and trying to get pregnant again. It took us nearly 11 months, but we finally did it ... and then, at five weeks, I miscarried.

Scott: That was tough. We tried again, but it just wasn't happening for us. So we saw a doctor who said that Lisa was too heavy — that she needed to lose weight in order to improve the chance of getting pregnant. In fact, the doctor said she wouldn't even look at our situation until she did.

We took that advice to heart and started running and paying attention to our nutrition. We were hoping it would be the elixir that cured everything.

Lisa: It was a tough thing to hear, but it was also a hopeful thing to hear. I thought, "Once I lose weight, I'll become pregnant and all will be right with world."

As we embarked on our healthier lifestyle, we saw a new doctor who put me on clomiphene (Clomid), a drug that helps stimulate ovulation. When three months went by and we still hadn't conceived, we were referred to a reproductive endocrinologist, a doctor who specializes in fertility issues.

Over the course of the next 15 months, we tried a procedure called intrauterine insemination (IUI) in which they took Scott's sperm, washed and spun it, then transferred it directly into my uterus.

Of the nine IUIs we tried, we had one pregnancy ... that we miscarried.

Scott: That was a hard time. I tend to be more positive, saying things like, "We'll just keep trying." But Lisa wasn't at that place. She asked how I could get over our miscarriages so quickly.

It's not that I "got over them." It's just that "moving on" is ingrained in me. From working in college athletics, I learned that even after the toughest games, there's always another chance. And that's how I approached this. No matter what happened, the dog still needed to be walked. The lawn still needed to be mowed.

Lisa: It bothered me. My way of coping was to lay in bed and cry. I would get mad at Scott and say, "How can you act like everything's fine?" Meanwhile, I felt like my world was ending.

After taking several months off to give ourselves a break, we started the in vitro fertilization (IVF) process. We were successful on our second try ... and then I miscarried that baby, too.

I was devastated. I thought, "When is enough enough?" The expense, the stress, the process — it's all so much.

Scott: I think the toughest part is that there was really no explanation to why Lisa was miscarrying. There was nothing we could do to make the problem better because we didn't know what the problem was.

We've taken every test, looked into every option. I wish they could say, "Scott, you're not producing sperm," or, "Lisa, you're not producing eggs." Then we could cry for a week and go through the grieving process instead of having this unknown.

Lisa: We've now suffered four losses, and we still don't have a baby. Despite that, I can't help feeling this little ray of hope that maybe the next time will be the one that works for us.

We're going to keep trying. Until someone tells me that there's something wrong, I feel like I have every right to get pregnant. I want to feel that child inside me. I want to experience labor. We still have four embryos left — why leave them hanging out in the freezer?

Scott: I can't wait to come downstairs and find Lisa throwing up because she has morning sickness. I want to experience that. I hope we will experience that.

Meanwhile, we're at the point where we broach the subject of adoption every two to three months, and we differ quite a bit on it. I'm all for it. I just want to have a child that we can raise, even if it's not a child we created. Lisa's in a different place. She wants to be told there's no chance she can have a baby; then maybe her mind will change.

Lisa: I do struggle with the thought of having to adopt. I feel like if we decide to adopt, I'm giving up the idea of having my own children. And I'm just not quite there, yet.

It's not that I'm against adopting. We have friends who've adopted, and it was the right thing for them. It's not that the idea of adoption bothers me. It's just that adopting means, to me, that I can't carry my own baby.

Scott: It's now been more than five years since we first started trying to have a family. We've watched so many friends and family members have babies over this time, and that's still hard for us, but it's made us stronger, too. And we definitely haven't given up hope. We have four embryos left, which will give us two more tries with IVF. One of those tries could give us a baby.

And if it doesn't, this journey has given us other things. I run every day now. Lisa runs five days a week. Since we started living healthier, I'm down 140 pounds and Lisa is down 85. If, God forbid, we aren't able to have a child, our healthier lifestyle is still a change for the better for us.

Lisa: If someone had told me two or three years ago, "Lisa, your marriage will be stronger because of this," or "You'll be a stronger person because of this," I never would've believed them. But that's exactly what has happened. I've learned that our experience is much more common than people know. No matter what happens, we're going to be OK.

Medications and surgery

So your fertility tests are finished. At this point, you know the proper medical name of the condition — or conditions — that are holding up your dreams of having a baby. Or maybe not. Maybe fertility testing helped your doctor rule out a lot of potential problems, but it didn't reveal any obvious reason for why you're having trouble conceiving. In either case, you're probably wondering: What's next?

Most couples choose to pursue some form of fertility treatment. Your treatment options will depend on your age and your partner's age, the specific causes of your infertility, how long you've been trying to have a baby, and many personal preferences — including financial and ethical or religious concerns.

Most couples choose to start with the least expensive treatment that's likely to work in their particular situation. They then move up the ladder of treatment options one rung at a time. It's generally recommended you give each option about three tries before re-evaluating and moving on. At any time, you can hop off the ladder — stepping on the first rung doesn't mean you're obligated to climb all the way to the top.

Where you begin — the initial treatment rung — varies from couple to couple, depending on the conditions that are identified during fertility testing. Most couples don't start at the top of the ladder with high-tech treatments, such as in vitro fertilization (IVF). Sometimes, however, because of pressing time issues or the manner in which their insurance covers infertility treatments, some couples will be aggressive from the start and begin with IVF.

Many couples can benefit from one of two simpler, more-economical baby-making approaches: The first is to stimulate the ovaries to produce more than one egg at a time. The second is to get the best sperm as close to the egg as possible at the right time.

In this chapter, you'll learn about medications and procedures that can accomplish both of these goals. You'll also learn about medications and surgeries that are used in special circumstances. The next chapter focuses on IVF and other assisted reproductive technologies.

MANY OPTIONS

There are a number of medications and surgical procedures that can help couples have a baby. Some are targeted at remedying specific medical causes of infertility. Others are a good bet for a particular category of conditions or unexplained fertility problems.

In most cases, women undergo treatment — even if the underlying cause of a couple's infertility is related to problems with the sperm. Researchers continue to look for treatments targeted at men, but few have been proved to work. You'll find out about a couple of surgical procedures for men at the end of this chapter.

During treatment, the fertility tests you learned about in the previous chapter may be used to monitor your progress. For example, the tests that were used to determine if you're ovulating properly may be used again to find out if you're ovulating in response to treatment.

In general, it's best to give a particular treatment roughly three menstrual cycles to work before moving on to something else. Research shows that if a treatment is going to work, it's likely to work sooner rather than later. Repeating the same treatment over and over and over isn't likely to change the result, and it may waste time and money.

If cost is a factor in your decision-making process, don't be shy to ask how much various medications and procedures cost and find out what — if anything — may be covered by your medical insurance. As you evaluate the cost of treatments, make sure you understand how many times you're likely to repeat them and whether monitoring tests, lab work and office visits are included in the cost of treatments. If not, ask about the price of these associated costs and get out your calculator.

It may seem unusual to discuss costs with your care provider, because that's not how other areas of medicine typically work in the United States. But fertility clinics are used to these conversations. Your doctor can help you spend your money wisely when he or she understands your financial plans. Some clinics even provide financial counseling or guidance to help you sort through the expenses related to fertility treatments.

FERTILITY MEDICATIONS

When people talk about "fertility drugs" they're often talking about ovulation-inducing medications. These medications induce your ovaries to develop and release an egg if you're not doing that normally. For women who do ovulate normally, using medications may stimulate your ovaries to release multiple eggs — rather than the single egg that normally develops each month — which increases your chances of getting pregnant.

This is the first line of treatment for many couples. It's the best treatment for most women who don't ovulate regularly (or at all), and it's often part of the treatment plan for couples with unknown causes of infertility. Since ovulation-inducing medications can be inexpensive and effective, they're also tried for a range of fertility problems before committing to assisted reproductive technologies. However, these medications are less likely to work if you have low ovarian reserve, severe problems with your uterus or fallopian tubes, or severe problems with sperm.

There are several medications that can be used for ovulation induction. Some are used in tandem.

Clomiphene For many women, this is the first medication a doctor is likely to prescribe. Overall, it's highly successful and inexpensive. It works by blocking the estrogen signals sent from your ovaries to your brain. This tricks the brain to signal the pituitary gland to release extra follicle-stimulating hormone (FSH) and luteinizing hormone (LH). As a result, the ovaries receive more consistent signals to grow eggs.

Clomiphene (Clomid, Serophene) is a pill that's typically taken for five consecutive days, starting on the third to fifth day after menstruation begins. A few days after you finish taking the pills, you may be advised to use an ovulation predictor kit to detect when you are about to ovulate. When your kit is posi-tive, you'll want to have sex that night. Or you may be encouraged to have sex approximately every other night on days 10 through 20 of your menstrual cycle, the most likely time during which ovulation will occur.

In some cases, your doctor will confirm that you ovulated with other tests — such as transvaginal ultrasound. During this procedure, an ultrasound wand is placed inside your vagina to view the nearby ovaries. The image produced allows your care provider to see the developing follicles within the ovaries or the ones that have recently released an egg.

Most women start with a 50-milligram tablet of clomiphene taken once a day. If that doesn't prompt ovulation, the dose can be increased by 50-milligram increments each month until ovulation occurs. Effective doses range from 50 to 150 milligrams — one to three tablets a day for five days. However, doses in excess of 100 milligrams aren't approved by the Food and Drug Administration (FDA).

Luckily, most women don't need that much. Studies show that when clomiphene is taken to treat ovulation problems it successfully triggers ovulation in 80 percent of women, and up to 50 percent of women who ovulate become pregnant. Of those who ovulate, about half do so when given a 50-milligram dose.

Side effects are common but tend to be mild. Hot flashes are most common. Some women report mood swings and irritability, especially at higher doses. This makes sense because clomiphene blocks estrogen levels in the brain, similar to what occurs during menopausal transition. Some women have significant symptoms and others none at all. Other side effects include breast tenderness, pelvic pressure or pain, and nausea.

There's also a chance that you'll become pregnant with more than one fetus — in fact, pregnancies involving more than one fetus occur in up to 10 percent of cases. In the cases involving the use of clomiphene, most often the woman is carrying twins. Triplets or higher gestations are rare. Being pregnant with more than one fetus poses higher risks to the mother and babies than does a single pregnancy, including premature birth and low birth weight, among other complications.

Aromatase inhibitors This class of medications, which includes letrozole (Femara) and anastrozole (Arimidex), is approved for treatment of advanced breast cancer. Similar to the medication metformin, aromatase inhibitors are increasingly being used off label to induce ovulation.

Aromatase inhibitors may be a preferable first line infertility treatment for women with polycystic ovary syndrome (PCOS). Like clomiphene, aromatase inhibitors are oral medications that temporarily block the signaling pathways between the brain and the ovaries. A recent large study of women with PCOS compared the effectiveness of letrozole versus clomiphene for fertility therapy. Women who took letrozole had significantly higher ovulation and live birth rates. There were no differences between the two treatments in rates of miscarriage, serious pregnancy complications or birth defects.

An early study of aromatase inhibitors as a treatment for infertility suggested the medication may increase the risk of birth defects. However, the complete study was never published due to several major methodology flaws, and the preliminary report has been discredited. Newer research doesn't show any statistical difference in birth defects.

Further analysis of the data showed that when it came to calculating the total cost of treatment for one live birth, letrozole also was more cost effective. The authors concluded that letrozole improved ovulation and live birth rates in women with PCOS and recommended that letrozole be used as a first line therapy.

Besides women with PCOS, aromatase inhibitors may be a good choice for women who don't get pregnant on clomiphene or who experience significant side effects to the drug, as well as women who may be at high risk of multiple pregnancies.

Gonadotropins These hormone shots contain synthetic versions of the two sex hormones produced by the pituitary gland that stimulate egg production and maturation — FSH and LH. Gonadotropins (Repronex, Menopur) are typically used when other less complicated, less costly methods have failed. They may also be used in preparation for intrauterine insemination or in vitro fertilization. They must be injected into the fatty layer of tissue under the skin or into muscle. Newer drugs (Gonal-F, Follistim AQ) contain more highly purified preparations of FSH and are generally easier to use, but they're more costly.

Unlike clomiphene, which works within the system to stimulate the pituitary gland to make additional sex hormones, gonadotropins override the delicate balance of the reproductive system to stimulate the ovaries directly. The result can be very quick and efficient, but it can also be too effective — sometimes creating 10 or more eggs. (This is a good thing if you're creating eggs for IVF, but it's not so good if you're just trying to trigger regular ovulation.) Much has been made of the "octomom" in the popular press. In most cases, quadruplets, quintuplets and greater multiples, come from the use of gonadotropins.

Gonadotropins are usually given as daily injections, starting on day two or three of your menstrual cycle and lasting for seven to 12 days. During this time, egg development is monitored with a combination of blood tests measuring estrogen levels and ultrasound exams to assess the size of the sacs the eggs grow in (follicles). When the eggs are mature, a shot of human chorionic gonadotropin (HCG) is given to trigger ovulation.

As with other fertility drugs, women typically begin with a low dose (75 IU a day) and then move on to higher doses, if needed. The biggest risk is too many babies. Some women also experience mood swings, bloating, mild nausea or abdominal discomfort. Your care provider will closely monitor your progress with transvaginal ultrasounds and blood tests to confirm when you ovulate and to help reduce the risk of multiple pregnancies.

Some women are terrified by the thought of giving themselves injections, but quickly discover that they aren't that bad. The injections can be given anywhere on the body, but most women find a site near the belly button is most comfortable and convenient. Your nurse or doctor will teach you exactly how to inject yourself safely and properly. Your partner also can learn how to do this for you. But he'll need to be available every time you need a shot if he's going to be in charge of injections. Some couples find that it's best for both people to get a tutorial. Then, you can decide which of you is best with the needle and what works best with your schedule.

Human chorionic gonadotropin This hormone shot is similar to luteinizing hormone but is longer acting. Unlike other medications, it doesn't signal the ova-

ries to grow an egg. Instead, it signals the ovaries to release a mature egg.

Human chorionic gonadotropin (Ovidrel, Pregnyl) is used in conjunction with fertility drugs. Typically, you'll take fertility drugs early in your cycle, as prescribed. And you'll have regular transvaginal ultrasounds, blood tests or both to track the growth of the follicles. When your care provider sees that at least one follicle has reached a specific size and is likely to contain a mature egg, you'll receive instructions on when to administer HCG and trigger ovulation.

Then it's time for you and your partner to get the sperm to the egg! In some cases, the next step is for you and your partner to have sex at the optimal time for fertilization. In most cases, the medication is used to prepare for intrauterine insemination and other advanced fertility procedures.

Metformin Metformin (Glucophage, Fortamet) is approved for the treatment of diabetes. It improves the sensitivity of body tissues to the hormone insulin. It also helps trigger ovulation when insulin resistance is a known or suspected cause of infertility, such as in the case of PCOS. However, the FDA hasn't approved metformin for this purpose. So using it as a fertility medication is an off-label use. And it's not appropriate for women who don't have insulin resistance.

Even for women who do have insulin resistance, metformin generally isn't the best drug on its own. However, for a woman who's significantly overweight, the medication can be beneficial because it's associated with weight loss and many women find it easier to limit the amount of food they eat when their insulin levels are lower. Therefore, metformin may provide a boost when taken with clomiphene.

Some doctors prescribe both medications right away. Others add metformin only if women don't ovulate with clomiphene citrate alone. Metformin does add extra costs and complexity to your treatment regimen.

The typical dose is 1,500 to 2,000 milligrams daily. Side effects include nausea, vomiting and diarrhea. They can be minimized by increasing the dose slowly, using sustained-release preparations, and taking the medication with a meal or at bedtime.

MEDICATIONS FOR SPECIFIC CONDITIONS

Medications aren't only used to induce ovulation. In some cases, they're used to treat underlying problems interfering with fertility — particularly hormone problems.

For example, if your care provider discovers that you have an underactive thyroid gland (hypothyroidism) or an elevated level of prolactin (hyperprolactinemia), you'll receive medications to treat these conditions. Getting your hormone levels under control will help you feel better if you're experiencing symptoms due to these conditions. In addition, restoring your hormone levels to normal will help regulate your menstrual cycles and may fix your fertility problems.

Medications may also be prescribed for men with hormone problems that are contributing to infertility, such as hypogonadism. In this condition, the body doesn't produce enough of the male sex hormone testosterone. Men may be born with the condition, due to a problem in the testicles (primary hypogonadism). Or it may develop later in life (secondary hypogonadism).

In secondary hypogonadism, the testicles are normal but function improperly due to an abnormality in the pituitary gland or hypothalamus. The abnormality may be the result of a harmless tumor on the pituitary gland or a condition called Kallmann syndrome. This type of hypogonadism can often be treated with hormone medications. When hormone levels are regulated, sperm production often resumes normally.

FERTILITY PROCEDURES AND SURGERIES

The remainder of this chapter describes the medical procedure intrauterine insemination (IUI), as well as surgeries used to treat infertility. IUI is a common infertility procedure that is often recommended for couples in many different circumstances. Surgical procedures, on the other hand, are generally used to repair specific conditions that are hampering fertility. Surgery is only recommended when a particular condition has been clearly identified by tests and diagnosis.

Intrauterine insemination When a couple has sexual intercourse, sperm-filled semen is ejaculated into the woman's vagina. As soon as this occurs, millions of sperm begin to swim up toward the opening to the uterus (cervix). They must travel all of the way through the uterus to the fallopian tubes and beyond, in search of an egg to fertilize. There are plenty of obstacles along the way — including acid levels in the vagina and cervical mucus. Most sperm get trapped, lost or die during the journey. (The odds of climbing to the top of Mount Everest are probably better!)

Q. WHY BOTHER WITH DRUGS? WHY NOT GO STRAIGHT TO IVF?

A. As one Mayo Clinic fertility specialist states, "In vitro fertilization is a very powerful hammer, but every couple isn't a nail."

In fact, many couples can have a baby using one of the less powerful, less aggressive, less life-disrupting tools in a fertility specialist's toolbox. Going straight to IVF may up your odds of having a baby more quickly, but it takes an incredible investment of time, emotion and money — often tens of thousands of dollars.

If you've been trying to have a baby for a long time, it's natural to be impatient. And it's normal to worry that you're wasting valuable time trying various treatments only to end up needing IVF in the long run.

Rest assured that IVF isn't necessary in every situation, so you're not spinning your wheels by attempting other options first. In fact, it's wise to consider simpler treatments before complex ones.

In most countries, the cost of fertility care is covered by insurance plans. With most plans, couples generally resort to IVF if they have severe problems that can only be treated with the high-tech procedure or they've failed other treatments. For some couples, however, their insurance coverage provides them with a set amount of money for fertility treatment. To increase their odds of becoming pregnant while staying within the amount of money they've been allotted, couples may seek more aggressive treatment sooner.

Give yourself time to slow down and make decisions with your head in addition to your heart. Weigh the success rate of something like IVF against the costs and the risks. Discuss all of your preferences and goals with your care provider, so you can develop a personalized treatment plan that feels comfortable for you.

Intrauterine insemination (IUI) shortens the sperm's trek through the female reproductive anatomy considerably. With this procedure, the goal is to place the best sperm into the uterus — as close as possible to the egg — at the time of ovulation. From there, it's a short swim into the fallopian tubes to fertilize the egg. IUI also pools all sperm in a single ejaculate and takes them past the obstacle course so that the best sperm end up near the egg and aren't left behind in the vagina or on the bedsheets. This procedure is sometimes referred to as artificial insemination (AI), although AI is really an older method where the sperm were simply placed in the vagina, similar to the old turkey baster method.

Often, fertility drugs are used in conjunction with IUI to ensure a better egg or an extra egg, which can increase your chances of getting pregnant. The combination of fertility drugs and IUI is more effective than either of the treatments alone among couples that have unexplained infertility, or in women with mild endometriosis or who are receiving drug treatment for ovulation problems and still are not pregnant.

Plus, it's a common, effective solution for various male infertility problems where some sperm may be abnormal, but within the entire collection there are enough good sperm that a viable sample can be placed in the uterus. IUI may also be used if a woman has had surgery to

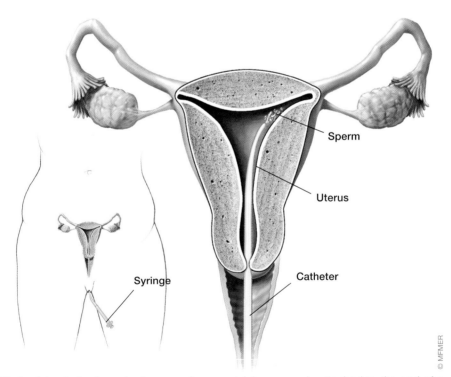

During intrauterine insemination, a syringe containing sperm is attached to the end of a thin, flexible tube (catheter) and the sperm are pushed to the tip of the catheter. The catheter is placed in your vagina and gently guided through your cervix and into your uterus, where the sperm are released.

her cervix and the mucus that the sperm need to swim in isn't optimal.

IUI, with or without the use of fertility drugs, can also help overcome problems getting or maintaining an erection or ejaculating the sperm effectively — such as in retrograde ejaculation, a condition in which semen ejaculates backward into the bladder instead of exiting out the tip of the penis. Rarely, IUI is used with frozen sperm when couples face timing or geographic obstacles, such as working opposite schedules or working in different cities.

IUI is less likely to work for women with moderate to severe endometriosis or significantly reduced ovarian reserve. Other treatments are better in these cases. The procedure isn't an option for women with blocked fallopian tubes.

How it works. Your partner provides a semen sample at the doctor's office or a fertility lab — following the same procedure used when conducting a semen analysis. This time, after the sperm are collected, they're washed with a special fluid for optimal sperm function. This reduces chemicals and bacteria that can cause infections, allergic reactions or other problems when the sperm are placed into the uterus. After washing, the sperm are collected and concentrated. This highly concentrated sample of healthy swimmers increases the likelihood of achieving a successful pregnancy.

It's key to place the concentrated sample into the uterus close to the time of ovulation. If you're using ovulation kits to predict when you're about to release an egg, IUI is typically done the day after the kit indicates a positive result — the day that ovulation is most likely to occur. Your care provider also may use transvaginal ultrasounds to determine when your ovaries are ready for ovulation.

If you're using medications to trigger ovulation, you'll administer them when a transvaginal ultrasound indicates the eggs appear to be ready. Often, an injection of human chorionic gonadotropin (HCG) is used for this purpose. About 36 hours later, you'll have the IUI procedure.

Typically, an intrauterine insemination appointment takes about 20 minutes and is done at your doctor's office. The procedure itself is similar to a Pap test or pelvic exam. You'll be asked to undress from the waist down and put on a gown. Then you'll lie on an exam table, with your legs in stirrups. Your doctor will insert a speculum — a plastic or metal-hinged instrument shaped like a duck's bill — to open your vaginal walls. A syringe containing the concentrated sperm sample is attached to the end of a thin, flexible tube (catheter) and the sample is pushed to the catheter's tip. Next, your doctor gently slides the catheter into your vagina, through your cervix and into your uterus. The sperm are released, the catheter and the speculum are removed, and the procedure is finished.

It's a fairly painless procedure, although it may not be the special conception story that you had in mind for your baby. It's perfectly normal to feel a bit disappointed about this aspect of the procedure. You may have heard your closest girlfriends tell stories about how their babies were conceived — on a romantic getaway or during the best sex of their lives. So you may feel angry or sad that you're stuck with this sterile, clinical approach to pregnancy.

On the other hand, IUI can be very effective. For many couples, the end result is worth the interruption to their private sex lives. Your partner can stay with you through the whole procedure, so you can be together during the moment when the sperm are released.

After the procedure. Immediately after the procedure, you'll be asked to lie on your back for a brief period. Then you may go back to work or go home and resume your normal activities. You may want to plan for some special time together after your appointment. Consider booking a dinner reservation at a favorite restaurant or picking up takeout food and snuggling up for a movie on the couch. This procedure is a momentous occasion, and you should celebrate, if you feel like it. If not, that's OK, too. Do what feels right for you and your partner.

Depending on your circumstances, your care provider may recommend that you begin taking supplemental progesterone to support the changes in the uterus needed to sustain an early pregnancy. Not all women require additional progesterone, however. Inquire if this is a step that would be beneficial for you.

After two weeks, you'll want to take an at-home pregnancy test. You may be tempted to take a pregnancy test earlier due to excitement and anticipation, but it's important to hold off. It will take two weeks for pregnancy hormone levels to reach a measurable level. Testing before the hormone levels are high enough may result in a negative reading when you're actually pregnant. (If you're using ovulation-inducing medications, such as HCG, testing too soon can produce a positive result when you're actually not pregnant. This is caused by the injected HCG that's still in your body.)

In some cases, your care provider may ask you to return to the office for a blood pregnancy test, which can confirm pregnancy earlier than a home test. If you don't become pregnant during your first IUI procedure, you can try again the following month.

Risks. For most women, the whole experience is no more uncomfortable or painful than a Pap test. Some women experi-

Q. ONCE A FERTILITY PATIENT, ALWAYS A FERTILITY PATIENT?

A. Not necessarily. Surprise pregnancies do happen. It's difficult to estimate how many couples have babies on their own after infertility treatment. However, it's not uncommon.

In one large study of fertility centers in France, researchers tracked down more than 2,000 couples that began IVF treatment seven to nine years earlier to find out how many had additional children on their own. They learned that 17 percent of those who had a baby through IVF had another baby without any help. In addition, 24 percent of couples that weren't successful with IVF treatment had a baby on their own. (Some couples in this group likely discontinued IVF treatment because they became pregnant on their own during treatment.)

It's unclear exactly why this happens. But it seems that some couples would eventually get pregnant without assistance, given enough time. Fertility treatments just accelerate the inevitable — possibly by years, not just months. In the French study, for example, the couples that had babies on their own did so over a seven- to nine-year period. For most couples, that's a long time to wait!

ence mild cramping of the uterus, similar to menstrual cramps, as a result of having the catheter inserted. In rare cases, infections occur after this procedure.

Surgical procedures for women
Historically, the first stop for many women undergoing an infertility evaluation was diagnostic surgery to determine if there were any visible impediments to pregnancy that could be fixed in the operating room. With improvements in imaging techniques, including ultrasound imaging and the development of newer and better fertility treatments, this is no longer true for most women. However, in certain situations, surgery is the best fix for treating infertility problems.

Surgery is often used to diagnose and sometimes repair blocked or damaged fallopian tubes. Surgery can also treat endometriosis in women with substantial pelvic pain or can remove a large ovarian cyst or uterine polyp. More often these days, surgery is used to further evaluate a problem or to increase the chances of successful in vitro fertilization (IVF).

If the thought of surgery scares you, remember that successful surgery has a big benefit: It may increase your odds of successful treatment. You also may be able to get pregnant on your own after surgery, rather than relying on your doctor for assistance month after month.

Today, most surgeries for infertility are laparoscopic or hysteroscopic surgeries. In laparoscopic surgery, the surgeon makes a small incision in the abdomen and then uses a tiny tube fitted with a camera (laparoscope) to conduct the surgery. With hysteroscopic surgery, there are no incisions; a similar tube and camera setup is placed inside the uterus by way of the cervix and vagina. Most laparoscopic and hysteroscopic surgeries are done as outpatient procedures, meaning you can go home the same day the procedure is done and be back to your normal routine soon afterward.

Obstruction of the fallopian tubes. If your fallopian tubes are blocked, opening the tubes sometimes improves your chances of becoming pregnant. Surgery may remove adhesions in or around the tubes, open (dilate) the tubes, or repair the tubes in other ways.

Sometimes a tube may be too damaged to repair. In that case, it's often better to remove it entirely. That may seem counterintuitive, but most studies show that pregnancy rates aren't that different for women with one healthy fallopian tube versus two. And having a damaged fallopian tube puts you at increased risk of developing an ectopic pregnancy, where the fertilized egg implants in the tube instead of within the uterus.

One type of a blocked and swollen fallopian tube, called a hydrosalpinx (see page 141), is also associated with a decreased chance of successful pregnancy. In this condition, a fallopian tube is blocked at the far end near the ovary, and the tube is typically filled with fluid. The fluid can leak back into the uterus and is potentially toxic to a developing pregnancy. Studies of women who undergo IVF show that the chance of success is reduced by almost half when there is a hydrosalpinx present. Surgery is performed to unblock or remove the damaged tube.

Tubal ligation reversal. Tubal ligation reversal is a procedure to restore fertility after a woman has had her tubes tied — when the fallopian tubes are cut or blocked to permanently prevent pregnancy.

During a tubal ligation reversal, the blocked segments of the fallopian tubes are reconnected to the remainder of the fallopian tubes, allowing eggs to move through the tubes and sperm to travel through the fallopian tubes to join an egg.

Tubal ligation reversal isn't appropriate for everyone. Your fertility specialist will consider a number of factors — including your age and weight, your ovarian reserve, the extent of damage to your fallopian tubes, and the type of tubal ligation you had — to determine if the procedure is likely to be successful. Your partner should also be tested and have a normal sperm count.

Sterilization procedures that cause the least amount of damage to the fallopian tubes, such as those that use clips or rings, are the most likely to result in successful tubal ligation reversal. Because of the way some procedures seal off the fallopian tubes with electricity, it may not be possible to reopen the tubes.

When tubal ligation reversal isn't an option or is unlikely to be successful, in vitro fertilization may be considered. Even if tubal ligation reversal is successful, it doesn't guarantee that you can become pregnant. Pregnancy rates following reversal of tubal ligation vary greatly, from 30 to 85 percent, depending on a woman's age and other factors.

Endometriosis. In this disorder, tissue that looks like the tissue lining the inside of your uterus (endometrium) grows outside of your uterus. The displaced tissue may be found on the ovaries or fallopian tubes, and it may coat the surfaces of structures throughout the pelvis. Rarely, it spreads outside the pelvic region.

Since the tissue isn't inside your uterus, it isn't shed during your regular menstrual cycle, so it has no way to exit your body. It becomes trapped and can result in ovarian cysts or scar tissue within the pelvis. This can interfere with your ability to have a baby. Some women also experi-

ence painful periods and discomfort during sex, urination or bowel movements.

Surgery may be performed to remove big collections of endometrial tissue or to remove patches of the tissue, while at the same time preserving your uterus and ovaries. However, nonsurgical approaches are increasingly being used to deal with endometriosis symptoms. Some women require fertility medications and intrauterine insemination to become pregnant after surgery for endometriosis, but removal of the displaced tissue helps pave the way for pregnancy.

If necessary, the surgeon also may remove scar tissue and restore normal pelvic anatomy, to improve the chances of conception.

Other conditions. Surgery is occasionally done to remove uterine fibroids, polyps or scarring, which can affect fertility (see Chapter 11).

Surgical procedures for men In men, surgery may help correct structural problems interfering with fertility. Surgery may be used for the following conditions.

Varicocele. A varicocele is an enlargement of the veins within the scrotum — the loose bag of skin that holds the testicles. It's similar to a varicose vein that can occur in your leg. A varicocele can prevent normal cooling of the testicle, which leads to reduced sperm count and fewer moving sperm. This condition can also cause the testicles to shrink.

Surgery can fix the damaged vein. However, it's unclear if surgery can restore fertility. Some studies show that repair of a varicocele can successfully treat infertility, but other studies show no clear benefit. Surgery may be worth a try for large varicoceles that appear problematic or if the varicocele causes testicular pain.

During surgery, the surgeon seals off the affected vein to redirect blood flow into normal veins. Most men are able to return to normal, nonstrenuous activities after two days. Pain is usually mild.

New, nonsurgical procedures to treat the condition block off the blood supply to the damaged vein using X-ray guided beads (embolization).

Obstruction of the epididymis or ejaculatory tract. Men can develop a blockage in the part of the testicle that stores sperm (epididymis) or a blockage within the ejaculatory tract. In both cases, the blockage interferes with the sperm traveling out of the body and decreases the number of healthy sperm that make their way into the vagina.

An obstruction is typically detected during a transrectal ultrasound — an ultrasound test in which a small, lubricated wand about the size and shape of a large cigar is inserted into the rectum to check for problems. Once an obstruction is detected, it can be treated with surgery. However, the chances that clearing the blockage will restore fertility depend on the reason for the blockage. In some cases, surgery can substantially improve sperm count and quality and result in a healthy pregnancy.

Vasectomy reversal. Vasectomy reversal is a surgical procedure to undo a vasectomy. It reconnects the tubes that carry sperm from the testicles into the semen. With successful surgery, sperm are again present in your semen and you may be able to get your partner pregnant.

Vasectomy reversal is more difficult than a vasectomy. The procedure may be performed even if several years have passed since the original vasectomy — but the longer it's been, the less likely it is that the reversal will work.

Reported pregnancy rates after vasectomy reversal range from 40 to 90 percent. Many factors affect whether a reversal is successful, including the type of vasectomy you had and the experience of the doctor doing the reversal surgery. Results are generally best when performed by a surgeon who has done the procedure many times.

When considering vasectomy reversal, keep in mind that the surgery may be expensive, and your health insurance might not cover it. So it's important to find out about costs ahead of time. Your doctor also will want to confirm that your partner is capable of having children, especially if she's never had a child or is older than age 35.

After surgery, your doctor will periodically examine your semen under a microscope to check for sperm. Unless you get your partner pregnant, this is the only way to tell if the surgery was a success. Sperm usually appear in the semen after a few months, but it can sometimes take a year or more.

LOOKING AHEAD

Many of the treatments in this chapter may take a couple of months to work, and you may need to try several options.

If a treatment isn't working, you'll reach a point where you may want to move on to another option. Keep in mind that throughout the process you're gathering information to help you determine your next step. Therefore, it's important not to be too hasty. Give each treatment enough time before ruling it out.

It's not easy to be patient with the fertility process. Try to remind yourself that practicing patience is good preparation for parenthood!

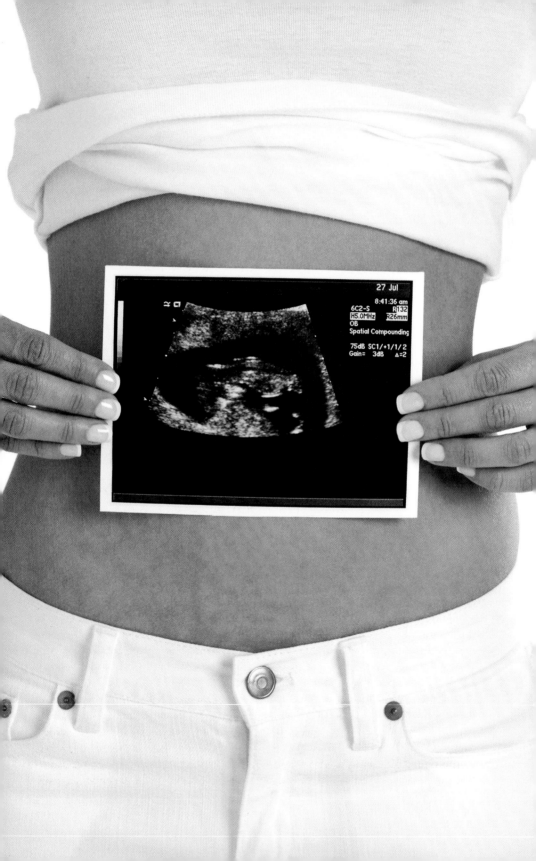

CHAPTER 15

Reproductive assistance

Now it's time to talk about in vitro fertilization (IVF) and other assisted reproductive technologies. With more than 35 years of experience, high-tech paths to parenthood such as IVF have gone from being viewed as producing "test-tube babies" to being recognized as accepted paths to help couples and individuals overcome fertility problems. Assisted reproductive technologies can make it possible to have a baby when other treatments aren't feasible or practical.

These procedures once were — and in a few cases, still are — considered controversial because conception typically occurs outside a woman's body. During IVF, the most common assisted reproduction procedure, mature eggs are collected (retrieved) from a woman's ovaries and fertilized by sperm in a highly specialized laboratory. One or more of the fertilized eggs (embryos) are then placed into a woman's uterus where they implant and grow.

Over the past several decades, the success rates and popularity of these high-tech procedures have soared worldwide, making pregnancy a possibility for many couples who struggled to have a baby on their own. Today, approximately 5 million babies have been born around the world as a result of assisted reproductive technologies. And as the procedures become more commonplace, more couples are opening up about their experiences.

WHAT IS ASSISTED REPRODUCTIVE TECHNOLOGY?

The term *assisted reproductive technology* (ART) is used to describe fertility treatments in which eggs are removed from a woman's ovaries, combined with sperm in a laboratory, and returned to the woman's body or donated to another woman. In addition to being the most common form of assisted reproductive technology, in vitro fertilization is the most effective. But there are other ART techniques, including gamete intrafallopian transfer

(GIFT) and zygote intrafallopian transfer (ZIFT).

All ART procedures can be done with your eggs and your partner's sperm — or with donor eggs, donor sperm or both, which is covered in the next chapter. Your chances of having a healthy baby with IVF or other forms of reproductive assistance depend on many factors, including your age and the cause of your fertility problems.

Getting pregnant with reproductive technology isn't exactly a walk in the park. Treatments can be time-consuming, expensive, invasive and exhausting. And it's common to transfer more than one embryo to your uterus, which can result in twins or, rarely, triplets.

The decision to try IVF or other technologies is a big one that requires careful thought and discussion. For many couples, though, this is the best chance of having a baby when other options have failed. With good planning, assisted reproductive technologies may help you have a healthy pregnancy, one baby at a time, until your family is complete.

The first test-tube babies The notion of making babies in laboratories might sound like a plot straight out of a modern-day science fiction thriller. But the idea of fertilizing an egg outside the body is nothing new.

Dating back to 1878, scientists in various parts of the world were conducting experiments involving rabbits, mice and hamsters that were centered on this very goal. In the United States, IVF research began on animals as early as the 1930s. Despite some reports of success, it's unlikely that very many eggs were actually fertilized in early experiments.

However, things heated up after a breakthrough in 1951. During this time, scientists discovered sperm "capacitation." They learned that sperm only become activated and develop the capacity to fertilize an egg when they reside for some time within the female reproductive tract. Scientists hypothesized that they needed to re-create this final step in the sperm-maturation process in order to fertilize an egg outside the body.

Bingo! In the 1950s and 1960s, the first convincing successes of IVF were reported in rabbits, mice, hamsters, rats and humans, as scientists found ways to "capacitate" the sperm. However, as news spread about these scientific advances, a great deal of controversy ensued. Scientists, religious leaders and politicians tangled over the idea of a "test-tube baby," conceived in a petri dish.

Amid the moral debate, a group of determined scientists forged on. British scientist Robert Edwards was one of them. By the 1970s, he and his colleagues were implanting fertilized embryos into

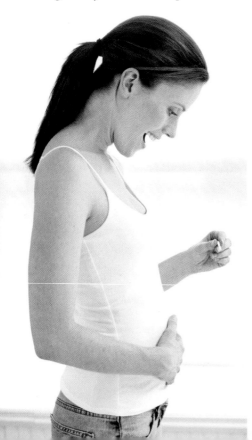

women's uteruses. For several years, they were unsuccessful. But, in 1978, Edwards' key collaborator gynecologist Patrick Steptoe delivered the world's first test-tube baby when little Louise Brown was born in England.

The first in vitro fertilization clinic in the United States opened in Norfolk, Virginia, in the early 1980s. Public opposition was considerable. People were worried about the unnaturalness of the procedure, the possibility that it would produce abnormal children and the fact that it was causing abortions because some fertilized embryos weren't expected to develop. For years, there were unfavorable editorials and letters to the editor in the local papers, as well as protests and picket lines. Yet, there were also many women clamoring for the clinic's services.

And so it was that the United States became the third country to produce an IVF baby, following England and Australia. When Elizabeth Carr was born in December 1981 at the Norfolk clinic, her birth made headlines. Eleven months later, the chubby-cheeked, diaper-clad Elizabeth appeared on the cover of Life magazine, pictured in the lab where she was conceived. The headline declared: "Test-tube baby boom."

IVF today With time and experience, the notion of a test-tube baby doesn't seem nearly so frightening to most people. There are still some people who object to in vitro fertilization for moral or religious reasons, but the conduct of this procedure is well regulated by many laws and governing organizations today. By and large, the field of reproductive medicine is now well established and accepted. In fact, British scientist Robert Edwards was honored with a Nobel Prize in 2010 for his pioneering role in the development of in vitro fertilization, before dying three years later at the age of 87.

The process of IVF is also a lot different today than its original form. In the earliest days of IVF, medications to produce multiple eggs weren't available, and doctors had to try to retrieve the lone egg developing in a particular menstrual cycle. Even if the egg was successfully recovered, it still needed to fertilize, divide, be implanted into the uterus, and continue to grow and develop. It could take dozens — or even hundreds — of attempts before a successful pregnancy was achieved.

Ways to monitor egg development were also much less sophisticated. Women were instructed to collect their urine every few hours to determine when they started the process of ovulation, and because the timing of ovulation can vary, many egg retrievals occurred in the middle of the night.

Fortunately, times have changed. Medications now allow multiple eggs to develop at once, and egg growth is carefully monitored through blood tests and ultrasounds. Medications to get the eggs to undergo their final steps to become mature are also commonly administered in a way that permits most egg retrievals to occur during daylight hours.

The role of IVF also has changed. Originally, it was viewed as a means to bypass blocked fallopian tubes that couldn't be surgically corrected. It then became a way for couples with low sperm numbers to achieve pregnancy. Putting sperm and eggs together in a small dish in a laboratory was more successful than having the sperm travel through a woman's entire reproductive tract on the chance of finding an egg. Today, with a three-decade track record of proven success, IVF is increasingly being made available to women with other causes of infertility.

In many cases, IVF is still a last resort, tried only when other treatments have failed. But it can be a primary treatment in some situations, such as when the fallopian tubes are completely blocked or there are severe problems with the sperm. Couples may also choose to opt for IVF right away because of age, budget or insurance considerations.

Your chances of giving birth to a healthy baby after using IVF generally depend on these factors:

Maternal age. Today, it's clear that the biggest factor in the success of IVF is the age of the woman producing the eggs that are being fertilized. The younger you are, the more likely you are to get pregnant and give birth to a healthy baby using your own eggs during IVF.

Among women who are younger than age 35, more than 40 percent of IVF attempts end in pregnancy and birth. Success declines significantly with each passing year. In women ages 35 to 37, the success rate drops to a little more than 30 percent. In women age 43 and older, less than 5 percent of IVF cycles have happy endings. It's possible for older women to prevail over these hard numbers by using donor eggs.

IVF success rates also appear to vary by ethnicity. IVF in black, Asian and Hispanic women in the U.S. is associated with lower live birth rates than in white women. The reasons aren't clear.

Infertility cause. If your only barrier to infertility is a physical one, such as a damaged fallopian tube or previous surgery to tie your tubes, you're likely to have success with IVF. The procedure has a higher success rate for women who have a healthy uterus and who respond well to fertility medications or who ovulate naturally. IVF can also help couples overcome male fertility problems, such as a low sperm count.

For women with untreated uterine abnormalities, such as uterine fibroids, uterine polyps, an abnormally shaped uterus or uterine adenomyosis — a condition in which the uterine lining grows into the muscular walls of the uterus — IVF success rates are lower. However, it's not always certain if the abnormality or a woman's age is the reason for the reduced success.

Lifestyle factors. Several lifestyle factors can impede your chances of success with IVF. The first is being overweight or underweight. You're considered significantly overweight (obese) if your body mass index (BMI) is greater than 30. If your BMI is less than 18.5, you're underweight (see the chart on page 17). Either extreme can make it difficult for you to get pregnant and have a baby with IVF.

Smoking is another factor that can lower your chances of success with IVF. Use of alcohol, recreational drugs, excessive caffeine and certain medications also can work against you. Doctors and scientists are researching other factors that may affect IVF success rates. For instance stress may reduce your chances of a successful outcome, while use of acupuncture may slightly increase it.

As experience accumulates and doctors learn more about the complex process of human reproduction, IVF success rates continue to climb. Today, women who undergo IVF have a higher chance of getting pregnant than healthy women who try to get pregnant the "old-fashioned" way. Granted, women who undergo IVF have an unfair advantage because the procedure typically involves the transfer of multiple embryos rather than the fertilization of a single egg. But this is a remarkable accomplishment, given the humble, controversial beginnings of this procedure.

HOW IVF WORKS

Undergoing in vitro fertilization is a process, not a singular event. During IVF, mature eggs are collected (retrieved) from your ovaries, and sperm is collected from your partner. The collected sperm and eggs then are combined in a laboratory for fertilization. A few days later, the fertilized eggs (now called embryos) are implanted in your uterus. The entire process — which takes about two to three weeks — is called an IVF cycle.

However, it will take several appointments before you're ready to begin the process. As part of your preparation for IVF, you may undergo specialized tests if they weren't part of your infertility evaluation. For example, your doctor may examine your uterine cavity and measure your uterus. This might involve sonohysterography — a special kind of ultrasound exam that includes the injection of fluid through the cervix into the uterus, which helps your care provider determine the size, shape and direction of the uterus. Or it might include a procedure called hysteroscopy in which your doctor inserts a slender device with a small camera into your vagina and through the cervix to view the inside of your uterus. The information gathered during these tests can be helpful later on when embryos are placed into the uterus.

If you haven't already done so, you may also have ovarian reserve testing to determine the quantity and quality of your eggs, as well as an ultrasound of your ovaries. These tests can help predict how well your ovaries will respond to fertility medications.

In addition, you and your partner will likely have blood tests to check for infectious diseases such as HIV and hepatitis B and C. These tests may be required to determine if special handling and storage conditions are required for your eggs, sperm or embryos.

After this testing is done, you'll discuss the results with your care provider and talk about your personalized IVF treatment plan. You can also expect a pile of paperwork, including consent forms for procedures that you will have and documents related to embryo storage.

Then the actual IVF process begins. It involves five basic steps — superovulation, egg retrieval, sperm collection, fertilization and embryo transfer.

Superovulation IVF is a numbers game. Given the high cost and the time commitment of IVF, most couples want to maximize their chances of success. One of the best ways to increase your odds is to induce your ovaries to make multiple eggs — rather than relying on the one lone egg that your ovaries normally release each month.

Increasing egg production is done using many of the same fertility medications discussed in Chapter 14. However, in IVF, the goal is to ripen several eggs at once — perhaps even 10 to 20 — rather than two or three. Hence the name superovulation.

Many couples don't think this sounds so super at first. Twenty eggs is a staggering amount of eggs. It's important to understand, however, that some eggs don't make it to the next hurdle during every step of the IVF process. So you need to start with extras to beat the numbers game.

Here's the math: At the time of egg retrieval, it's unlikely that all of the eggs harvested will be at the right stage to attempt fertilization. The goal is to have the majority of eggs mature at the time of retrieval, but it's typical that some may still be immature and others may be overly mature (atretic). In most cases, fertilization is only attempted on eggs that are at the right stage of development.

Typically about 70 to 80 percent of the retrieved eggs will be at the right stage to attempt fertilization, and of these mature eggs, about 70 percent will successfully fertilize. Beyond that, some of the fertilized eggs won't continue to develop normally and won't be suitable for transfer into the uterus. It's also unlikely that all of the embryos that are transferred into a woman's uterus will properly implant themselves and become healthy babies. That's why it's not uncommon to have more than one embryo transferred into a woman's uterus in the hopes of creating one healthy pregnancy.

In addition to increasing the quantity of eggs produced, medications can also help your doctor control when ovulation occurs. Superovulation usually relies on a combination of different medications. These may include:

Medications for ovarian stimulation. Hormones called gonadotropins are typically used to stimulate the ovaries to develop multiple eggs at once. The hormones, administered by way of a shot (injection), contain synthetic versions of follicle-stimulating hormone (FSH) or a combination of FSH and luteinizing hormone (LH). Examples of synthetic FSH include Gonal-f, Follistim and Bravelle. Combination medications include drugs such as Menopur and Repronex. The medications stimulate more than one egg to develop at a time and are described in more detail on page 186.

While undergoing hormone shots, you'll likely have regular blood tests and transvaginal ultrasounds to measure your response to ovarian stimulation and to track the growth of the small sacs (follicles) in which the eggs develop. This helps your doctor decide when the eggs are ready for retrieval. Typically, most women need eight to 14 days of ovarian-stimulating medications until their eggs are mature enough to proceed to the next step.

Medications to prevent premature ovulation. The reproductive process starts in the brain where your hypothalamus gland releases a hormone called gonadotropin-releasing hormone (Gn-RH), which prompts your pituitary gland to release two more hormones — FSH and LH. FSH primarily controls egg development and LH the release of mature eggs from the ovaries.

However, when you're recruiting more than one egg the last thing you want to have happen is for LH to kick in when the first egg is ready. Shutting off LH alone is difficult, so medications that affect the production of Gn-RH, called Gn-RH agonists or Gn-RH antagonists, are used for this purpose. Depending on the protocol your doctor uses to stimulate egg development and how your ovarian reserve looks, you may start these hormone-suppressing shots at the beginning of your menstrual cycle, several days into the cycle or even during your previous menstrual cycle. You'll probably be instructed to administer the shots once a day for a few days to up to several weeks, until you're ready to take a shot of human chorionic gonadotropin (HCG) to trigger ovulation.

Medications for oocyte maturation and release. When your doctor can see that the follicles have reached the right size and are likely to contain mature

A MORE GENTLE APPROACH

Some couples wonder if it's possible to try IVF without using strong ovarian-stimulating medications that create so many eggs. The answer is yes. However, not using any ovary-stimulating medications with IVF can cut your likelihood of success by more than half if you're young. And if you're older, such an approach may not be very effective.

It's very rare for IVF to be performed without any fertility drugs because the odds of success with one natural egg are simply too low to justify the cost and invasiveness of the procedure. Some clinics do offer IVF with "gentle" ovulation stimulation, using clomiphene (Clomid, Serophene) instead of more powerful gonadotropins.

This less potent medication might produce two or three eggs instead of 10 or more. As a result, IVF with clomiphene can be a good option for couples that have strong ethical or religious beliefs against creating too many embryos. Another option is to use the normal dose of medication and create a large group of eggs, but only fertilize a few of them. The remaining unfertilized eggs can be frozen and stored for future use, if needed.

A less-potent approach may also be reasonable for older women who have a low chance of making a lot of eggs no matter what medications they use. This may sound counterintuitive, but the logic makes good sense: Why spend thousands of dollars on expensive gonadotropin medications if they're not likely to work any better than $20 worth of clomiphene? Many fertility clinics, however, don't offer this option because of the low success rates.

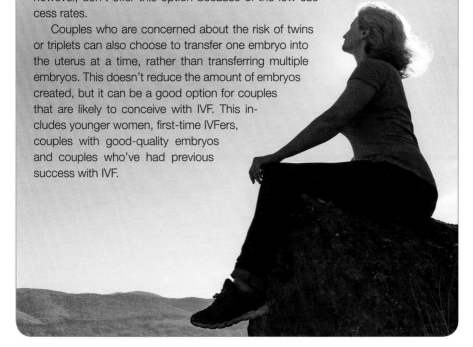

Couples who are concerned about the risk of twins or triplets can also choose to transfer one embryo into the uterus at a time, rather than transferring multiple embryos. This doesn't reduce the amount of embryos created, but it can be a good option for couples that are likely to conceive with IVF. This includes younger women, first-time IVFers, couples with good-quality embryos and couples who've had previous success with IVF.

eggs, you'll be instructed to inject a hormone shot that matures the eggs similar to how LH does naturally. Often the hormone HCG is used, but Gn-RH agonists are another option. These medications are often called ovulation triggers. They start the countdown clock for release of the eggs from the ovary. Don't worry, though. Your doctor will remove the eggs from the ovaries before they're released on their own.

All of this may sound confusing and complicated. But you'll know what to do when you get to this point in the process. Your health care team will provide you plenty of instruction and a personalized calendar that shows all of your medications and when to use them. You'll receive information about how to administer each medication, and you'll have plenty of opportunities to ask questions along the way.

Sadly, 10 to 20 percent of IVF cycles are stopped (canceled) before egg retrieval. The most common reason for cancellation is that not enough eggs are developing. On the flip side, the process can also be stopped if you have too many egg follicles developing, which can lead to ovarian hyperstimulation syndrome. In this condition, the ovaries become swollen and painful and can leak fluid into the belly. In some cases, women taking fertility drugs can develop a severe form of the syndrome, which causes rapid weight gain, abdominal pain, vomiting and shortness of breath if fluid also leaks into the lungs. This can require hospitalization and surgery. Ovarian hyperstimulation syndrome is temporary and usually gets better on its own, but it can cause serious health problems when it occurs. Therefore, it's important to prevent the condition.

A canceled IVF cycle is often a heartbreaking disappointment, but it can provide your doctor with information to make the next attempt more effective. If your cycle is canceled, your doctor may recommend changing medications or altering their doses to promote better responses. In some cases, you may be advised to consider an egg donor instead of trying again with your own eggs.

Egg retrieval Once the eggs are mature and the ovaries are close to being ready to release them, it's time for egg retrieval. This process usually happens about 36 hours after the HCG injection. It must be timed very carefully so you don't miss the opportunity to retrieve the eggs. The procedure is often scheduled early in the morning to avoid operating room delays and to give laboratory staff the rest of the day to separate out and fertilize the healthy, mature eggs.

In the early days of IVF, laparoscopic surgery was used to retrieve the eggs, but this type of surgery is rarely used today. Most clinics now use transvaginal ultrasound aspiration. The procedure is simpler, less invasive and less expensive than laparoscopic surgery and is generally done as an outpatient procedure.

When you arrive at the location where the procedure will take place, you'll be asked to undress and put on a hospital gown. Then you'll lie on your back on a table in a procedure room. You'll be given a combination of sedation medications through an IV that will make you feel sleepy and relaxed, as well as a pain medication. The procedure generally isn't painful, but it may cause some cramping or discomfort.

To begin a transvaginal ultrasound aspiration, an ultrasound probe is inserted into your vagina to locate the ovaries. Using the ultrasound as a guide, your doctor then passes a thin needle through your vaginal wall and into the adjacent

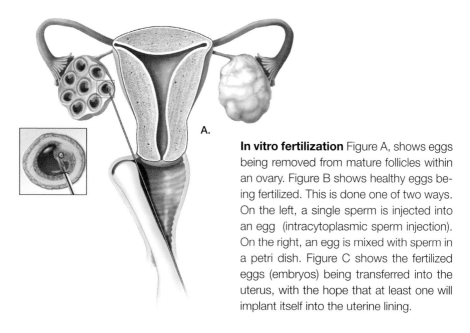

In vitro fertilization Figure A, shows eggs being removed from mature follicles within an ovary. Figure B shows healthy eggs being fertilized. This is done one of two ways. On the left, a single sperm is injected into an egg (intracytoplasmic sperm injection). On the right, an egg is mixed with sperm in a petri dish. Figure C shows the fertilized eggs (embryos) being transferred into the uterus, with the hope that at least one will implant itself into the uterine lining.

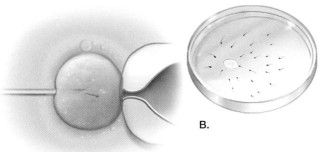

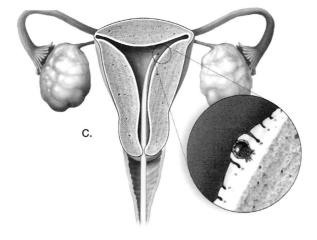

ovary to retrieve the eggs from the follicles. The follicular fluid that contains the eggs is removed through the needle, which is connected to a suction device (aspiration). The same procedure is then performed on the other ovary. The whole process takes about 15 to 30 minutes.

The follicular fluid containing the eggs is taken immediately to a nearby laboratory. Here, it's placed in a sterile dish so that the eggs can be located using a microscope. The eggs are then placed in a nutrient-rich solution (culture medium) and stored in an incubator for a few hours at a temperature that's close to the natural temperature of the fallopian tubes. Eggs that appear healthy and mature will eventually be mixed with sperm to create embryos. However, not all eggs are successfully fertilized.

Shortly after the egg retrieval and prior to the time of embryo transfer, you may begin taking progesterone to cause the lining of your uterus (endometrium) to thicken and be more receptive to egg implantation. Your body naturally secretes progesterone after ovulation in preparation for pregnancy, and this hormone is an important part of early pregnancy development.

Progesterone may be administered in several ways, including injectable shots, a vaginal gel you insert with a plastic applicator, similar to a tampon, or a vaginal suppository. You may need to take progesterone from shortly after egg retrieval until about seven weeks of pregnancy.

Sperm collection or retrieval At this point in your fertility journey your partner becomes actively involved. During your initial evaluation, your partner will have undergone an evaluation to assure that he's producing sufficient numbers and quality of sperm (semen analysis). A male evaluation provides additional information that can improve ART outcomes and assist the fertility laboratory in tailoring the type of fertilization to be performed.

If the sperm are within normal ranges, a fresh sperm sample is collected on the morning of your egg retrieval. In cases where sperm numbers are low, or your partner isn't available the day of the retrieval, frozen sperm may be used as a backup.

If a semen analysis finds no sperm in the semen, there are still some options available. It's possible to retrieve sperm directly from a testicle or epididymis to be used in the fertilization process. The following techniques may be performed in a doctor's office or an operating room:

Microsurgical epididymal sperm aspiration (MESA). This technique involves retrieving sperm directly from the epididymal tubules in the operating room under sedation. A powerful microscope is used to identify specific tubules likely to contain sperm, after which sperm-rich fluid is taken from these regions with a needle and syringe. If no sperm are seen, the surgeon may be able to perform a testicular sperm extraction (TESE) at the same time without need for a separate procedure.

Percutaneous epididymal sperm aspiration (PESA). PESA is similar to MESA except that it's performed in a doctor's office without an operating microscope or sedation. The skin and a testicle are numbed with a temporary local anesthetic. A needle is then inserted into the epididymis and fluid retrieved.

Testicular sperm extraction (TESE), including microsurgical. In this technique, a doctor makes an incision in the testes with or without an operating microscope to extract the sperm. TESE is often used if sperm cannot be identified in the epididymides or in cases where a testicular biopsy is needed for diagnostic purposes at the time of sperm retrieval.

Testicular sperm aspiration (TESA). With this method the skin is numbed with a local anesthetic, a needle is inserted into the testicle, and sperm is aspirated into a syringe. Similar to PESA, this minimally invasive technique doesn't require an incision. However, less sperm and tissue are obtained compared with other procedures.

No matter how the sperm are collected, fresh or frozen sperm can't fertilize an egg until the sperm has undergone capacitation, discussed at the beginning of this chapter. The sperm must be incubated in a special culture medium for a few hours — right after ejaculation, upon retrieval or upon thawing.

Fertilization Here's where the magic happens. During fertilization, incubated eggs may be fertilized one of two ways (see figure B on page 205). They may be mixed together with the sperm in a process called standard insemination, or each egg may be injected with a single sperm, in what's called intracytoplasmic sperm injection (ICSI).

ICSI. In the earliest days of IVF, fertilization was performed the same way for everyone who had the procedure — sperm and eggs were mixed in a petri dish. However, this process requires several hundred thousand sperm for success. For couples with low sperm numbers, this meant their

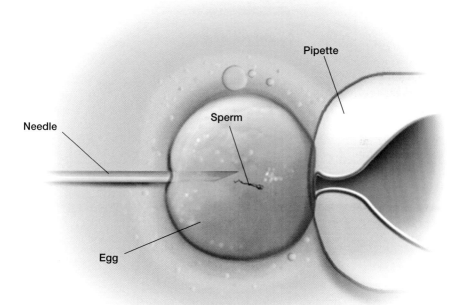

During intracytoplasmic sperm injection (ICSI), a mature egg is held with a specialized tool called a pipette. A very delicate and sharp needle picks up a single sperm. The needle is inserted through the shell of the egg, and the sperm is injected into the egg's cytoplasm. The needle is then removed. The egg is checked for signs of normal fertilization before it's placed in a woman's uterus.

Q. HOW ARE EMBRYOS SELECTED?

A. Choosing the best embryos to transfer to the uterus involves both art and science. Embryos are graded on several parameters to determine which ones appear to be the healthiest and thus the most likely to create a successful pregnancy. Grading early-stage (cleavage) embryos is also different from grading those that have reached the blastocyst stage.

Parameters for selecting an embryo to be transferred include how it looks, the number of cells in the embryo, their relative sizes, and whether any irregular pieces leftover from cell divisions (fragments) are present within the embryo. Each embryo is given a score, and the ones with the highest scores are considered for transfer or freezing for possible future use.

For example, the highest score for a cleavage stage embryo would be given to one in which the cells are of equal size and there's no fragmentation. Since blastocysts are older than cleavage stage embryos, they've had longer to divide. As more cells become present with each division, the blastocyst starts to take on a different shape, similar to a beach ball or a globe with a cluster of cells in the middle. The outer portion of the ball (trophectoderm) will eventually become tissue needed for pregnancy such as the placenta. The inner cell cluster — the inner cell mass — will become the fetus. Separate grades are given for the appearance of the trophectoderm, the inner cell mass and the fluid-filled space between them. The highest grade would be given to a blastocyst with a well-formed trophectoderm and inner cell mass, as well as a nicely expanded space between them.

Keep in mind, though, that embryo-grading systems are largely subjective. Although experience with grading thousands of embryos allows embryologists to make educated guesses about an embryo's pregnancy potential, there are many cases of embryos with poor grades resulting in successful births and perfect embryos failing to produce a pregnancy. The appearance of the embryo also doesn't tell the whole story about its genetics.

In order to improve identification of embryos with the highest potential for pregnancy, newer techniques sampling the culture medium the embryos are grown in or using incubators with time-lapse imaging to more precisely study cell division are being used in some centers.

---

only option was to use donor sperm. Plus, even with good sperm numbers, some couples have low fertilization rates or no fertilization when the eggs and sperm are left alone with the lights out.

Intracytoplasmic sperm injection (ICSI), is an alternative method of fertilization. Rather than mixing sperm and eggs together in a dish, in this procedure a single sperm is injected directly into each mature egg. ICSI is a very common addition to in vitro fertilization in the United States and is now used in more than 60 percent of all IVF cycles.

ICSI is most often used when sperm quality or quantity is a problem. This includes men with low sperm counts. It may also be used if examination of sperm under a microscope shows even a slight abnormality or if the eggs fail to fertilize normally with standard insemination. ICSI also is a common form of fertilization in cases where sperm harvesting techniques had to be used to obtain sperm, or in men who banked their sperm before cancer treatment.

In many of these situations, ICSI can increase the likelihood of pregnancy. Some fertility clinics use ICSI for all couples, but that means performing the procedure more often than may be absolutely necessary.

Once the eggs are fertilized — by way of either standard insemination or ICSI — they're called embryos.

Embryo transfer The next step in the IVF process is called embryo transfer. Two to six days after egg retrieval, the embryos are graded according to their health, and the best embryos are readied for transfer into your uterus.

As with other fertility procedures, you'll be asked to undress from the waist down and put on a gown. The transfer is performed in a procedure room, but is much more like having a Pap test or other simple office procedure. You'll lie on a procedure table with your feet placed in footrests. Many women are given a mild sedative to help them relax. You'll still be awake and may be able to watch the procedure on the ultrasound with your partner.

Your doctor will use a speculum to view the cervix. He or she will pass a swab through the speculum to clean your cervix and then place a catheter containing the embryos into your vagina, through your cervix and into your uterus. Within the catheter, the embryos are suspended in a small amount of nutrient-rich fluid. The catheter, in turn, is attached to a syringe.

The last step is to gently inject the fluid containing the embryos into your uterus. Many physicians perform the transfer using ultrasound guidance. Although the embryos are too small to see on the ultrasound screen, you may be able to detect the path they travel as the fluid and embryos are injected into the uterus. The entire procedure takes about five to 10 minutes. If successful, an embryo will implant in the lining of your uterus a few days after the transfer.

Timing. Embryos can be cultured for several days before transfer. The time between egg retrieval and embryo transfer depends on the quantity and quality of your embryos and the cause of your infertility.

Embryo transfer can occur as early as day two — 48 hours after egg retrieval — for couples with a low number of embryos. However, day three is preferred if you have enough embryos. An extra day of growth in the lab can identify and sort the more vigorous embryos from those that stop dividing and aren't viable. This slightly increases the chances of success.

Embryos can also be transferred on day five or six. At this point, embryos typically reach the blastocyst stage of development where the embryo has started to mature so that certain cells are committed to become the embryo and other cells the placenta. At the blastocyst stage, the embryos are ready for implantation into the uterus without further dividing. If your doctor is transferring embryos at this stage, he or she will likely recommend transferring fewer of them because they have a greater chance of success.

Although uncommon, there's a chance a blastocyst embryo can divide into identical (monozygotic) twins. The exact reason why this happens is unknown, but it seems to be related to some of the laboratory conditions associated with longer embryo culture. Identical twins occur 1 to 5 percent of the time following blastocyst transfer. This is one of the reasons why fewer blastocysts are transferred than earlier stage embryos.

Number. Remember, all embryo transfers don't take. Transferring more than one embryo increases the chances at least one embryo will implant into the uterus and a baby will be born nine months later. But transferring multiple embryos also increases the risk of multiple babies, which can lead to complications for mom and the babies.

The exact number of embryos transferred in any given IVF cycle depends on the number of embryos produced, the quality and stage of the embryos, your age, your overall health, and your personal preferences. Typically, one to three embryos are transferred.

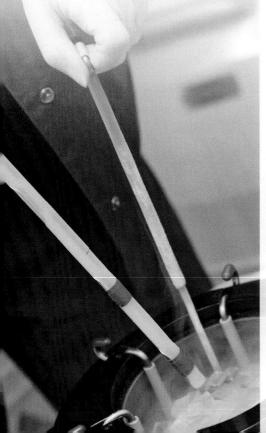

Because successful implantation declines with age, more embryos are often transferred in older women. Clinical guidelines from the American Society for Reproductive Medicine recommend that no more than two embryos be transferred in women younger than age 35, no more than three embryos in women ages 35 to 37, and no more than three to four embryos in women ages 38 to 40. At the highest end of the guidelines, women ages 41 and 42 cap out at no more than five transferred embryos. However, some doctors suggest a max of two transferred embryos, no matter what your age.

There's a fine balance between increasing your odds of pregnancy and rolling the dice on quadruplets. If too many embryos implant, it may be possible to use a procedure called selective fetal reduction to terminate one or more of the pregnancies. But some couples aren't comfortable ending pregnancies after they fight so desperately to create them. Others won't do so for moral or religious reasons.

One of the reasons why the current trend in the U.S. is toward blastocyst transfer is that the more advanced the embryo, the better its chance of implanting. It has already cleared more hurdles, suggesting it has the stamina to continue. So, by transferring blastocyst embryos, you can get good pregnancy rates with fewer embryos.

Talk to your fertility doctor about the number of embryos to transfer long before you get to this point in the process. Discuss the pros and cons of various philosophies with your partner and your doctor. Make sure your doctor is aware of your preferences on this issue so you can make decisions accordingly.

After transfer. Women are sometimes wheeled into a recovery room after the transfer, where they're encouraged to rest for several minutes or up to several hours. Other women are allowed to get up and walk out the door. It's becoming clear that bed rest after IVF isn't necessary in any way, shape or form. In fact, it's possible that bed rest can contribute to increased stress, which isn't good for success.

Try to resume your normal daily activities. Your ovaries may still be enlarged, so it's best to avoid vigorous activities that could cause discomfort. At the same time, there's no need to tiptoe around the house. Try to relax. You'll need to wait nine to 12 days to take a pregnancy test to see if pregnancy occurred.

Many women experience mild bloating, mild cramping, constipation or breast tenderness due to high estrogen and progesterone levels. It's also common to pass a small amount of clear or bloody fluid shortly after the procedure, due to the swabbing of the cervix before the embryo transfer. This is normal — it's not a sign of trouble or of miscarriage.

IVF can take several attempts to work. If you don't become pregnant — or don't stay pregnant — during your first cycle, your doctor will carefully evaluate your progress and refine your treatment plan to increase your chances of a better outcome in the next cycle.

It can be terribly disappointing and distressful if pregnancy doesn't occur. Take heart, and remember that IVF pregnancies are sometimes similar to great inventions. They can take great perseverance, and often result after failure.

Freezing extra embryos Healthy embryos that aren't transferred to your uterus during an IVF cycle can be frozen using a process called cryopreservation. This preserves the embryos for later use. If you don't become pregnant during your first IVF cycle, you can try IVF again with the frozen embryos. If you do become pregnant but want more children at a later date, the frozen embryos can be used months or years later.

The stage the embryo is at when it's frozen can make a difference as to how effective it may be with later use. Best results often occur when the embryo is still a single cell (pronuclear embryo) or when it has reached the blastocyst stage.

Frozen embryos are typically stored in a commercial long-term facility. When you store frozen embryos, you don't have to repeat the ovarian stimulation and egg retrieval process. The embryos can be thawed and transferred into your uterus.

Freezing protocols have improved significantly over the years, so there's no disadvantage to freezing your embryos. In fact, new research indicates that in some cases when IVF is performed with frozen embryos pregnancy rates may be higher than those of IVF cycles using fresh embryos. Researchers believe this is due to the medications used with fresh embryo transfer causing problems with the development of the lining of the uterus, not the state of the embryos themselves.

Ovarian hyperstimulation is generally necessary to produce enough eggs for a successful IVF cycle, but the process creates a higher level of estrogen in the body than normal, which may interfere with implantation. Since IVF with frozen embryos is done without ovarian stimulation, there's a more natural environment in the uterus that may be more receptive to implantation.

Freezing embryos also has another advantage: When embryos are frozen, they're frozen in time. And that's a good thing for future IVF cycles. For example, say you undergo IVF at age 36, become pregnant and freeze the extra embryos. Three years later, when you want a second baby at age 39, you'll be able to try

IVF again, using embryos made with your 36-year-old eggs. You're more likely to have a successful IVF cycle with your 36-year-old eggs than your 39-year-old eggs. Risks for chromosomal problems in the baby, such as Down syndrome, are also those of a 36-year-old mother, even if you're now older.

Risks of IVF Generally, the risks associated with IVF are low, but, as with most medical procedures, there is some risk. Using fertility medications during IVF can create side effects, including hot flashes, moodiness, irritability, breast tenderness, fatigue, and bruising and tenderness at your medication injection sites. These risks are the same if you use fertility medications alone or use them before intrauterine insemination.

There are also risks associated with the later steps in the IVF process, some which also exist in natural pregnancies. However, IVF can increase the risk of certain complications.

Ovarian hyperstimulation syndrome. Fertility drugs used to induce ovulation, such as human chorionic gonadotropin (HCG), can cause ovarian hyperstimulation syndrome. In this condition, your ovaries become swollen and painful. Signs and symptoms typically last a week and include mild abdominal pain, bloating, nausea, vomiting and diarrhea. If you become pregnant, however, your symptoms might last several weeks. Rarely, it's possible to develop a more severe form of the syndrome that can cause rapid weight gain and shortness of breath.

Women with polycystic ovarian syndrome, with high estrogen levels or having a high number of eggs retrieved are at increased risk of the problem. If ovarian hyperstimulation syndrome occurs before embryo transfer, your embryos may be frozen and the transfer delayed until your ovaries return to normal.

Multiple births. If more than one embryo is implanted in your uterus, there's a risk of multiple births. About 30 percent of births after IVF are multiple births. The large majority of these are twins, but about 2 percent of moms who deliver babies after IVF have triplets or greater numbers of multiples.

Pregnancy complications. There's an association between IVF and complications such as placenta previa, placental abruption, preeclampsia and cesarean delivery. In general, women who undergo IVF are older and may have underlying conditions contributing to their infertility and to pregnancy complications. It's not clear if IVF is a direct cause of the complications or if other factors are present.

Premature delivery and low birth weight. Premature delivery and low birth weight are more common in multiple births, but even single babies born after IVF are more likely to be born slightly early or at a lower birth weight than those conceived naturally. Again, the reason for this isn't clear. It may be associated with medications, underlying causes of infertility, stress, intense pregnancy monitoring or other factors.

Miscarriage. The rate of miscarriage for women who conceive using IVF with fresh embryos is similar to that of women who conceive naturally — about 15 to 20 percent — but the rate increases with maternal age. Use of frozen embryos during IVF may slightly increase the risk of miscarriage.

Ectopic pregnancy. Women who undergo IVF have an increased risk of ectopic pregnancy, a condition in which the fertilized egg implants outside the uterus, usually in a fallopian tube. A fertilized egg can't survive outside the uterus, so the pregnancy must be discontinued. This occurs in about 2 percent of pregnancies after IVF.

Birth defects. Since the beginnings of IVF, there have been concerns the procedure would lead to birth defects and genetic abnormalities. Researchers have studied — and continue to study — this carefully. Scientists agree that the age of the mother is the primary risk factor in the development of birth defects, no matter how the child is conceived. There is some evidence the age of the father may play a role as well.

There may be a slight increase in birth defects among couples who have a baby using IVF, but the increase is likely due to risks associated with the parents' age or genetics — not the procedure.

Stress. Undergoing IVF can be financially, physically and emotionally draining. Don't underestimate the impact this type of stress can have on all facets of your health and wellness. And don't be afraid to seek out support from counselors, family and friends to help you and your partner through the ups and downs of infertility treatment. See Chapter 17 for more information.

ADVANCED ART

IVF is the most recognized and most common assisted reproductive technology. In the United States, it's used in 99 percent of assisted reproductive procedures. However, there are other technologies that can be used to have a baby.

Zygote intrafallopian transfer (ZIFT) In ZIFT, fertilization occurs in the laboratory, just like with IVF. However, the embryos are transferred to a fallopian tube instead of the uterus. This procedure is also called tubal embryo transfer and is performed in an operating room.

A normal fallopian tube is considered a better environment for the fledgling embryo to develop, as compared with the uterus. This is where the sperm and egg would naturally unite. However, getting the embryos into the fallopian tube is more complicated, requiring laparoscopic surgery.

Because of improvements in laboratory culture methods that have increased the success of IVF, ZIFT is rarely used. It may be considered in rare cases when it's not possible to place the embryos in the uterus through the cervix.

Gamete intrafallopian transfer (GIFT) Similar to ZIFT, during the GIFT procedure the eggs are transferred into a fallopian tube. This time, though, the eggs aren't fertilized. Unfertilized eggs and sperm are placed together in a fallopian tube. This allows fertilization to occur in a woman's body — not in a laboratory. This is a key difference between the GIFT procedure and IVF and ZIFT procedures.

The GIFT technique was very popular in the late 1980s and early 1990s. However, it's more invasive than IVF and it typically requires more than two eggs to be placed in the tubes, which can backfire in the form of triplets or greater multiples. As laboratory techniques have improved, IVF has almost completely replaced GIFT. But some clinics still offer GIFT to couples with moral or ethical concerns about fertilization taking place outside the body. This procedure is accepted by some religious groups that don't allow IVF.

MARCUS OR MICHELLE?

In addition to providing important genetic information, preimplantation genetic testing can determine which embryos will grow up to be girls and which embryos will grow up to be boys. As you might imagine, this part of the technology is controversial.

Preimplantation genetic screening (PGS) can create an ethical predicament when the procedure is used for non-medical reasons. PGS can be used to test and transfer only embryos of a particular, desired sex into the uterus. This essentially allows parents to choose whether they want to send out blue birth announcements or pink ones.

The friendly euphemism for this procedure is "family balancing." Proponents say it's a perfectly legitimate choice that's in the best interests of the family and the child. Opponents argue that using PGS in this manner is sexist, inappropriate and unethical. They worry it could skew the male-to-female ratio among the general population and put fertility clinics on the slippery slope to creating "designer babies."

Sex selection is only offered at some fertility clinics in the United States. Most clinics transfer the healthiest embryos, no matter what their sex. However, the technology is becoming more commonly used in other countries where there's a desire to have sons to continue the family lineage and to bring honor and security to the family. As technologies improve, sex selection is likely to be a continuing topic of discussion.

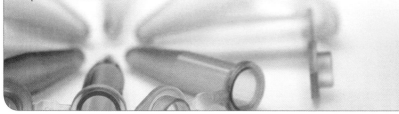

Assisted hatching About five to six days after it has been fertilized, an embryo "hatches" from its surrounding membrane (zona pellucida), which allows it to implant into the lining of the uterus (endometrium). Assisted hatching is a laboratory procedure in which the shell-like protein coating that surrounds the egg is mechanically or chemically opened before embryo transfer to help the embryo hatch.

This technique may be used because there's evidence the zona pellucida thickens as you age. It may also be performed if you have poor quality embryos or you've had several unsuccessful attempts at IVF.

Preimplantation genetic testing Preimplantation genetic diagnosis (PGD) and preimplantation genetic screening (PGS) have been around since the early 1990s but are becoming increasingly more common. In these procedures, a biopsy of the embryos is performed, removing a cell or a few cells during the time between egg retrieval and embryo transfer. DNA is then harvested from the cells to be able to detect genetic problems that the embryos may carry.

In the case of PGD, the sample is tested for a specific genetic disease known to be carried by one or both of the parents. With PGS, all of the chromosomes (genes) are screened to look for the presence or the absence of abnormal amounts of genetic material. With both techniques, the goal is the same: to identify healthy embryos for transfer to the uterus.

The technology behind these techniques is rapidly changing and can be controversial because of how the tests may be used. These procedures aren't intended to help parents select babies of a certain sex or with certain characteristics. Rather, the goal of PGD is to help parents who are carriers of genetic diseases, such as cystic fibrosis, sickle cell anemia or Huntington's disease, prevent passage of

INTERPRETING IVF SUCCESS RATES

In the United States, fertility clinics are required to report every assisted reproductive technology cycle to the Society for Assisted Reproductive Technology and the Centers for Disease Control and Prevention (CDC). More than 400 clinics do this each year. This provides helpful information for couples that are looking for a successful fertility clinic. But it's important to interpret this data carefully.

The success rates at a particular IVF center depend on a number of factors, including the number of patients accepted, the age of patients accepted, the underlying causes of these patients' fertility problems, the number of canceled cycles and the number of embryos transferred. Clinics that accept older couples with complex fertility problems will naturally have lower success rates than clinics that weed out difficult cases. You may also notice a difference in success rates among states that mandate insurance coverage of IVF. This mandate allows many women to undergo the procedure before they get to the point of last resort, which tends to decrease the average age and level of complexity of cases in covered states.

As you review published success rates, remember that assisted reproduction is a very competitive industry — not just a medical procedure. There is a big financial incentive for clinics to publish good success rates, and there are ways to bend the rules without breaking them. For example, clinics can cancel a cycle if it's not going well, so that cycle doesn't count in their statistics.

Arm yourself with information about the clinics you're considering, and scrutinize the details of success rates. Ask questions to help you understand the numbers. Inquire about any numbers that seem especially high or low compared with other clinics.

Also, make sure you understand the various terms used in success rate reports and marketing materials. Some clinics boast about their success based on the percentage of IVF cycles resulting in pregnancies. But only about 80 percent of pregnancies result in a live birth. So pregnancies aren't necessarily the best measure of success. The live birth rate — the "take-home baby" rate — is what matters the most to those undergoing the procedure.

the disease to their children. PGS may be helpful for couples with known genetic problems called chromosomal translocations or couples with a history of multiple unexplained miscarriages.

PGD and PGS aren't foolproof. They can't totally eliminate the risk of having a baby with a medical condition, but they can reduce the likelihood.

THE SUCCESS OF ART

IVF is a difference-maker for many couples that struggle with infertility. In one trial, couples about to start their first IVF cycle were randomly assigned to receive IVF within 90 days or to have no treatment for 90 days. The difference was significant. Twenty-nine percent of couples that were assigned to the IVF group delivered babies, compared to just 1 percent of those who didn't receive treatment.

Overall, IVF success rates are on the rise. In the United States, more than 400 fertility clinics report data on the outcomes of all of their ART cycles. In 2012, more than 165,000 ART cycles were performed at more than 400 reporting clinics, resulting in the birth of 61,740 babies. As mentioned earlier, more than 40 percent of IVF cycles end in a live birth among women younger than age 35. That number drops to about 30 percent

for women ages 35 to 37 and to about 20 percent for women ages 38 to 40.

Of course, success depends on other factors besides age, including the cause of your fertility problems and the clinic performing your procedure.

All in all, though, IVF is no longer a long shot. And it's important to put these numbers in perspective. The success rate for natural pregnancy isn't 100 percent. The average fertile couple only has about a 20 to 25 percent chance of success in making a baby on their own each month.

Costs In the United States, most people aren't used to comparison shopping and paying out of pocket for medical treatment. In that regard, fertility medicine is different from other medical specialties.

IVF is only covered by health insurance in a few states where there's a state mandate to cover fertility care like other medical treatments. As a result, many couples must take on a tremendous amount of personal expense to fund IVF procedures. According to the American Society for Reproductive Medicine, the average cost of an IVF cycle in the United States is $12,400 — and many couples undergo multiple cycles.

In response to this financial burden, some clinics offer financing options and "affordable treatment packages." This may include multicycle discounts for couples that buy two or three (or six) IVF

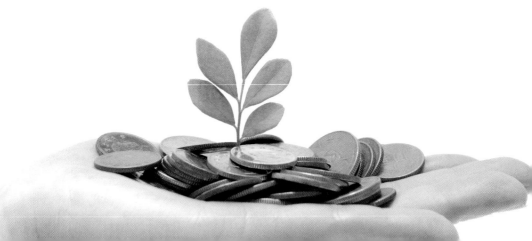

cycles upfront, rather than purchasing one IVF cycle at a time. In this scenario, you pay one fixed fee for multiple tries at IVF. The multicycle package is complete when you deliver a baby, whether you used all of the cycles or not.

Some clinics also offer refund plans, which may be called "shared risk plans." Couples prepay for several IVF cycles upfront, but the clinic will refund a percentage of the costs — 70 to 100 percent — if IVF is unsuccessful at the end of the purchased cycles. If you get pregnant on the first IVF cycle, you probably paid more than you needed to. If you don't get pregnant until the third cycle, you may end up getting a deal. If you don't get pregnant at all, the clinic assumes the bulk of your costs.

What's the catch? Typically, couples only qualify for refund packages or multicycle packages if they're likely to have good success with IVF.

Always make sure you understand exactly what you're purchasing and whether you need everything you're buying.

Extra embryos There is a cruel irony of IVF. Some couples go from desperately wanting to have one baby to a situation in which they have too many potential babies. After conceiving the number of children they desire, the couple is left with extra embryos that they can't support.

There are steps you and your doctor can take to prevent this possibility. But despite the best of planning, you may end up with excess embryos. It's up to you to determine the future of these embryos. The medical term for this is "embryo disposition."

Excess embryos can pose a difficult dilemma, but there are several options:

▶ *Freeze the embryos.* This is a good option if you may want to have more babies in the future, but you'll pay a monthly, quarterly or yearly storage fee. And you'll need to wait at least six months after delivery to get pregnant again. Most programs want you to use the embryos within 10 years of the time they were created.

▶ *Donate the embryos to an embryo donation agency.* When you do this, another couple can use your embryos in their IVF cycle. Many couples begin the IVF process thinking this is what they want to do with the extra embryos. But some couples get cold feet when they're holding their new baby in their arms and they realize that the embryos that remain would be biological brothers or sisters to this baby.

▶ *Discard the embryos or donate them to fertility research.* Donating your embryos to research can help advance the science of fertility medicine and give other couples an opportunity to have a healthy baby.

▶ *Have a disposal ceremony.* You can take your embryos from the fertility clinic and dispose of them as you see fit. You can say goodbye in a personal ceremony or dispose of the embryos in a place that's special to your family.

▶ *Undergo 'compassionate transfer.'* With this option you have the embryos transferred into your uterus in a way that's unlikely to result in pregnancy. This option is attractive to couples that have religious or ethical concerns about disposing of the embryos. The embryos are thawed and transferred into your uterus during the wrong time of your menstrual cycle, so it's extremely unlikely that you'll become pregnant.

Leaving your embryos frozen indefinitely, with no plans for using them, can cause angst and guilt. Most couples experience a sense of closure when they take action, no matter what action they choose.

TREATING INFERTILITY
A summary of the treatment process

Treatment of infertility isn't a straightforward path. The route you follow depends on the cause of your infertility, your age, how long you've been trying to have a baby and your personal preferences. The graphic on page 165 outlines the steps in evaluating infertility. Below, are possible treatment scenarios based on the outcome of an evaluation.

Most couples start with the least expensive, least invasive treatment that's likely to work in their particular situation. If pregnancy doesn't occur, they proceed to the next step

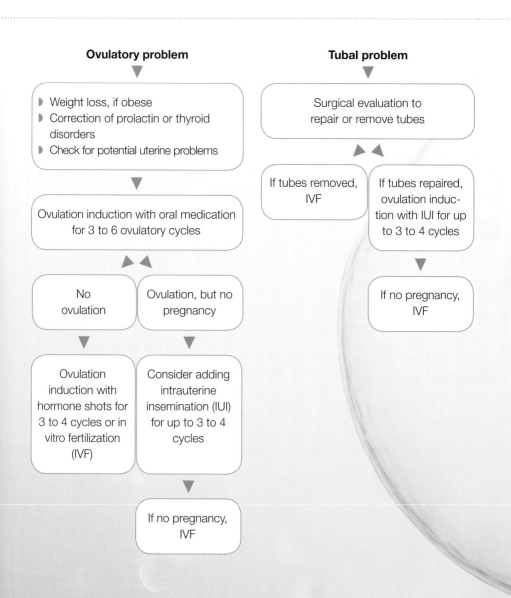

Ovulatory problem

- Weight loss, if obese
- Correction of prolactin or thyroid disorders
- Check for potential uterine problems

Ovulation induction with oral medication for 3 to 6 ovulatory cycles

No ovulation

Ovulation, but no pregnancy

Ovulation induction with hormone shots for 3 to 4 cycles or in vitro fertilization (IVF)

Consider adding intrauterine insemination (IUI) for up to 3 to 4 cycles

If no pregnancy, IVF

Tubal problem

Surgical evaluation to repair or remove tubes

If tubes removed, IVF

If tubes repaired, ovulation induction with IUI for up to 3 to 4 cycles

If no pregnancy, IVF

in the treatment process. It's generally recommended you give each option about three tries before moving on.

Most treatment paths eventually end with in vitro fertilization (IVF). Some couples prefer to take a more aggressive route and they begin with IVF. But it's not necessary that you do so. Many couples have babies using less powerful, less disruptive and less expensive medical options.

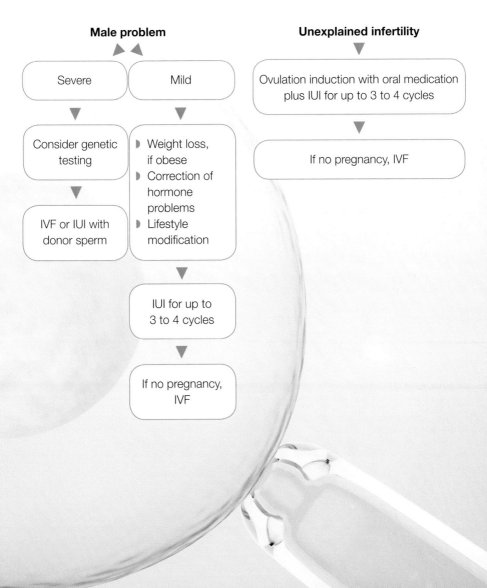

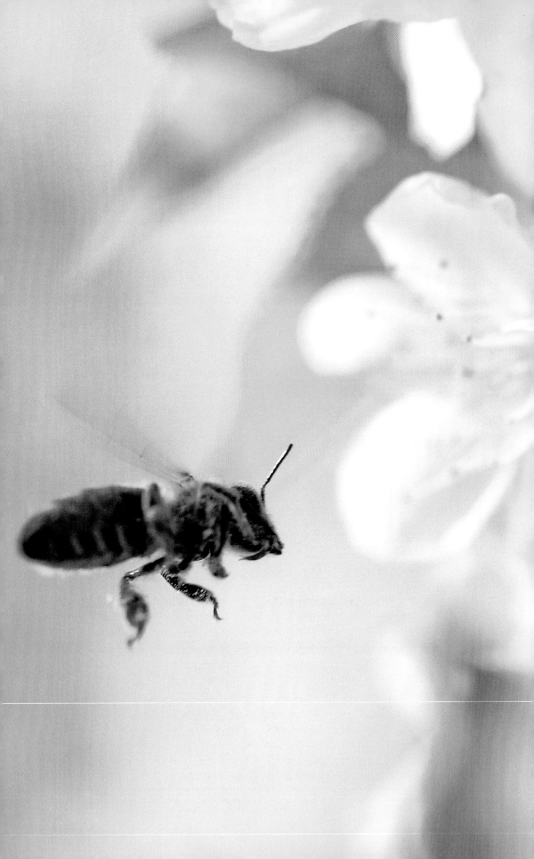

CHAPTER 16

Third party reproduction

If you think it takes just two people to make a baby, you might have to change your thinking. In the real world of modern fertility medicine, that isn't always the case. Today, making a baby may involve assistance from others.

Third party reproduction refers to a donation by a third person — in the form of donor sperm, donor eggs, donor embryos or a gestational carrier — to enable an infertile individual or couple or a same-sex couple to become parents. Third party reproduction is routine at most fertility clinics in the United States.

Donor eggs or embryos are used in more than 18,000 attempts at pregnancy using in vitro fertilization (IVF) in the United States every year. Most women younger than age 40 still use their own eggs for IVF. But 37 percent of women ages 43 to 44 — and 73 percent of women older than age 44 — opt for donor eggs from a younger woman to increase their chances of success. Donor sperm and gestational carriers also play an important role in present-day pregnancies.

Third party reproduction generally isn't anyone's preferred path to parenthood. The process often is complex, difficult and expensive. And it may mean that one parent isn't genetically related to the baby.

But third party reproduction offers the hope of a healthy baby to:

▶ Couples that can't have a baby with their own sperm, eggs or uterus
▶ Couples that have a genetic disease that could be passed onto their baby
▶ Couples in which a pregnancy could be dangerous to the mother
▶ Same-sex couples wanting to have a family (You can read more specific information pertaining to pregnancy in same-sex couples in Chapter 19.)

Third party reproduction relies on many of the same medications and reproductive techniques discussed in the last two chapters. The difference is that the eggs, sperm or embryos — or the uterus where the baby lives and grows during pregnancy — are provided by another person.

DONOR EGGS

All of the assisted reproductive technologies described in the last chapter can be performed with donor egg cells (oocytes). The most common of these is in vitro fertilization (IVF), a fertility treatment in which mature eggs and sperm are combined outside the body in a specialized laboratory.

When donor eggs are used for IVF, the egg donor undergoes the first two steps in the IVF process — ovarian stimulation and egg retrieval. The male partner's role is to provide sperm, which are used to fertilize the donor eggs in a laboratory. The fertilized embryos are then transferred into the female partner's uterus to implant and develop. In some cases, donor sperm is used along with the donor egg to create embryos.

Do you need donor eggs? Fertility treatments using egg donation have been around for more than 30 years. Donor eggs were originally offered to women with dysfunctional ovaries, due to disease or surgery, or to women who were known carriers of significant genetic diseases. Assisted reproductive technologies with donor eggs are still an effective treatment in these cases.

Today, donor eggs are also an option for women with a normally functioning uterus who are unlikely or unable to conceive using their own eggs. This includes:
▶ Women with diminished ovarian reserve
▶ Women who have consistently produced poor-quality eggs or embryos during previous fertility treatments
▶ Women who have tried fertility treatments with their own eggs without success
▶ Women who are unable to tolerate ovarian stimulation and egg retrieval
▶ Older women

Donor eggs are increasingly used for the latter group, who may have delayed having children due to school or a career, or who didn't find a partner until later in life. For these women, donor eggs can reverse the decline in successful IVF outcomes that come with each passing birthday.

In general, eggs produced by older women face several hurdles. They form embryos that are less likely to implant and more likely to result in miscarriage if they do implant. They also are more likely to have chromosome abnormalities that can affect the chances of having a healthy baby. IVF success rates drop sharply with age for women who use their own eggs — from more than 40 percent among women younger than age 35 to less than 5 percent among women age 43 and older.

In contrast, the female uterus can respond normally at any age. Given the right amount of estrogen and progesterone, women can successfully carry pregnancies even when they have entered menopause and their ovaries are no longer producing eggs. When donor eggs are used, the percentage of embryo transfers that result in live births remains consistently high — generally above 50 percent — among women at various ages.

The bottom line is this: The likelihood of a fertilized egg implanting during IVF is related to the age of the woman who produced the egg, not the age of the woman having the embryos implanted into her uterus. For older women, donor eggs can result in pregnancy rates comparable to women in their 20s. Most couples willing to undergo IVF with donor eggs end up with a successful pregnancy.

How egg donation works The donated egg may come from someone you know or someone you don't. In a known donor egg program, couples receive healthy eggs from someone they have recruited — often a good friend, sister or other relative. In an anonymous donor egg program, couples choose an unknown young woman recruited and screened by a fertility clinic or agency specializing in egg donors. These women are typically between the ages of 21 and 34 and have volunteered to donate their eggs to other couples. The anonymous donor doesn't know the identity of the couple that receives her eggs, and the couple doesn't know her identity. Another option increasing in popularity is to purchase frozen eggs (see page 225).

Remember, the egg donor is the genetic mother of the baby. So if you use a known donor such as a younger sister who donates her eggs to an older sister, the younger sister will be both the baby's aunt and true genetic mother. Some couples are elated to accept such a gift from a favorite sister, while others squirm at the thought of living with this unusual family dynamic for the rest of their lives.

You and your partner will need to evaluate which choice is best for you.

Your doctor or a fertility counselor can help you work through your feelings and concerns. Many fertility clinics require meeting with a trained professional to talk about your feelings and potential issues before the process occurs.

Whether you recruit a known donor or select an anonymous donor, the medical process is the same. All donors must submit to a comprehensive series of tests. Once you have selected a donor, that person will begin a regimen of fertility drugs to stimulate her ovaries to produce multiple, mature eggs that can be retrieved and used for in vitro fertilization. The medications your donor will take (or did take if you buy frozen eggs) are similar to the ones that you would have used if you were using your own eggs for IVF.

When the donor's follicles have reached the right size and are likely to contain mature eggs, a final hormone shot is given to help mature and release the eggs. About 36 hours later, the eggs are retrieved. Most doctors use transvaginal ultrasound aspiration to insert a needle through the donor's vaginal wall and into the ovaries to suction out the follicular fluid containing the eggs. At this point

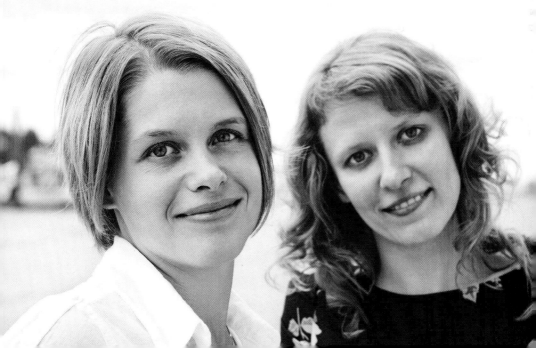

in the process, your donor's job is done, and yours begins in earnest.

However, you and your partner aren't sitting idly by through the first part of the process, waiting for the baton to be passed! Before the time of egg retrieval, your uterus needs to get in sync with your donor's ovarian stimulation cycle so that you're ready to carry the transferred embryos. Embryos implant only if the uterine lining is at the right stage of development, so this is a critical part of the process.

If you have regular menstrual cycles, you may need to take a birth control pill or other medications to suppress your own menstrual cycle before the donor cycle begins. Once your donor starts taking ovary-stimulating medications, you'll likely need to take estrogen to synchronize your cycle with hers and to help prepare the lining of your uterus (endometrium) for pregnancy. Finally, after the embryo transfer, you'll take progesterone supplements to encourage the lining of your uterus to thicken and be more receptive to embryo implantation.

As for your partner, on the day of egg retrieval, he'll need to provide a sperm sample that will be used to fertilize the donated eggs in the laboratory. Three to five days after fertilization, the embryos will be transferred into your uterus. Similar to standard IVF treatments, the timing of and number of eggs transferred into your uterus depend on many factors, including your moral and religious beliefs.

You may continue taking hormone medications after the embryo transfer to help foster a healthy pregnancy. And you'll probably know if you're pregnant about 10 to 14 days after the transfer.

Similar to standard IVF with your own eggs, the biggest risk of IVF with donor eggs is multiple babies. If you have a surplus of fertilized embryos made up of the donor eggs and your partner's sperm, you'll also need to determine what to do with the embryos. The embryos belong to you and your partner. You can freeze them for a future IVF treatment or use them in some way (see page 217).

DONOR SPERM

Sperm donation is a procedure in which a man donates semen — the fluid released during ejaculation — to help an individual or couple conceive a baby. Donor sperm can be used for in vitro fertilization (IVF) or intrauterine insemination (IUI), the most commonly used type of donor insemination. Donor sperm is typically obtained from a regulated sperm bank, but it may be collected from a known individual, such as a friend, brother or other close relative.

Artificial insemination with donor sperm has likely been taking place for centuries. Published reports referring to this practice date back to 1945. Since the 1980s, when concerns surfaced about AIDS and the unethical selection of sperm donors in many hospitals, it's become a highly regulated industry.

Today, donor sperm are largely available through large commercial sperm laboratories regulated by the Food and Drug Administration (FDA). Before being allowed to donate his sperm, a man must undergo medical, psychological, genetic and infectious disease screening. If approved, he provides one or more sperm samples, which are frozen (cryopreserved) and kept in quarantine for at least 180 days. The donor is then tested again for infectious diseases, such as HIV. The sperm are only released for donation once all tests are complete and all results come back negative.

FROZEN DONOR EGGS

For decades, scientists have successfully been freezing sperm, using a process called cryopreservation. However, until recently, it wasn't possible to freeze eggs in the same way without the quality of the eggs deteriorating. So all donor eggs used in IVF had to be "fresh."

In recent years, the freezing (cryopreservation) of eggs (oocytes) has improved dramatically. Eggs can now be frozen, stored, shipped and thawed, as needed. IVF cycles with fresh donor eggs are still more common than those with frozen donor eggs. But success with frozen eggs is increasing, and this technique is gaining popularity. Of the 18,000-plus IVF cycles performed with donor eggs in the United States in 2010, more than 9,800 of these involved fresh donor eggs, while the remainder used frozen eggs.

There are several advantages of IVF with frozen donor eggs:

◗ During IVF with frozen donor eggs, there is no need to synchronize your uterus with the donor's cycle. This may eliminate the need for some hormone medications and allow IVF to take place on your timeline.

◗ When you use frozen eggs, you typically minimize the number of embryos that are created. This is important for couples that have ethical concerns about extra embryos.

◗ Frozen eggs can be shipped to locations where egg donors are in short supply or to provide more racial or ethnic diversity than is present in a particular community.

◗ Frozen eggs may be less expensive, because there's no need to initiate an ovarian stimulation and egg retrieval process for each donor IVF cycle.

If success with frozen eggs continues, it may dramatically affect the supply chain for donor eggs. Right now, donor egg programs are typically managed by fertility clinics. Large fertility clinics can help match egg donors and recipients and provide medical care for women on both sides of the donation equation.

This same type of transition occurred in the 1980s with frozen sperm. Specific programs no longer recruited their own donors locally. Instead, national, independent, certified sperm banks took over the process. If the market for frozen eggs continues to grow, it's possible that the egg donor selection process could become similar to the sperm donor selection process.

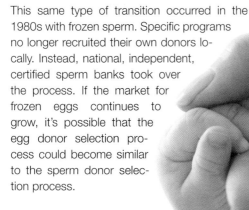

Do you need donor sperm? Artificial insemination with donor sperm may be recommended if:

▶ The male partner has a very low sperm count (oligospermia)
▶ The male partner has a complete absence of sperm (azoospermia)
▶ There are other significant sperm problems
▶ The male partner has ejaculatory conditions, such as retrograde ejaculation
▶ The male partner has significant genetic disorders or sexually transmissible infections that he doesn't want to pass on to his children
▶ There is no male partner

In some cases, intrauterine insemination or in vitro fertilization with donor sperm may be considered for couples that have tried assisted reproductive technologies with their own sperm without success. IVF with donor sperm and donor eggs may be recommended for couples that can't use their own eggs or sperm but in which the woman is able to carry the transferred embryos. Artificial donor insemination is also used by single women or same-sex couples who don't have a male partner.

Generally donor insemination with IUI is the first step for single women or lesbian couples where there's no evidence of an infertility problem — just a need for sperm to fertilize an egg. However, if you've completed a number of IUI cycles without achieving pregnancy or there's a factor that may reduce the chances of successful IUI in the woman attempting pregnancy, taking the IVF route sooner may be a reasonable strategy.

The role of donor sperm has changed over the past decade, as intracytoplasmic sperm injection (ICSI) technologies have become a popular and successful add-on to IVF treatments. Before ICSI, use of donor sperm was often the only treatment

option for many male fertility problems. For a good chance at pregnancy using IVF, you needed millions of active sperm.

Today, with the use of ICSI, all you need is one good sperm for each egg. This allows men with certain fertility problems to use their own sperm. The procedure increases the chances of successful IVF among men who don't produce much sperm and men who produce sperm with abnormal shapes or movement that may have trouble penetrating the egg. In vitro fertilization with ICSI is more expensive than is a single cycle or a few cycles of artificial donor insemination, but it allows the male partner to be the genetic father of the baby.

How donor sperm works Using donor sperm for intrauterine insemination or in vitro fertilization doesn't change either medical procedure dramatically. The sperm used in your procedure simply comes from a vial of frozen donor sperm that has been thawed and prepared, rather than from your partner.

Artificial donor insemination. With artificial donor insemination, the donor sperm is placed into your uterus close to the time of ovulation (see page 190). Your care provider may use transvaginal ultrasounds to time the intrauterine insemination procedure correctly.

Often, fertility drugs are combined with this procedure to induce your ovaries to develop and release multiple, mature eggs to increase your chances of getting pregnant. You may also take medications to prepare your uterine lining for pregnancy.

IVF with donor sperm. In the case of in vitro fertilization, after eggs have been retrieved from your ovaries, the prepared donor sperm are mixed with your incubated eggs in a laboratory dish. The resulting embryos are then transferred into your uterus.

In some cases, ICSI — in which a single sperm is isolated and injected into an egg for transfer — may be used to fertilize your eggs, even with donor sperm. ICSI can increase the chances of successful fertilization, but it's more expensive. The added expense may not be warranted, since donor sperm are usually high-quality sperm and generally have no trouble fertilizing eggs using traditional procedures.

Some women wonder whether the use of thawed, frozen sperm — rather than fresh sperm — will impact the chances of success with these procedures. (Remember, all anonymous donor sperm are frozen due to testing regulations.) In general, the use of frozen sperm doesn't seem to affect the success rates of IVF. But frozen sperm may be less effective than fresh sperm for intrauterine insemination. That's because freezing can decrease motility and sometimes the sperm count. Although the IUI procedure puts the sperm as close to the egg as possible, the sperm still needs to swim to the egg to fertilize it. Your doctor can try to gauge the donor sperm's motility before the procedure.

DONOR EMBRYOS

Some fertility clinics allow couples to donate their unused frozen embryos to other couples struggling to have a baby of their own. This type of donation may make sense for couples that have untreatable male and female fertility problems or those that have experienced recurrent pregnancy loss that seems to be related to a problem with the embryos.

Embryo donation may also be an option for couples with serious genetic disorders that could be passed on to their children.

From a medical perspective, donor embryos actually simplify the IVF process, since the ovulation induction, egg retrieval and fertilization stages are already complete. However, from a moral and legal standpoint, there's nothing simple about donor embryos.

This type of third party reproduction is much more complicated and controversial than is egg donation or sperm donation. The baby will not be genetically related to either of the parents. In addition, the baby may have full genetic siblings that are being raised by other parents — the couple that donated the embryos.

Some couples have no interest in the concept of embryo donation. However, others view it as an opportunity to "adopt" unused embryos that may otherwise be discarded. This can be very satisfying to couples with certain religious and ethical beliefs.

Donor embryos are quarantined for six months — similar to donor sperm — while the donors undergo all of the established guidelines for screening and testing. Psychological counseling also is recommended for the donors, to make sure they are emotionally prepared for the decision to part with their embryos. It's also a good idea to involve legal counsel because the laws governing embryo donation aren't always clear.

SURROGATES AND GESTATIONAL CARRIERS

A traditional surrogate is a woman who donates both her eggs and her uterus to help another couple have a baby. She can become pregnant through intrauterine insemination or assisted reproductive techniques. The surrogate is the genetic mother of the baby.

A gestational carrier is a woman who agrees to carry a baby for a couple who is unable to carry a baby to term. Unlike a traditional surrogate, a gestational carrier doesn't supply her eggs for this arrangement. The gestational carrier has no genetic relationship to the baby — she is simply the carrier of the child.

Gestational carriers are used in less than 1 percent of IVF cycles in the United States. But they can be a huge help for women who can't carry a baby themselves. Traditional surrogates, on the other hand, are becoming almost obsolete. This is mostly due to a few high-profile legal cases in which the surrogate mother sued for custody of the baby and prevailed. Because of these lawsuits, very few, if any, fertility clinics offer this option.

The term *surrogate*, however, is still commonly used. The media or lay public will often refer to a surrogate when what they are really referring to is a gestational carrier.

Do you need a gestational carrier?

At most fertility clinics, gestational carriers are only recommended when there's a legitimate medical reason that a woman can't carry a baby on her own or if pregnancy would pose significant risks to the woman or her baby.

Candidates for this option include:

▶ A women who had a hysterectomy to treat cervical cancer or for other reasons

---

UNTRADITIONAL OPTIONS

Third party reproduction is generally quite expensive. Some couples can't afford the costs but are desperate to conceive a child. This has created a market for private online donations (especially sperm donations), home fertility treatment products and other untraditional strategies for having a baby.

A quick search of the Internet will result in many offers for free or discounted sperm, donor sperm home delivery kits, home insemination kits and instructions on how to perform a vaginal insemination by yourself. You'll also find ads from sperm donors who are willing to deliver their sperm sample to your home or meet you at a public location.

If you're struggling to have a baby, you may be tempted by the promise of these nontraditional reproduction techniques. Be aware that they pose significant health and legal risks. It's important to be cautious and careful.

When you work with a certified sperm bank and a licensed fertility specialist, extensive health regulations and legal protections are woven into the process. If you opt for a private arrangement, it's your responsibility to screen and verify donors and research legal implications in your area.

Mayo Clinic doesn't recommend any of these untraditional options. It's better to work with your care provider to determine proven treatments that are most likely to work for your particular situation. If you can't afford certain treatments, your care provider can help optimize treatments you can afford.

- A woman with a medical condition that makes pregnancy dangerous, such as primary pulmonary hypertension
- A woman with several late pregnancy losses
- A woman with an incompetent cervix, birth defect of the uterus or severe scarring of the uterus
- A woman born without a uterus

How gestational carriers work With a gestational carrier, in vitro fertilization is almost always used. You provide the eggs to be used in the procedure by way of ovulation induction and egg retrieval. Your eggs are fertilized with your partner's sperm to create embryos that are transferred into the uterus of the carrier.

Your gestational carrier will need to take medication to prepare her uterus for implantation and get her menstrual cycle in sync with your stimulation cycle. When pregnancy occurs, she is responsible for making healthy choices to carry your baby to term.

The relationship between gestational carriers and the biological parents varies. You may be in close contact with your gestational carrier and be in the delivery room when the baby arrives. Or you may not have a great deal of contact with your gestational carrier over the nine months of pregnancy. The exact arrangement should be determined in advance with the help of your fertility doctor and an attorney familiar with gestational contracts.

SELECTING A DONOR

When you select an egg donor or sperm donor, you will want to consider the donor's health history. You may also consider his or her family history, eye color, hair color, race, ethnicity, height, weight, blood type, education level, occupation and hobbies. If the donor's eggs or sperm have been used in previous fertilization attempts, you might inquire into the outcomes of their previous donations. However, due to privacy concerns, not all clinics may be able to or willing to share this information. Most couples hope to find a donor that appears to be similar to them — both in terms of physical characteristics and lifestyle.

Blood type and certain infectious disease testing, such as the presence of prior cytomegalovirus (CMV) infection, also can play a role in finding a donor. Incompatibility relating to these factors can make pregnancy more complicated for mom and baby. Your care provider will make sure that the test results of all three parties — you, your partner and your donor — are compatible.

Egg donor Egg donors are often recruited by egg donation programs or agencies. Many large fertility clinics have their own egg donation programs and provide medical care for their donors. If your clinic doesn't have its own program, it may work with an independent, private egg donor agency. These agencies typically don't provide medical testing or care. They simply match egg donors with couples that need them. Once selected, the donor candidates undergo the fertility clinic's screening and assessment protocol before being approved for use as donors.

In order to maintain donor anonymity, clinic-based programs often release only a limited amount of information about an egg donor. There are only so many egg donors in a particular geographic area, so giving away a complete biography could compromise privacy.

In contrast, independent, unaffiliated egg donation agencies may offer hundreds of egg donor profiles from candidates all over the country. These profiles may include much more detailed information than a clinic would offer, including photographs. However, if you choose to work with an independent agency, you typically pay thousands of dollars in agency administration fees and travel expenses for your donor to travel for egg retrieval, in addition to the costs of the screening tests, clinic visits and standard fees associated with IVF.

Sperm donor Strict laws surrounding sperm donation make it difficult for fertility clinics to maintain their own sperm donation programs. Many fertility clinics work with independent, commercial sperm banks. You and your partner can browse, search and filter through the available online profiles at accredited sperm banks to choose the ones that interest you. Sperm banks provide varying levels of information about their donors. Some provide a basic profile (race, height, weight, eye color, religion) for free, but charge extra if you want to see baby pictures, current photos or more detailed information (such as education, occupation, hobbies, even a handwriting sample or voice recording). Some can even match you with a donor that looks like you or your favorite celebrity. Since sperm is frozen from donors all over the country, anonymity isn't as much of an issue.

Gestational carrier The ideal gestational carrier is typically a healthy woman between the ages of 21 and 45 who has successfully delivered at least one baby but not more than five — or more than three by cesarean section. Unlike egg and sperm donors, the gestational carrier isn't contributing to the biological makeup of your baby. So hair color and height aren't so important. Instead, you're likely looking for someone who is healthy, takes good care of herself and

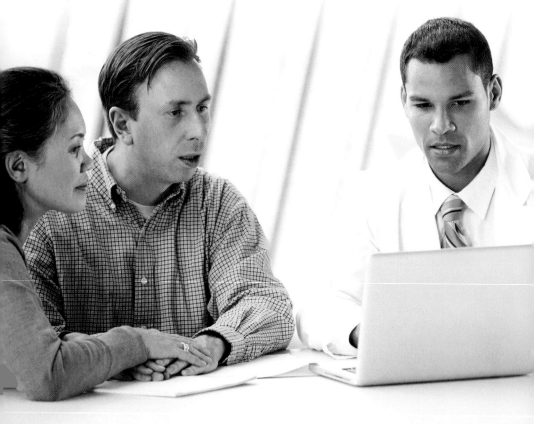

TALKING TO YOUR CHILD ABOUT DONOR EGGS OR SPERM

If you become a parent with the help of a sperm or egg donor, you will at some point confront an unavoidable question: Should you share the details of your child's conception with him or her? The decision of whether to disclose this information — and how much to disclose — is an extremely personal one for a parent or a couple to make.

Your particular circumstances and beliefs may lead you to choose to not disclose any information to your child about your use of a donor. On the other hand, you may be firm in your desire to openly share your child's conception story. If you're unsure or wavering, it may be worth noting that sharing your child's conception story is thought to be best for his or her well-being. Bringing the subject out into the open avoids the risk of your child learning about his or her background in an unplanned way. It also avoids the potentially negative impact that maintaining a secret can have on you and your family.

Your child's future access to his or her family medical history may be another reason to consider disclosure. Each fertility program, sperm bank and egg donation agency will have its own policy regarding the sharing of such donor information, and that policy will come into play should you choose to raise the subject with your child.

Along with the question of what to share with your child comes the related decision of what to disclose to others in your life. The general rule of thumb is either to be completely open about your use of a donor or else to tell no one. Telling only selected people while keeping the secret from others can lead to unintended consequences.

If you're facing these choices as a couple, it's important to discuss all of the issues upfront so that you can reach an agreement you both feel comfortable with. If you find yourself struggling with any of these decisions, seek the counsel of a health professional who specializes in this area of family counseling.

---

lives in an environment that will be safe for your baby — for example, an environment void of toxins or secondhand smoke. Your fertility clinic may help you find a carrier or refer you to an agency that can do so.

Known donor If you want to use a known egg or sperm donor or gestational carrier, there's a whole other set of criteria you'll need to consider: Which friend or family member would you feel comfortable asking to help you have a baby? Could you live with this unique relationship for the rest of your lives? (Would your sister want to tell you how to raise the baby if she's the genetic mother?) Will your arrangement cause strain, tension or unrest among other members of the family?

Like anonymous donors, known donors are subjected to a thorough battery of medical tests and screens. This may include a complete physical exam, blood testing, drug testing, sexually transmitted infection testing, psychological testing and more. If you choose a known donor, he or she will need to be cleared before you can continue with treatment.

COSTS AND CONTRACTS

Third party reproduction is often an expensive proposition. You and your partner are responsible for all of the usual costs of in vitro fertilization or other assisted reproductive technologies, as well as the costs associated with donors.

Whether you use a known donor or an anonymous donor, it's important that compensation is determined and documented in advance. It's generally best in all cases of third party reproduction that you seek the advice of legal counsel.

Donor sperm Fees for donor sperm vary by sperm bank, donor characteristics, the amount of information provided about the sperm donor and how the sperm was prepared — washed or unwashed. Prices may range from $125 to $600 per vial. One vial is typically required per pregnancy attempt. Plan for additional storage and shipment fees.

Donor eggs The ovulation induction and egg retrieval procedures require a significant amount of time, inconvenience and discomfort, compared with a simple sperm donation. So egg donors are compensated accordingly. Most donors receive about $5,000 per cycle. But payments may range from $2,500 to $8,000. Paying more than $10,000 is generally considered inappropriate.

Some fertility clinics offer two ways to reduce the cost of donor eggs by splitting expenses with another couple. The first option is called a shared donor program or split donor program. In this scenario,

two or three couples are matched with one anonymous egg donor, and they split the eggs — and the costs — of the cycle. In most cases, there are plenty of high-quality eggs to go around.

The second option involves another woman who is trying to get pregnant, as opposed to an anonymous donor. Some fertility centers allow a woman to undergo IVF at a reduced cost in exchange for providing some of her eggs to another couple. You may be paired with this type of egg donor at a reduced cost because you'll be splitting the eggs she creates. This type of situation is only offered to young women with high-quality eggs who are using IVF for other reasons.

Donor embryos Embryo donors typically receive no compensation for their donation. Payment for excess embryos is viewed as unethical.

Gestational carriers Gestational carriers are typically reimbursed for all the expenses involved in fulfilling this role. This may include medical bills, insurance bills, legal fees, transportation, maternity clothes, lost wages and pregnancy vitamins. In addition, carriers are paid a fee for their time, effort and inconvenience. Fees vary greatly, depending on your location, the carrier, procedures performed and other factors. Using a gestational carrier can add tens of thousands of dollars to the cost of assisted reproductive technologies.

Legal advice is particularly important if you're using a gestational carrier. You and your carrier should each be represented by an attorney with experience in reproductive law. These professionals can help draw up a comprehensive contract, stipulating all of the expectations and possible complications, before you proceed. This includes how many embryos will be transferred, how many babies the carrier will carry, who makes decisions about discontinuing a complicated pregnancy, who is allowed in the delivery room and what happens in the case of miscarriage.

Laws surrounding reproduction also vary by state. For example, in some states the gestational carrier and her legal spouse may be required to be listed on the birth certificate, with a later adoption-like process performed to permit the intended parents to be listed instead. In other places, the intended parents can be listed on the birth certificate from the start. Having an attorney familiar with the laws in the state where your gestational carrier intends to deliver is crucial to avoid legal headaches later on.

Known donors The financial agreement between parents and known donors is as personal as those of anonymous donors. Many known donors don't expect any compensation, but receive a thoughtful gift from the grateful parents at the end of the process. In other cases, this arrangement becomes an opportunity for a couple to provide financial help to a sister or a friend who agrees to serve as an egg donor or gestational carrier.

TAKE YOUR TIME

This is a lot of information to wrap your head around. Third party reproduction is the right choice for some couples, but it doesn't sit well with others. Consider your personal situation and take some time to understand exactly how all of these scenarios work. Don't be afraid to discuss them with a medical professional, such as a doctor or counselor.

If you don't know of anyone who has become a parent through third party reproduction, you may feel alone in unchartered waters. But there are plenty of other couples like you. Consider connecting with others that have been through this process, either through online fertility message boards or support groups in your area. Successful parents are often willing to share their experiences. Hearing what they have to say may help you decide what's best for your family.

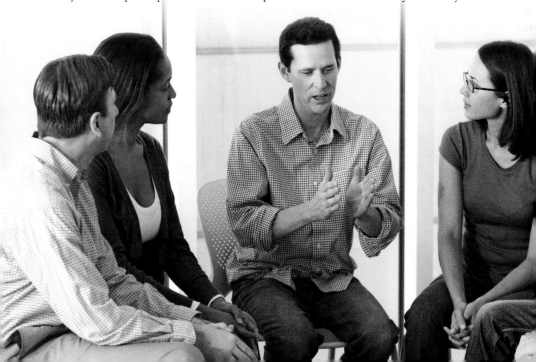

Ashley and Susie's Story

Ashley: When I was 2 years old, I was diagnosed with primary pulmonary hypertension (PPH), a condition that affects the heart and lungs. Throughout my childhood and adolescence, my PPH didn't cause any real problems. It was when I got married, at age 21, and wanted to start a family that it affected me the most.

People with PPH aren't supposed to get pregnant — and there's a good reason for that. Women who have PPH and get pregnant face a 70 percent risk of death during pregnancy.

Clearly, my husband and I weren't going to play the odds. Still, having a family was important to us. So four years after we got married, we decided to look into adoption. We had just started the process of applying to an agency when my mother approached us with another possibility.

Susie: I'd been watching a talk show on TV, and the guest was a woman who had served as the gestational carrier for her daughter, meaning that the mother had carried her daughter's baby in her uterus. I thought, I wonder if I could do that for Ashley?

I didn't want to get their hopes up or offer something that I couldn't do, so I talked to my doctor first. I asked, "Am I crazy to think this could work?"

My doctor didn't see a reason why it couldn't. Neither did our local OB-GYN. That's when I mentioned the idea to Ashley. I told her to take her time and talk it over with her husband. I told her that she wouldn't hurt my feelings if they

said no. But I also said, "Why don't you let me do this for you?"

Ashley: I told her she was crazy! She was pushing 50, and I thought she was too old for that. At the same time, I was excited. It took some debating — and some convincing when it came to my husband. It's a little awkward for your mother-in-law to carry your child. But, he, too, really wanted his own, biological child, if possible. We knew that it might not work, but that can happen with adoption, too. We decided to go for it.

Our doctor in Iowa, where we lived, arranged for us to see a reproductive specialist two hours away. They explained that my mom would carry the embryo from my egg and my husband's sperm so that the baby would be biologically ours. My mom would essentially be the vessel that carried it.

The process is long. Nine months before the embryo transfer to my mom, we had many appointments. We all had to go through infectious disease testing, psych evaluations and counseling. My mom and I both had to get hormone shots at regular intervals. For me, the shots helped boost egg production so there would be more eggs to retrieve. For my mom, the shots helped prepare her uterus for the transfer and, ultimately, to carry a baby. Sometimes this preparation was tiring or painful, but it was all worth it: The pregnancy was a success on our first try.

Susie: It was pretty amazing. It really was. I might've been more tired than when I was pregnant with my own children at age 20, but otherwise the pregnancy wasn't any harder than what I remembered.

It actually might've been harder on my husband who was concerned about both of us. He was worried that I was too old to carry this baby, and that something could happen to me. And he was worried about the drugs Ashley would have to take to donate eggs, and about her being heartbroken if this didn't work.

And then, of course, there was the social part of it — his 49-year-old wife being pregnant. In our small community, people know us and they understood what we were doing. But outside of our town, people probably wondered what the heck was going on!

Ashley: All four of us — my mom and dad, my husband and I — were in the delivery room when our little girl, Harper, was born. It happened so quickly: We hit the labor and delivery area, and within 40 minutes Harper was born. It was so emotional for all of us. My dad, who was standing next to my mom, had to ask three times whether we'd had a boy or a girl!

The experience was truly amazing. We had waited so long to get to that point, and it just felt like a dream come true. I felt so grateful.

The nurse said, "Who wants to hold her first?" And I said, "Mom, do you?" She answered, "No, I just want to see her in your arms."

Susie: When Harper was just over a year old, we decided to try again. That time it didn't work. The transfer didn't result in a pregnancy. It was hard to go through the process and not get a baby out of it. We always said that we would "expect the best and prepare for the worst," but when it happened, there was definite heartache.

Ashley: We were sad, and we spent our time mourning. But we tried again — and now we're expecting twins in about six weeks. The pregnancy is going wonderfully. Our babies are due two days before Harper turns 2, and just days before my mom turns 52. I think these will probably be our last children, but I don't know. We'll see how these twins wear me out!

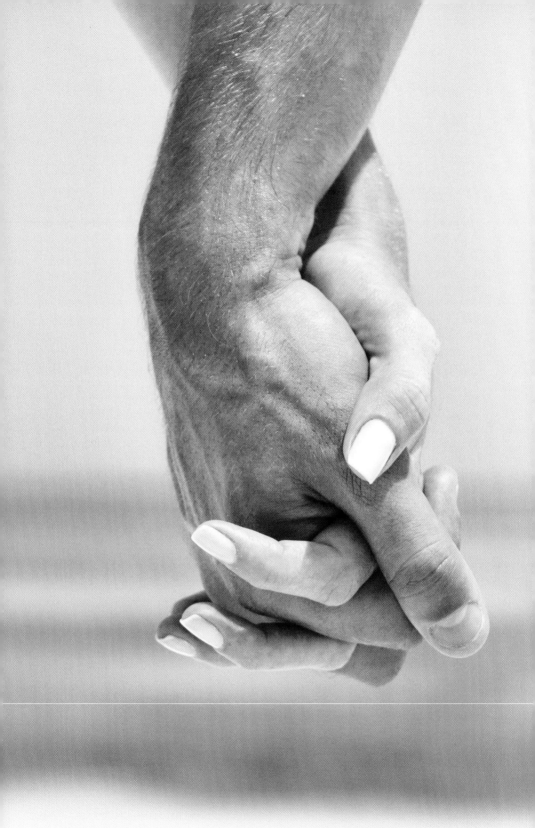

CHAPTER 17

Coping and support

If you're in the midst of treatment for fertility problems, you probably don't need a bunch of medical studies and research to tell you that infertility can be very stressful. You're likely all too familiar with the emotional roller coaster that repeats every month — from hope and anticipation that you might be pregnant to disappointment, grief and anger when you're not. You may also experience feelings of loss, denial, shock, numbness, guilt and shame.

All of these feelings are normal. Treatment for infertility is physically, emotionally and financially exhausting. Not to mention time-consuming! Still, it's important not to let infertility consume your entire life. (Read that last sentence again. Slowly.)

How do you do that? Start by learning more about the sources of stress that are associated with fertility treatments so that you can understand what you're feeling. Honor these feelings and acknowledge that they're real. Then, experiment with different coping techniques that help you keep these feelings in balance.

Also don't be afraid to let your care providers and others know how you're feeling, and talk about what generally works best for you to relieve stress. Remember that there isn't a one-size-fits-all solution. Some of the things your care providers may do or suggest are designed to decrease stress for most couples, but they could be the exact thing that drives you crazy. Similarly, friends or family members may say things that in a different context are fine, but when you're experiencing infertility, the words are painful. This is especially true, if you haven't shared your fertility problems with them.

It's also important not to forget the rest of your life — the rest of your relationships with your partner, your family and friends, and the rest of what's core to you being you. Hold on to normalcy as much as possible as you go through the treatment process. Give yourself a break by doing things you enjoy.

STRESS AND INFERTILITY

Research shows that many women who are being treated for infertility experience as much stress as women who have cancer or heart disease. And women don't suffer alone.

Infertility is associated with significant distress, anxiety and depression for both men and women who are trying to conceive. Stress and anxiety usually increase throughout the course of each menstrual cycle, peaking as you wait to hear the results of that month's attempt at conception. This peak can set you up for great elation or great disappointment and grief.

If you don't become pregnant, the stress cycle repeats again the following month. And you don't know how it will end or when it will end. Sometimes, you don't even have any clear answers about what's going wrong. The whole cycle is fraught with uncertainty and unpredictability that you simply can't control.

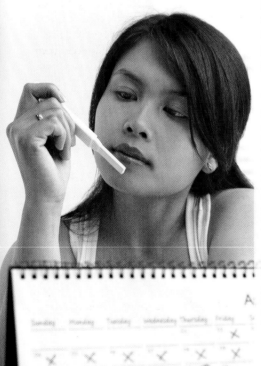

It's normal to experience very high emotions throughout this process. Give yourself space to grieve or swear or stomp or cry — whatever feels right to you. Allow yourself to feel whatever you're feeling. There is a tendency to underestimate the stress that's caused by infertility, rather than accepting it and facing it head-on.

Causes of stress Struggling to have a baby is a big deal. Try to resist the urge to minimize or hide your feelings. There are many very real causes of stress and anxiety that are inherent in infertility:

Physical discomfort. Diagnosis and treatment procedures for fertility problems can be long, intrusive, embarrassing and, frankly, not so pleasant. Common medications and procedures can cause physical pain, cramps, fatigue, bloating, muscle tension, a change in appetite or mood swings. All of these physical side effects of treatment can be grueling, especially when treatment lasts for many months. Women are usually more physically involved in reproductive technologies, so they may feel greater physical stress than do their partners.

Time burden. Diagnosis and treatment of fertility problems require a high level of participation from you and your partner. From ovulation testing and semen samples to injections and timed sex to egg retrievals and embryo transfers, there's a lot of time and effort that goes into fertility treatment. You are truly working to have a baby.

One study estimates that couples spend an average of 125 hours pursuing care for fertility problems, with some spending well over 160 hours. Not surprisingly, stress seems to rise as time spent on fertility care increases.

This is partly because dedicating time to fertility treatments can disturb your daily routines and intrude on important relationships. You may have to skip lunch with your girlfriends to go to a doctor's appointment. You may miss your favorite exercise class or a family get-together on the evening of a scheduled injection or procedure. You may fall behind on work projects and assignments or be unable to travel for work due to your treatments. All of these things can magnify your stress and anxiety and make it difficult for you to focus on anything else besides having a baby.

Financial drain. Fertility treatments can cost tens of thousands of dollars. Some couples have to scrape together their life savings for a chance at having a baby. Some couples can't afford as many chances as they want. If you're in this boat, a negative pregnancy test can be particularly nerve-racking.

Even if you can afford fertility treatments, knowing how much each attempt costs can add stress to the process. If you and your partner are arguing about how much money you should spend to have a baby, your disagreements can add even more tension.

Emotional loss. From a very young age, most people expect to start a career, get married, have children, retire and enjoy their retirement. When you discover that you can't have children without assistance, it can put a huge hitch in your entire life plan.

Being a parent is a very important role in our society. The threat that you may never achieve that role is no small thing. It can cause significant distress.

Infertility is really a loss. When you discover the loss of your fertility, you may also feel a loss of your plans and dreams for your future. And you may experience this loss every month, as you mourn the child you were so desperately hoping to meet. Some couples also experience miscarriage before or during fertility treatment.

All of these losses bring about a lot of grief and bereavement that isn't well understood in our society. It's common to receive bereavement cards and words of encouragement if you lose a relative or close friend, but people rarely realize the losses associated with infertility. Even those who understand this intangible loss may not know how to recognize it.

As a result, infertility can feel very lonely. This is especially true if you feel surrounded by friends, family members, co-workers and neighbors who all seem to be focused on children.

Sense of failure. If you always imagined that you'd have children, your inability to do so on your own may make you feel like a failure. Even worse, you may deal with this feeling month after month after month. And no matter how hard you work at it, you may not be able to fix the problem. If you're used to achieving success through your own hard work, your inability to control the outcome of this situation can be maddening.

Not being able to experience something that seems so natural can also feel shameful. You may feel inadequate or defective. You may question your masculinity or femininity. You may feel guilty that you aren't able to give your partner a baby or that you're being punished for something you did in the past. You may believe that you're failing your parents, in-laws and siblings, as well as yourself. These feelings can erode your self-esteem and cause great sadness or depression.

Relationship problems. If you and your partner deal with the stresses of infertility in different ways, it may cause you to grow apart, which can fuel the stress you're already feeling. In general, men and women tend to cope with fertility problems and treatment in different ways. Women tend to want to talk about their feelings — sometimes a lot! — and reach out to others for support. Men may not want to talk about the issues as much. Instead, they may channel their emotions into work or researching possible treatments and solutions.

Of course, the roles may be reversed, too. Every couple is different. Sometimes, the man is more vocal about his struggles, while his wife is quiet, private and less willing to discuss the situation.

No matter what the case, different ways of coping can lead to conflict. For example, you may argue over an invitation to a good friend's baby shower, if one person wants to get out of the house and forget about infertility for a bit, while the other is too upset and emotional to attend.

Infertility can also affect your sex life. When you're focused on having a baby, sex can seem like a chore, rather than a flirty, fun rendezvous. Ovulation kits and semen samples aren't so sexy either. Some couples lose their interest in sex during fertility treatments. Sexual dysfunction also is common. Either way, problems in the bedroom can put a wedge between you and your partner that adds to the stress on your relationship.

Your quest to become pregnant can also take a toll on other relationships. If you're spending a lot of time on fertility treatments, you may naturally spend less time with family and friends. Or you may intentionally avoid siblings and friends who are pregnant if it's too painful to be around them. You may also be dealing with family members or friends who make hurtful comments or don't agree

SYMPTOMS OF STRESS

Even if you don't feel stressed or anxious, you may be experiencing the physical effects of infertility stress. These include:

 ▶ Lack of energy
 ▶ Headaches
 ▶ Irritability
 ▶ Insomnia or difficulty sleeping
 ▶ Inability to concentrate
 ▶ Extreme sadness

If you experience any of these common signs and symptoms — especially on the day of a doctor's appointment or when you know you're going to see a pregnant friend or after an unsuccessful treatment cycle — you may need to focus on coping techniques.

When you're in the throes of artificial hormones and stimulated treatment cycles, it can be difficult to identify what you're really feeling — and why. Try to stay in touch with your body and look for signs of stress. Then you can do something about it.

WHEN TO SEEK HELP

Chronic stress can put your health at risk. If you can't stop thinking about having a baby or talking about having a baby, you may be constantly activating your body's stress-response system — constantly revving up your body's adrenaline and cortisol levels, your heart rate and your blood pressure. This can put you at increased risk of health problems. It may be time to talk to a counselor about how you can better manage your stress.

It's also possible to become depressed while undergoing fertility treatment. This is especially true if you've been treated for depression previously or have a family history of depression.

If you feel as if your emotions are careening out of control, it's important to seek treatment. High emotions are a common part of fertility treatment, but if your emotions are keeping you from going to work or participating in regular activities, you may benefit from discussing your feelings with a counselor. Your fertility clinic may have a psychologist on staff that specializes in fertility counseling. Or your care provider may be able to refer you to someone in your area.

Be sure to seek help if:

▶ You're consumed by the idea of having a baby
▶ You're consumed by anger, guilt or shame that you can't have a baby
▶ Your anxiety or stress is interfering with your relationships or your ability to participate in your regular activities
▶ You have strong emotions all the time, not just during stressful times of your treatment cycle
▶ You feel sad or unhappy most of the time
▶ You're often irritable or frustrated, even over small matters
▶ You experience loss of interest or pleasure in normal activities

If you're experiencing an extremely high level of stress or anxiety, you may need to take a break from the fertility process. You can always pick up where you left off.

---

with your treatment choices. All of these changes in your social circle can weaken your support network, which can be another source of stress.

The bottom line is that infertility is very stressful for very good reasons. The physical, emotional and financial burden can be almost overwhelming. It's important to recognize this challenge and seek out ways to cope.

Sexual dysfunction It's common for men and women to experience sexual problems during fertility treatment. And it's really no wonder.

The constant focus on making a baby instead of making love can zap your passion and pleasure. Months of forced timing — dictated by menstrual cycles and medication schedules — don't help either.

Many couples report that sex becomes mechanical, purposeful and robotic during diagnosis and treatment. If you and your partner are fighting or growing apart, your emotional distance can also contribute to problems in the bedroom.

For all of these reasons, you may experience low libido, low satisfaction during sex, trouble becoming aroused or trouble achieving orgasm. Infertility is also associated with erectile dysfunction. These sexual side effects of fertility treatment can be embarrassing and frustrating, particularly if they occur on a fertile day or a day when you need to produce a semen sample.

The good news is that these sexual problems are usually temporary. Most couples resume a healthy sex life when fertility treatment is over.

However, you may need to work with your doctor or a counselor to overcome these issues during treatment. There are also coping techniques that can help mend strife in your personal and sexual relationship.

COPING TECHNIQUES

Experiment with different coping techniques and stress management strategies to see what works best for you. Support groups aren't for everyone. Neither is journaling or yoga. Every couple's formula for coping with stress is unique.

Moderate exercise is good for improving your mood, but remember that vigorous exercise can be a double-edged sword when it comes to fertility and conception.

Try out a few different coping techniques and see what sticks. If you don't like a particular technique, ask yourself why. Try to learn from your experience and move on.

The techniques that work best for you may depend on the sources of your stress. For example, if you're experiencing a lot of physical stress or discomfort, relaxation techniques are a good bet (see page 23). If you're having relationship troubles,

you might need to prioritize solutions that involve your partner.

In general, try to focus on the things you can control — and how you react to the things you can't control. Put your trust in your fertility team to handle the rest.

Support groups and counseling

There's good evidence that social support can help reduce the stress and anxiety associated with infertility. If you have a core group of friends and family members who understand and support you, that's great. But many couples benefit from connecting with other couples that are struggling with infertility.

A professional- or peer-led infertility support group may help you feel less lonely and isolated and help validate your feelings. A support group can also provide valuable information and real-life experience when you're facing a difficult decision or looking at new parenting options.

You don't have to share the intimate details of your sex life with a group of strangers if you choose to try a support group. You can decide exactly how much information you're comfortable sharing with the group. Whether you choose to open up or not, you may benefit from the stories, experience and empathy of others who understand what you're going through.

Your doctor may be able to refer you to a group in your area. You may also be able to find Resolve support groups, offered by The National Infertility Association, in your area (see page 274). The association also offers online support groups.

Try not to judge a group based on one meeting. It often takes a few meetings to relax and feel at ease. You may also need to try a few groups before you find one that's right for you. It's important to connect with the group leader and the other participants. You'll naturally gel with some groups more than others.

Other coping techniques Most couples rely on a combination of coping techniques to help them get through the stress of infertility. If you already have some stress-busting strategies that work for you, keep them up. Consider adding others, as needed.

Read up on infertility. For some people, knowledge really is power. If you're one of them, do your research. Ask your care provider if you need help finding reliable sources of information on infertility.

Understanding the nitty-gritty details about your particular diagnosis and treatment options may help you feel more in control and more prepared to make good decisions. Knowing the facts can also help you evaluate advice from others and educate your loved ones about your situation.

Talk it out. Set up weekly meetings with your partner. It can be over Wednesday night dinner or Saturday morning coffee or a Sunday afternoon bike ride. Use this time to discuss how things are going and how you feel. Make up your minds on important decisions. Review any upcoming milestones, appointments or schedules. It's important that you and your partner stay on the same page about your infertility.

Having a weekly meeting about infertility is particularly helpful for couples with differing views on how much they want to talk about their infertility. A dedicated meeting provides a clear opportunity for the person who wants to talk to do so. He or she can look forward to the opportunity and plan the agenda. For the

person who doesn't like to dwell in discussion, a dedicated meeting time means that infertility talk is limited to one time of the week. Then, he or she doesn't have to worry about the constant threat of a lengthy discussion throughout the rest of the week.

Recognize your different coping styles. Every person copes with difficult circumstances in his or her own way. It's important for you and your partner to acknowledge your differences in coping and to find ways of supporting one another.

Take the example of the person who doesn't like to talk about infertility issues. If that's your partner, you may think his closed mouth is a sign of callousness. You may assume he isn't bothered by infertility if he doesn't want to talk about it. However, if you take the time to understand his coping preferences, you may learn that talking about the situation all the time makes him feel like a failure. He prefers to focus on the future, and it's difficult for him to do when you want to re-hash last month's treatment.

Rather than trying to get your partner to cope in the same way that you do, give him permission to cope in his own way. Figure out what works best for both of you, and talk about it candidly. Don't expect your partner to be able to comfort you without some instruction. You may also need to look outside your relationship for solace, and that's OK. Remember, it may be the differences between you and your partner that attracted you to each other at the start of your relationship.

If you really need to talk about your feelings, for example, it may be helpful for you to meet with a support group, a counselor or a good friend on a regular basis. Your partner may not be able to handle your drawn-out deliberations, but he or she can understand how important this is to you and prioritize your time to talk with others. Perhaps the two of you can meet afterwards for a long walk or some ice cream — and you can vow to talk about other things.

Rekindle your romance. Find something to do with your partner that doesn't involve sex. At the end of the day, if your treatments don't work, you will still have each other. So it's important to stay connected and keep enjoying one another.

Buy tickets to a concert. Play tennis. Go canoeing. Book a table at your favorite restaurant. Make a special meal at home. Hold hands. Take an impromptu trip out of town. Stay up late playing board games. Drink coffee and discuss the Sunday paper.

After you've spent some time reviving your relationship outside the bedroom, bring the sexy back. Kiss. Give your partner a massage. Have sex at least once a month when there's no chance of creating a baby — just for the opportunity to be intimate and affectionate.

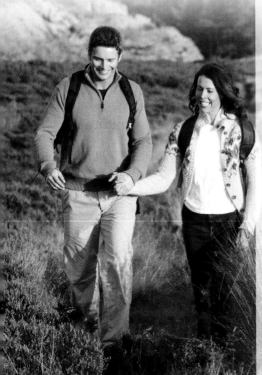

Learn stress-reduction techniques. This includes practices such as meditation, guided imagery or deep breathing. When practiced regularly, relaxation techniques can reverse your stress response, reduce your heart rate, lower your muscle tension and help you focus your thoughts on the present moment. You can perform these techniques with an instructor as part of a yoga or meditation class. Or you can learn these techniques on your own with an online class or demo. Experiment with different techniques to see which are most comfortable for you. Then use them regularly. For more information on relaxation techniques, see page 23.

Be honest with family and friends. Your inner circle may not know a lot about infertility. You may need to explain what you're going through, so they can commiserate with you and prop you up during difficult times.

You don't have to provide a play-by-play of your diagnosis and treatments. Tell your friends and family members whatever you want them to know. Then, explain how stressful it is and how they can help. Let them know if you're looking for advice and recommendations or just reassurance and encouragement. Tell them if you're sensitive about certain topics, if you want to talk about your struggles or if you'd prefer to banter about other things.

If a well-meaning friend or family member isn't providing the support you need, let him or her know. Distance yourself from that relationship for a little while if it's causing you a great deal of stress. People who've never struggled with infertility are sometimes critical or hurtful without realizing it.

Avoid difficult situations. If you find it difficult to be around painful reminders of your infertility, such as attending a baby shower or having dinner with kids at a friend's house, give yourself permission to stay away. Be honest about your feelings, if you're comfortable doing so.

This can be particularly difficult if the event involves a dear friend. Tell her you're really happy for her. Explain that you're trying really hard to have a baby and it's difficult to be around reminders that it's not working. Let her know that you may not be around for a little while, while you figure things out, but your absence isn't a reflection on your relationship.

Think about how you can sustain important relationships while avoiding painful situations. Try scheduling a coffee date or movie night if you turn down a shower or dinner invitation. That way, you can stay connected without putting yourself in an uncomfortable situation.

Keep a journal. Writing about your emotions and experiences can help you process them. Putting your struggles on the page may also help you see patterns in your stress level and uncover insights you didn't recognize before. You can keep your journal to yourself or share important ideas and entries with your partner or care provider.

Give yourself a break. If you're trying to become pregnant, you may be cautious about lifestyle habits that could affect your baby. You may be vigilant about everything you eat and drink. In theory, this is a good idea. But it may be unsustainable month after month. You don't have to turn yourself into a martyr. You can't beat yourself up for every cup of coffee or glass of wine you drink.

Be kind to yourself. Take time to focus on everyday activities that you enjoy. Keep your life as normal as possible, amid the chaos that you're feeling. It won't last forever.

Q. CAN STRESS AFFECT FERTILITY TREATMENT SUCCESS?

A. *If you would just relax, you would get pregnant. If you would just stop worrying about having a baby, it would happen.*

If you've ever heard this type of "advice" from a well-meaning family member, friend or acquaintance, you may wonder if it's true. (You might even worry about this, if you weren't worried about worrying.)

The truth is that stress alone doesn't cause infertility, although there's some evidence that lower stress levels may increase natural fertility.

But what about fertility treatments? Can stress affect your chances of a successful IVF cycle? More than a dozen studies have attempted to answer this question with mixed results. Some research shows that high stress levels may be associated with lower pregnancy rates. Other research shows no significant effect.

In the end, no one can guarantee you that practicing stress-reduction techniques will up your chances of having a baby. But learning to cope with the stress of infertility will surely make you feel better, and it may improve your relationship with your partner.

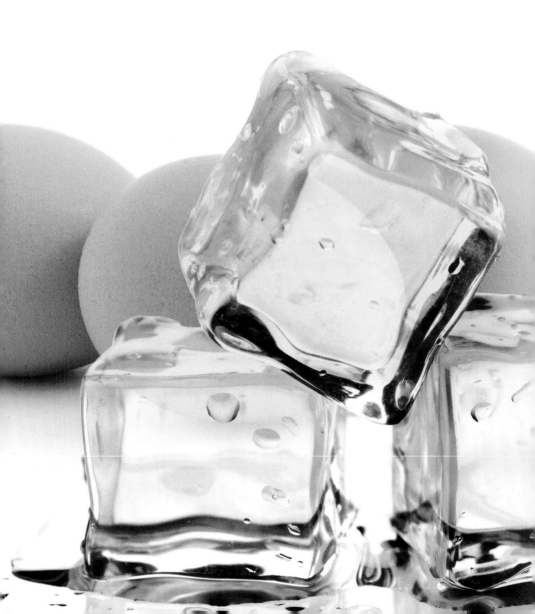

PART 5

Special Considerations

CHAPTER 18

Fertility preservation

Sometimes an event can occur in a person's life that may jeopardize his or her future fertility. Perhaps this has happened to you. You hope to one day have children and raise a family, or maybe to have more children, but a health condition such as cancer has you wondering if your dreams are at risk. Fortunately, there are ways to preserve your fertility and keep your hopes of future parenthood alive.

It's not uncommon if you have a serious health condition to learn that some of the therapies to treat the illness could possibly leave you infertile. Treatment of certain cancers is the most common example. Fortunately, before treatment begins, steps can often be taken to preserve your eggs or your partner's sperm, making it possible for you to become a biological parent after your treatment — or your partner's — is complete. This is known as fertility preservation.

Advances in assisted reproductive technology, such as embryo cryopreservation and in vitro fertilization, have made fertility preservation possible. And it's not just for individuals facing a health crisis that steps to preserve fertility are considered. Fertility preservation is increasingly being used by women wanting to have a family, but at a later point in their lives — such as when their careers are on track or they feel they're ready for motherhood.

REASONS FOR FERTILITY PRESERVATION

A new diagnosis of cancer is the most common reason for undergoing fertility preservation. This is because certain cancer treatments — mainly chemotherapy and radiation — can impair fertility to varying degrees. Fertility problems may be temporary or permanent, and they may occur immediately or at a later point in life.

Cancer Cancer-associated infertility may result from surgery to remove the cancer, as in the case of testicular or prostate cancer in men or ovarian cancer in women. Infertility may also be a side effect of cancer treatment. Chemotherapy medications and radiation treatment can both lead to infertility, depending upon the medications used or the location of the treatment.

Chemotherapy. The effects of chemotherapy on a man's or a woman's fertility depend on a variety of factors: the type of drug used, the dose, the type and extent of disease, and whether the drug was administered orally or intravenously.

Cancer drugs known as alkylating agents — including the medications ifosfamide, procarbazine, chlorambucil, cyclophosphamide, busulfan, carmustine and lomustine — and the drug cisplatin have been shown to be the most damaging. In women, the medication cyclophosphamide, which is used to treat breast cancer as well as leukemia and lymphoma, is a common source of fertility impairment. These medications may not destroy your fertility, but they can significantly reduce the odds of bearing healthy sperm or eggs.

The age at which a person receives chemotherapy is an important factor to be considered. Younger men seem to be somewhat protected from the toxic effects of chemotherapy on their sperm in comparison with older men. The same is true for women. Women younger than age 30 who receive chemotherapy are less likely to become infertile than are older women.

Other cancer medications. Hormone therapies used to treat certain cancers, including prostate cancer in men and breast cancer in women, can affect fertility. However, the effects are often reversible. Once the treatment is stopped, fertility may be restored.

The effects of newer cancer medications on fertility, such as cancer vaccines, immune therapies and biological response modifiers, aren't yet known.

Radiation. Radiation can be equally if not more damaging to fertility than chemotherapy. Research has shown it takes only small amounts of radiation to the male testes to have a negative impact on sperm health. Men most at risk of irreversible damage to their sperm-producing abilities include those being treated with radiation therapy for early-stage testicular cancer and those undergoing total body irradiation before a bone marrow or stem cell transplant.

For women, radiation therapy also has the potential to be more damaging to fertility than chemotherapy, depending on the location and size of the radiation field, the dose of radiation given, and the woman's age. Radiation is particularly toxic to immature egg cells in your ovaries (oocytes). It can also damage the uterus, putting you at risk of experiencing fetal growth restriction or preterm birth should you become pregnant after radiation treatment.

Other medical conditions Beyond cancer, other illnesses and their treatments also can impair fertility. Stem cell transplantation used to treat blood disorders such as thalassemia major, aplastic anemia, Fanconi anemia and myeloproliferative diseases can harm reproductive function.

In women, autoimmune diseases including diabetes mellitus, multiple sclerosis, thyroid dysfunction, Addison's disease, myasthenia gravis, Crohn's disease, lupus erythematosus, autoimmune thrombocytopenia and rheumatoid arthritis have all been associated with premature ovarian failure. Infertility may also result from the genetic abnormalities Turner's syndrome, trisomy X syndrome and fragile X syndrome.

Personal reasons Sometimes, women — and even some men — who are in good health will seek out fertility preservation. Why? They want to have children of their own some day, but they're not ready to do so right now — the timing isn't right. If this is the case for you, you may worry that when you have your education complete, your career in order or other aspects of your life in place, your biological clock may not be in your favor — you may be trying to have children too late in life. To increase the chances of having a biological child later on, a woman can take steps to preserve her eggs. So, too, a man can preserve his sperm.

Fertility preservation for personal reasons is more of an issue for women than for men. Unlike men who are continually producing sperm, women experience an age-related decline in the quantity and quality of their eggs. This decline makes conception and pregnancy more difficult with age. Infertility in women increases significantly after age 35. By age 45, upwards of 99 percent of women are infertile, whereas men can produce viable sperm much longer.

When fertility preservation is performed at a relatively early age, a woman may be able to beat these odds and become a biological mother later in life since the uterus can respond to hormones normally at any age.

SEEING A SPECIALIST

If you're in a situation where your fertility may be at risk and you're considering fertility preservation measures, one of the first steps you should take is to meet with a fertility specialist. During what may be an already trying time, a fertility specialist can help you understand your situation and your possible options. He or she can answer important questions to help lessen the uncertainty and stress. And he or she can serve as your fertility advocate in discussions and decisions regarding upcoming treatment.

Studies suggest that women with cancer are less likely to be given information about preserving their fertility than are men. If you would like to have children in the future, you may need to be the one who starts the conversation with your medical team.

If the medical center where you're receiving your care doesn't have a fertility specialist or reproductive endocrinologist, an obstetrician-gynecologist (OB-GYN) or oncologist can often help you with questions and decisions regarding fertility preservation or refer you to a center nearby for this special aspect of your care. This person will work with your existing medical team to help ensure your wants and needs are considered and implemented.

For women and men who want to delay pregnancy for personal reasons, a fertility specialist can review existing options and important factors to be considered.

OPTIONS FOR WOMEN

Women hoping to preserve their fertility have more options available to them than do men. If you're considering fertility preservation, the option you choose will depend on your individual situation, including the type of illness you may have, the recommended treatment and how quickly this treatment needs to occur. Discuss your options with your doctor before your treatment. In some cases, you and your doctor might decide to try more than one option.

Keep in mind that many fertility preservation procedures require additional steps later on in order for a woman to become pregnant, such as intrauterine insemination or in vitro fertilization and embryo transfer. These procedures are discussed in detail in Chapters 14 and 15.

It's important to remember, too, that you may become pregnant spontaneously, without the help of assisted reproductive technology. Some women and their partners do beat the odds, despite the threats to their fertility from their medical treatments.

Embryo cryopreservation Embryo cryopreservation is the most common and successful method of preserving a woman's fertility. It involves creating and freezing embryos to be implanted at a later date. Research shows that embryos can survive the freezing and thawing process up to 90 percent of the time. Successful pregnancy rates vary from one medical center to the next, but pregnancy rates have been reported to be as high as 60 percent in some studies, if multiple embryos are available. In fact, successful pregnancies have occurred in embryos that have been frozen for almost 20 years.

The process. Embryo cryopreservation involves stimulating a woman's ovaries to produce multiple eggs so that the mature eggs can be retrieved. In most

---

PRESERVING OVARIAN TISSUE

Researchers continue to look at different ways to preserve fertility. One procedure being evaluated is known as ovarian tissue freezing. In this procedure, all or part of an ovary is removed during minimally invasive surgery. The ovarian tissue is cut into small strips, frozen and stored. After a woman's treatment is complete, the tissue is thawed and transplanted back into the body, often near the fallopian tubes but occasionally in sites like the skin of the abdomen or even in the forearm.

Studies have shown the transplanted tissue can grow a new blood supply and produce hormones, but these ovarian tissue grafts may only last for a few months. In a few situations, the transplanted tissue was able to produce eggs, which were collected and fertilized in a lab.

So far, the process has produced very few live births, but researchers continue to study the approach to see if they can improve its success. Researchers are experimenting with laboratory techniques to get immature eggs in the ovarian tissue to fully mature and be capable of fertilization outside of the body.

For women with cancers that originate in the ovary or could spread to the ovaries, ovarian tissue freezing generally isn't an option. Because it involves surgery to remove the ovarian tissue, it may also not be an option for women who will be undergoing surgery as a part of their medical care. Some fertility centers don't want to subject these women to additional surgery.

women, this requires approximately two weeks, during which egg development may be monitored with vaginal ultrasounds and blood tests. Once mature, the eggs are removed, fertilized with sperm and kept in frozen storage. For more information on embryo cryopreservation, see Chapter 15.

Issues to consider. Although embryo cryopreservation is the most well-established means of fertility preservation for women, it does have some disadvantages. There's concern that some medications used to stimulate egg development may increase a woman's estrogen level, which could potentially impact estrogen-sensitive cancers. Doctors have responded to this concern with an ovarian stimulation regimen that includes estrogen lowering drugs known as aromatase inhibitors, and most oncologists feel comfortable with the short duration of stimulation even for estrogen-sensitive breast cancers. The levels of estrogen reached with fertility preservation procedures are low compared with the levels seen in normal pregnancy.

Another issue for some women is the need for sperm. For women who aren't in a relationship with a man or who don't want to use a sperm bank, embryo cryopreservation may not be a viable option. It can also be an emotionally difficult decision for a woman in a relationship in which she and her partner haven't committed to having children together and suddenly have to make a decision. Negotiating this difficult decision while undergoing medical treatment can be very stressful.

Oocyte cryopreservation Another method of fertility preservation that's becoming more common involves freezing a woman's eggs (oocytes) rather than

embryos. The process of egg stimulation and retrieval is similar to that of embryo cryopreservation. The difference is the eggs aren't fertilized before they're frozen.

Issues to consider. Oocyte cryopreservation offers some major advantages over embryo cryopreservation. Most importantly, it doesn't require a male partner or a sperm donor. It also avoids the problem of what to do with excess frozen embryos once the number of pregnancies you desire have been achieved.

On the downside, human eggs don't survive freezing as well as human embryos do. While human eggs are very different from chicken eggs, the two resemble each other in certain respects. They're both very big and specialized, containing not only the same amount of DNA as sperm but many other components that the embryo uses for early development. Because eggs contain a lot of water, they're prone to damage from ice crystal formation. The machinery that helps cells divide (mitotic spindle) also may be damaged during the freezing process.

So, just like it would be difficult to freeze a chicken egg by itself, but easy to freeze a cake or cookies in which parts of the egg have been transformed, it's more difficult to freeze and thaw a human egg compared with freezing an embryo.

However, the process continues to evolve and improve. In the near future, the survival rate for frozen oocytes may resemble that of frozen embryos.

Radiation shielding Radiation to a woman's ovaries can result in infertility. For this reason, women who need to undergo radiation to their abdomen or pelvis to treat cancer or another illness may have the option of radiation shielding, also known as gonadal shielding. In this procedure, small lead shields are placed over the ovaries to reduce the amount of radiation exposure they receive.

Radiation shielding can be successful for some women, but it has limitations. It generally works best in women whose radiation field — the area to receive radiation — is farther away from the ovaries. And it requires expertise to ensure the shielding doesn't interfere with getting sufficient radiation delivery to affected areas.

Ovarian transposition Some women facing a cancer diagnosis may receive radiation therapy as part of their treatment but not chemotherapy. Or, they may be given chemotherapy in addition to radiation, but not the type of chemotherapy that's harmful to fertility. These women may be candidates for a fertility-preserving surgical procedure known as ovarian transposition, or oophoropexy.

The process. With this procedure, the ovaries are surgically repositioned in the pelvis so they're out of the radiation field when radiation is delivered to the pelvic area. After treatment, the ovaries are left in their new position; they're not repositioned unless a woman has trouble conceiving. Ovarian transposition may be an option for some gynecologic cancers requiring radiation therapy, as well as for spinal, colon, rectal and anal cancers.

Ovarian transposition can be performed with one large abdominal incision (laparotomy), but laparoscopic surgery is generally the preferred option because it has fewer complications and a shorter healing time. This often means that doctors can begin radiation therapy for the underlying cancer more quickly. Radiation therapy may begin within just a day or two after laparoscopic surgery. In fact, the shorter the time between the surgical procedure and radiation therapy, the lower the chances that the ovaries will migrate back into the pelvic radiation field.

When performed properly, ovarian transposition can reduce by up to 95 percent the amount of radiation exposure the ovaries receive. In addition, studies show that ovarian function remains intact after transposition in 60 to 89 percent of women under age 40 with cancer. When the procedure isn't successful, it's most often due to scatter radiation that reaches the repositioned ovaries, damage to the blood vessels that supply the ovaries or high doses of radiation.

Issues to consider. As with other preservation options, ovarian transposition does have drawbacks. It's not a good option for women older than age 40. Older women are already at high-risk of ovarian failure and ovarian transposition only increases the risk. Ovarian transposition can also cause ovarian dysfunction leading to ovarian cysts. In addition, because the ovaries are repositioned within the pelvic area, it can be difficult for a doctor to detect ovarian cancer when examining the pelvis.

Conization and radical trachelectomy
For women facing a diagnosis of cervical cancer, treatment most often is surgery to remove the cancer as well as a hysterectomy. Depending on the location and stage of the cancer and how much tissue needs to be removed, treatment typically leaves a woman infertile. For some women with small, localized tumors, it may be possible to preserve fertility, especially if the cancer is in the early stages. The goal, if possible, is to leave the uterus intact so that the woman can carry a pregnancy.

The process. During a procedure called cervical conization, a large cone-shaped section of the cervix, including the cancerous area, is removed, leaving the remainder of the cervix and the uterus intact. This is generally an option only for women with the earliest type of cervical cancer. In a similar type of surgery, called radical trachelectomy, a surgeon either partially or completely removes the cervix and the connective tissues next to the uterus and cervix known as the parametria.

Radical trachelectomy is moderately successful at preserving fertility. Reports put the incidence of infertility after vaginal radical trachelectomy at between 14 and 41 percent. Of pregnancies that result after a radical trachelectomy, about two out of three are successful. Cancer recurrence after the procedure is similar to that following a radical hysterectomy.

Issues to consider. Radical trachelectomy does have several potential side effects, including chronic vaginal discharge, irregular bleeding or absence of menstrual periods, deep menstrual cramps, and erosion of the opening made to replace the cervix. Both radical trachelectomy and conization can lead to cervical narrowing. Surgery may also impair a woman's ability to form an adequate mucous plug or have the cervix remain closed during pregnancy, putting mother and baby at risk of infection or premature labor.

It's recommended women who have conization wait two to three months before attempting to become pregnant. After radical trachelectomy, you should wait at least six, preferably 12, months. Because of the higher risk of complications associated with such pregnancies, it's recommended you seek care from a maternal-fetal medicine specialist. Babies born after radical trachelectomy are generally delivered via cesarean section. This is because a tear in the surgically altered cervix during a vaginal delivery could cause massive bleeding.

OPTIONS FOR MEN

A man faced with a medical condition that could affect his ability to father children in the future generally has two options for preserving his fertility: sperm freezing (cryopreservation) and gonadal shielding. Gonadal shielding is a procedure to protect the testicles against the harmful effects of radiation therapy.

Sperm cryopreservation In a process similar to freezing female eggs, male sperm can be frozen and stored at a fertility clinic or sperm bank for use at a later date. Sperm cryopreservation is a fairly easy and successful procedure that's routinely offered to younger men before they go through cancer treatment. But it's an option for any man facing a threat to his fertility who thinks he might want children in the future, but isn't sure. By storing his sperm, he doesn't have to make the decision now. He can decide later. Samples can be stored for years, even decades, and can still yield viable sperm. If the sample isn't used, it can be discarded or donated for research.

The process. Masturbation is the most frequently used method for gathering a semen sample for cryopreservation. The sample is generally collected in a private room at a fertility clinic or sperm bank. It's often recommended that men provide three samples, each collected about 48 hours apart. Results generally indicate that sperm counts are improved if the samples are gathered at least two days apart. However, samples can be collected closer together if necessary. Before providing a semen sample, a man may be asked to abstain from sexual activity that involves ejaculation for at least two days, but not more than five days.

For men facing cancer treatment, sperm is often collected as soon as possible so that treatment can begin. It's also essential the collection be done before beginning any therapy that could potentially damage sperm, such as radiation or chemotherapy. Even a single treatment session can compromise sperm DNA.

Men who are unable or unwilling to masturbate may use a special nontoxic condom to collect semen during sexual intercourse. Commercially available condoms sold in stores can't be used because they contain chemicals that kill sperm.

For men who have problems ejaculating semen naturally, there are several options. One is penile vibratory stimulation, which involves placing a vibrator on the head of the penis, resulting in ejaculation. In a procedure called electroejaculation, a probe that generates electrical impulses to stimulate ejaculation is placed in the rectum. Sperm can also be obtained directly from testicular tissue using a technique called testicular sperm extraction (TESE). The procedure is generally performed in an office setting with local anesthesia.

The collected sperm are evaluated in a laboratory and frozen. A fertility doctor will review your results and provide you with preservation options. The options depend on how much sperm is frozen and whether you and your partner have other infertility risk factors. When you're ready, the sperm are thawed and placed into a female partner during intrauterine insemination or used as part of in vitro fertilization. In general, pregnancy rates involving sperm that have been frozen and preserved are comparable to pregnancy rates achieved with use of fresh sperm, although pregnancy rates for individual cycles are often higher with fresh sperm than with frozen.

Before recent advances in assisted reproductive technology, sperm banking was considered an option only among men with normal sperm counts. Today, with the advent of intracytoplasmic sperm injection (ICSI), conception is possible using a single sperm that's injected into an egg. This makes sperm cryopreservation a viable option even for men with extremely low sperm counts.

Issues to consider. Similar to embryo and egg freezing, sperm banking can be expensive. However, it's much less expensive than the fertility options for women because there are no medications involved and only minimal laboratory use. If you're concerned about the costs, compare plans at different centers and check if your insurance will cover some of the expense. Many sperm banks offer financing and payment plans for cancer patients.

Radiation shielding Men who need to undergo radiation therapy to the pelvic area to treat cancer, especially testicular cancer, may opt for gonadal shielding of their testicles to help preserve their fertility. The shields reduce the amount of radiation delivered to the testicles. Gonadal shielding may also be used in other situations involving radiation to the pelvis, including treatment for prostate cancer, bladder cancer or certain types of colon cancer.

LOOKING FORWARD

If you're facing cancer or another illness that could jeopardize your fertility, the good news is that in many cases you can still become a biological parent once your treatment is complete. It might not happen the way you had planned, but if you can be flexible, you'll find there are options open to you.

If you're thinking about fertility preservation because you're not ready to become a parent yet but you want to have the option in the future, you can also take comfort in knowing help is available.

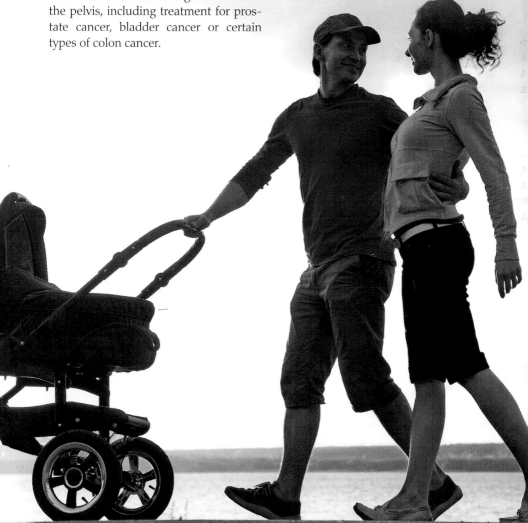

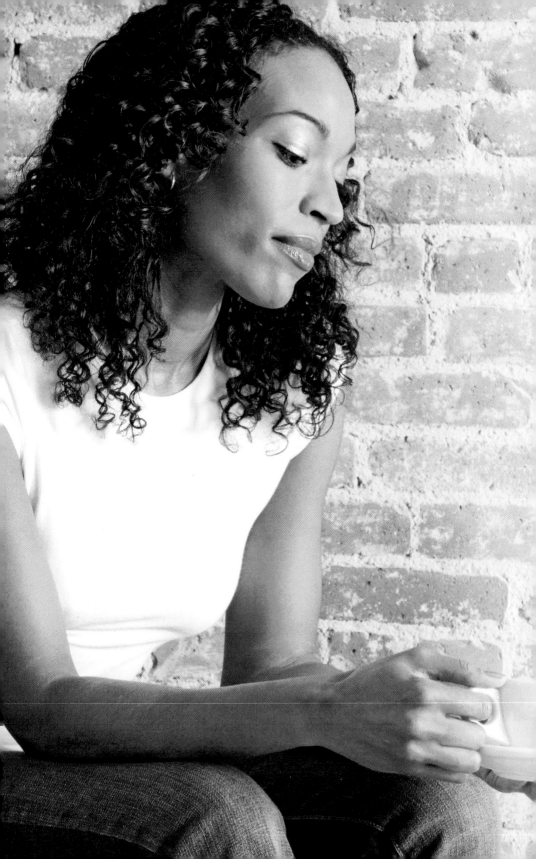

CHAPTER 19

Unique circumstances

Perhaps you're a single woman or man who feels a strong desire to have a baby but aren't in a committed relationship. Or maybe you're part of a lesbian or a gay couple and yearning to start a family of your own. If so, you're in good company. Today's families are not one size fits all. They encompass an evolving and diverse array of possibilities, all of which can successfully support and nurture a child. At the same time, modern medical practices have opened the door to single individuals and same-sex couples who may not have had the option of starting a family in the past.

Regardless of your particular circumstances, your success as a parent will have less to do with your family structure or sexual orientation and more to do with the nurturing relationship you create with your child. Your child's emotional, physical, and psychological health will be closely linked to your sense of competency and security as a parent, your financial stability, and your access to a supportive social network.

CHOOSING SINGLE PARENTHOOD

The past three decades in the United States have seen an increase in the number of children living in single-parent households. While some of these mothers and fathers may not have planned to be single parents, others made an intentional decision to have a child on their own.

Single parents by choice often come to parenthood later in life, and the number of older single parents in the United States is growing. While teenage single mothers are decreasing, more women age 35 and older are having children outside of marriage. In fact, in 2010, 1 in 5 births to women age 30 and older in the United States were to unmarried women. Figures representing single fathers by choice are harder to come by, but evidence points toward a growing trend.

As a single parent, you're likely to face the same joys and struggles as any other new parent, married or otherwise. But parenting a newborn on your own presents its own set of challenges, not the least of which is the fact that nearly all parenting responsibilities rest ultimately on the physical, mental, emotional and financial resources of one person: you.

Issues to consider If you're thinking about becoming a single parent by choice, you're probably asking yourself a lot of questions about whether single parenthood is right for you. That's a good thing. Taking time to carefully explore your hopes and fears will help you make this potentially life-changing decision. Before setting off on the path to pregnancy, review these key questions:

▶ *Have you considered both the advantages and disadvantages of raising a child alone?* Take the time to think through the positives and negatives of raising a child on your own. It can be helpful to talk to other single parents to get a realistic picture of single parenthood. For example, as a single parent, you will be empowered to raise your child based on your values and principles, without having to make compromises with a partner. On the other hand, you won't have the input of another person when it comes to difficult child-rearing decisions.

▶ *Can you afford to raise a child on your own?* The costs associated with conceiving and having a baby as a single woman or man can be considerable. And once your baby is born, you'll be the sole provider for yourself and your child. Make sure you understand the financial investment involved, and assess whether you are in a secure enough place in your life and career to meet those financial needs.

▶ *Do you have a solid social network?* As a single parent, there will be times when you'll need to lean on others for support, both for yourself and your child. Having a strong social network is essential. That network could consist of friends, siblings and other family members. It can also include other single parents. Make a list of all the people in your life who might be able to offer support. Take time to get to know your neighbors, join a religious community or participate in groups dedicated to single parents.

▶ *Have you come to terms with your current situation?* In the past, you may have dreamed of getting married before starting a family. Are you ready to move forward knowing that you're letting go of some of your dreams? By the same token, have you taken the time to examine why you want to be a single parent? What experiences in your life have led you to make this decision?

▶ *Are you prepared for possible judgment by others?* It's possible that some people will be critical of your decision to become a single parent by choice, or they may not understand why you've decided to take such a step. Maintaining a positive and confident attitude in the face of such criticism will benefit you and your child.

REPRODUCTION OPTIONS

Whether you're a single woman or man or part of a same-sex couple, having a baby is well within your reach. The path you choose will depend on your personal preferences and circumstances. Here are some choices to consider.

Women without a male partner As a single woman or a lesbian couple, your options for getting pregnant will likely involve donor sperm and intrauterine insemination. Detailed information about donor sperm and insemination procedures can be found in Chapter 16.

Many women choose to work with sperm banks, which provide sperm from anonymous donors who are medically screened and tested for infectious disease that can be transmitted by insemination. Some women use sperm donated from a friend or family member that's screened in the same way through a fertility center.

Some women try to inseminate themselves on their own at home. We don't recommend home insemination, and we feel it's important to point out that recruiting a donor on your own or doing home insemination can bring into play a variety of legal, emotional, and medical considerations (see page 260).

There are several advantages to working with a fertility doctor to perform intrauterine insemination. A reproductive specialist can help you:

▶ *Find an appropriate donor.* Knowing the sperm donor's height and eye color is an obvious advantage, but figuring out if a particular donor's blood type or cytomegalovirus (CMV) status has implications for a healthy pregnancy is an area in which a fertility clinic has helpful expertise.

▶ *Identify other factors.* Lack of a male partner might not be the only concern when it comes to achieving pregnancy. Before you invest time and money

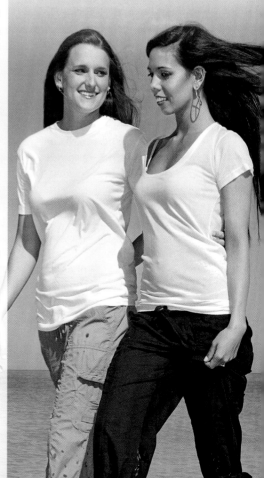

trying to get pregnant, it's important to identify any other potential roadblocks, such as a medical problem.

- *Track your fertility.* The simplest way to get pregnant using donor sperm is to track your fertility cycle, as described in Chapter 6. Once you reach your time of ovulation, your doctor can perform the insemination procedure at the clinic.

- *Increase your chances.* To increase your chances of getting pregnant, your doctor may suggest that you take one of several fertility medications. These medications stimulate your body to release multiple eggs at a time. An insemination procedure is more likely to result in at least one egg being fertilized, leading to a successful pregnancy.

- *Explore fertility treatment options.* Because many single women and lesbian couples choose to pursue pregnancy later in life, reduced fertility can sometimes be an issue. If insemination alone isn't leading to the results you're hoping for, don't lose heart. Depending on your situation, your doctor may recommend medication, surgery or assistive reproductive technology. These options are described in more depth in Chapters 14 and 15.

Men without a female partner Having a baby as a single man or a gay male couple can be a complicated undertaking, but it's entirely possible. It requires donated eggs and someone who will carry the baby to term (gestational carrier). Many men seek the help of a fertility clinic along with an egg donor and gestational carrier agency to guide them through the process. These agencies generally recommend that you work with two separate parties: an anonymous egg donor and a gestational carrier.

USING A KNOWN DONOR

For certain reasons, you may be considering using a known sperm or egg donor, perhaps a friend or relative. Before going this route, make sure to educate yourself about the potential risks involved. In particular, using a known donor can open up legal and emotional issues concerning parental rights that are not in play with an anonymous donor. If you go forward with a known donor, you'll want to work closely with an attorney who specializes in this area of reproductive law.

Single women or lesbian couples have the additional option of performing the insemination procedure at home without the involvement of a health care provider. If you're contemplating this do-it-yourself approach, be aware that this type of donor isn't required to undergo tests and screenings required by the Food and Drug Administration (FDA). In the United States, all anonymous sperm bank donors must be screened and tested for risk or evidence of communicable infections and diseases such as HIV and hepatitis B and C. Most sperm banks also conduct extensive genetic, medical and psychological screens and tests on donor candidates. A fertility clinic will likely conduct similar medical tests and screenings on known donors.

WHO WILL BE LISTED ON THE BIRTH CERTIFICATE?

This is a question single parents or couples often don't think about until they're facing the situation. Pregnancies involving donors or gestational carriers must take into account complex legal considerations, including parental rights. Laws regarding who will be listed on the birth certificate in these types of births vary from state to state. For that reason, it's essential that you work with an attorney who is knowledgeable about the reproductive laws in your state, in the state of your donor or gestational carrier, and in the state in which the baby is delivered. An attorney can also advise you on the necessary steps to be recognized as your baby's legal parent or guardian.

Unlike a surrogate, who both donates her own egg and carries the baby, a gestational carrier has no genetic relationship to the baby she is carrying. A clear division between egg donor and gestational carrier can avoid potential emotional and legal complications down the line. In this scenario, your sperm is used to fertilize an egg from an egg donor through the process of in vitro fertilization. The embryo that results is then implanted in another woman, a gestational carrier. Chapter 15 contains further information about in vitro fertilization. Detailed information about working with egg donors and gestational carriers can be found in Chapter 16.

Although using an anonymous egg donor from a donor agency is a common route to take, you may choose to use a known egg donor, such as a relative or friend. If you're considering this option, make sure to explore the legal, emotional, and medical considerations.

There are two options for selecting a gestational carrier. You can use the services of an agency that specializes in gestational care, or you can find a carrier independently, without the help of an agency. The independent approach often involves a friend or family member who acts as the gestational carrier. Having someone you know be the gestational carrier can significantly reduce the cost of having a baby, but it also places the burden of all financial, administrative, legal, and medical issues squarely on your shoulders. For that reason, the independent route is less commonly taken.

Same-sex couples If you're planning to have a baby as a couple, you'll be part of a growing number of lesbian and gay parents in the United States. In 2010, the U.S. Census Bureau reported that 646,464 households identified themselves as belonging to same-sex couples. Of those households, at least 115,000 reported raising one or more children.

A substantial number of lesbian and gay individuals who are single also are raising children. In all, it's estimated that nearly 2 million children in the United States are being raised by same-sex couples or single gay or lesbian parents. In many cases, the children are from previous relationships. However, more and more gay and lesbian adults are choosing to conceive or adopt children.

As a same-sex couple seeking to have a baby, you'll face some unique decisions. One of those decisions can be particularly emotional: For lesbian couples, it's who will carry the baby. Or maybe you each plan to carry a pregnancy but at different times. For gay couples, it's which partner's sperm will be involved in conceiving a baby. You may find the decision comes easily — one of you prefers to take on the role of pregnant mom or sperm donor. It's not uncommon, though, for couples to struggle with these choices.

Here are some options that address these and other concerns specific to same-sex couples.

Lesbian couples. As a lesbian couple, there are several routes you can take on the journey to pregnancy:

▶ You may opt for one partner's male relative, such as a brother, to serve as the sperm donor while the other partner carries the baby. In this way, both of you will be genetically linked to the baby.
▶ You can choose to use the same donor sperm for multiple pregnancies over several years. Frozen donor sperm can be stored at your fertility clinic and is usually viable for 10 years or longer. When you and your partner are ready to conceive again, using the same donor sperm insures that your children will be biologically related, regardless of which one of you carries the second child.
▶ If you need to use in vitro fertilization, one of you can donate your eggs and the other can carry the baby. The donated eggs are fertilized with donor sperm, and the embryo is placed in

the other partner's uterus. Chapter 15 contains additional information about in vitro fertilization.
▶ You can both try to get pregnant at the same time using the same donor sperm. Whoever becomes pregnant first carries the child. However, having both partners undergoing fertility care at the same time generally isn't recommended.

Gay couples. Several options may appeal to you as a couple hoping to start a family:
▶ Some fertility clinics may be able to use both of your sperm to fertilize separate batches of a donor's eggs through in vitro fertilization. This technique can result in two embryos that are both genetically related to the same egg donor, but one embryo is related to one partner while the other is related to the other partner. The two embryos are then placed in a gestational carrier's uterus with the goal of giving birth to both babies. If only one baby is born, a DNA test will be needed to determine which of you is the father.
▶ You may opt for one partner's female relative, such as a sister, to serve as the egg donor while the other partner donates his sperm. In this way, both of you will be genetically linked to the baby.
▶ You can choose to use the same donor eggs for multiple pregnancies over several years. Frozen donor eggs can be stored at your fertility clinic and may be viable for up to 10 years or longer. When you and your partner are ready to conceive again, using the same donor eggs insures that your children will be biologically related, regardless of which one of you donates your sperm.

CULTURAL AND RELIGIOUS CONSIDERATIONS

For some people, the hope of having a family with the use of assisted reproductive technologies is complicated by cultural or religious considerations. Perhaps this may be your situation.

Before assuming that infertility treatments aren't an option for you, speak to your care provider. Most doctors are sensitive to religious and cultural issues, and they want you to feel free to raise any concerns that might influence your fertility care. Fertility technology has evolved and continues to evolve, and there could be treatment options you aren't aware of that may work for you.

It's possible to address your concerns while still adhering to specific cultural or religious principles.

Concerns about in vitro fertilization

In vitro fertilization involves harvesting multiple eggs from a woman's ovaries and fertilizing those eggs outside the body. For religious reasons, this process may not be an option for some people. While there have been some attempts to work around the issue, such as placing an egg and sperm in a capsule in the vagina for fertilization, these approaches haven't been widely accepted.

For others, the key issue is creation of many embryos, some of which may be preserved and stored. The concern is what happens to the unused embryos. If this is an issue for you, talk with your doctor about possible options. Rather than fertilizing a large number of eggs, your doctor can fertilize a small number, perhaps two or three, and use all of the embryos created at that time to help you get pregnant. The rest of the harvested, but unfertilized eggs can be frozen and used at a later time if needed. This approach is widely used in other parts of the world but less often in the United States.

Intercourse restrictions

A potential concern for an Orthodox Jewish couple trying to get pregnant is the prohibition of intercourse during vaginal bleeding, such as menstrual bleeding, and for the seven days that follow.

If a couple is fertile, and the wife's menstrual cycle lasts 25 to 28 days, this doesn't generally present a problem. However, about one-fifth of women of childbearing age experience shorter cycles lasting from 21 to 25 days. If you fall into this category, it can be more difficult to get pregnant. That's because ovulation — the time when you're most fertile — is likely to be occurring during the days in which sexual intercourse is prohibited.

Fortunately, there is a relatively easy way to address this concern. A fertility doctor may be able to prescribe a medication to delay ovulation and lengthen your menstrual cycle.

Sperm collection

For couples having difficulty getting pregnant, both the female and male partners are generally tested for fertility concerns. For a man, this often involves having his sperm tested. This can be particularly problematic for men of certain religious backgrounds. The most common way to collect a man's semen for medical testing is to have the man masturbate in a room at the clinic designed for this purpose. Masturbation, however, goes against some religious practices, including Orthodox Jewish law, which prohibits ejaculation outside of the vagina.

Ask your fertility doctor if the medical facility permits special testing conditions where sperm are collected during intercourse at home using a special condom made specifically for this purpose.

Melissa's Story

As the only child of an only child of an only child, having a family wasn't a priority for me when I was young. At the time, I didn't want children. I wanted a career, and I chased that dream instead.

Then, when I was in my mid-30s, I got married and my thinking changed. My husband and I started to talk about having a family. Unfortunately, I had a strike against me. I'd recently had an ovary removed due to a large cyst that was feared to be cancerous.

The doctor had told me that if I wanted to have children naturally, I should get on it. So my husband, who'd had a vasectomy, went in to have it reversed. Unfortunately, our marriage didn't work out, and we divorced after just nine months.

I threw myself back into work. By this time, I was 36 years old. I hadn't given up the idea of having a family, but I knew that time wasn't exactly on my side.

That's when my ex-husband called. Back when he'd had his vasectomy reversed, he chose to store some sperm tissue in case the reversal didn't work. He'd been paying storage fees for the tissue and wasn't interested in storing it anymore. He told me that he knew I'd make a good mother and that the tissue had always been meant to share with me. "Do you want it?" he asked.

After much thought, we agreed that he'd transfer ownership of the sperm tissue. I decided I'd store it until I was 42, and if I hadn't met someone I wanted to start a family with by then, I'd go through with in vitro fertilization (IVF).

My body, however, had another timetable. When I went in for some preliminary blood tests, I was told that some of my hormone levels didn't look good. My doctor told me that if I wanted to have a baby through IVF, I shouldn't wait. As I was processing this, I was thrown another wrench: The doctor discovered that my tissue donor was my ex-husband and not a current partner, and refused to perform the IVF procedure. I was told that I'd have to use an unknown donor.

I was uncomfortable using an unknown donor, and I didn't have time to fall in love. So I contacted another fertility clinic and shared my story. After some debate, they agreed to perform IVF. I was overjoyed. I was going to have a baby! At the same time, the situation was complicated. The clinic was nearly 250 miles from my home. Both my ex-husband and I had to make trips for blood tests, to meet with a psychologist and to attend other appointments.

When it came time for my first round of IVF, though, I went alone and did everything myself. For three weeks, I stayed in a nearby hotel. When I gave myself the shots required before the IVF procedure, I cried because it hurt so much, but also because I was scared and alone. I felt wrecked, while at the same time feeling empowered. I thought, "If I want a child, I can do this."

If I thought I was emotional when we did the transfer, it was nothing compared with how I felt when it failed. I cried for days. I'd had three of my embryos transferred, and now I had lost each of those babies. I felt like I'd miscarried.

About six weeks later, I tried again. Again, it failed. I went through every emotion you can imagine — from thinking that it wasn't meant to be to deciding that God hated me.

I decided that I wouldn't try anymore. But then I got a call from my doctor. He said that we could try something different — something more aggressive now that I was nearly 38 and classified as an older candidate. He told me about "assisted hatching" and steroids they could give me so that my body didn't reject the embryos. Despite my earlier hesitation, I decided to go for it.

This time felt different. I was more relaxed, and less worried. I felt like, whether it worked or not, I had given it my best shot.

My doctor transferred three embryos on a summer day, and then I drove back home. With my first two IVF treatments, I'd taken pregnancy tests every day following each transfer. But this time, it wasn't until I returned for my post-transfer appointment that I learned the good news: I was pregnant.

Five weeks and two days later, I had my first ultrasound. That's when I was told that I'd been blessed with not only one, but two babies. I cried with joy … and then I became filled with fear. How was I going to handle two babies by myself? I wondered how I'd ever manage it all.

Because I wanted to deliver my babies with my fertility doctor, I moved to an apartment near the hospital when I was in my seventh month. It was a difficult time. Now I wasn't only alone but feeling fat and ugly, too. There were times when I wondered if I'd made the right decision. But when I saw my babies for the first time — a boy and a girl, Michael and Mariah — it was overwhelming joy. I knew I'd done the right thing.

That doesn't mean it's been easy. I thought that because I'd gone through the IVF process alone that I'd be able to handle being a parent alone. But I had never even held a newborn before, much less diapered or fed two of them. I could rock a man's business world, but I couldn't care for a baby. Fortunately, the nurses were fantastic and taught me everything they knew.

Still, as much as I love my children — and as happy as I am that I'm their mother — our road has been tough. Even though I have a nanny, parenting twins as a single woman is a challenge. Sometimes I feel guilty that I brought children into this world without a father present. In the end, though, I feel like I did the right thing.

Still, I'd caution another woman against using a known donor. It complicates things. I've vacillated between gratitude and resentment. My ex-husband helped me have these two wonderful children. And while he has no legal rights to them, he also has no responsibilities. On days when being a mother feels overwhelming, I find myself resenting that he doesn't have to do any of the work.

Most days, however, I feel deep gratitude. Gratitude that I was able to have my children, and deeper gratitude yet that I had twins. My children are not the only child of an only child of an only child. They will have each other.

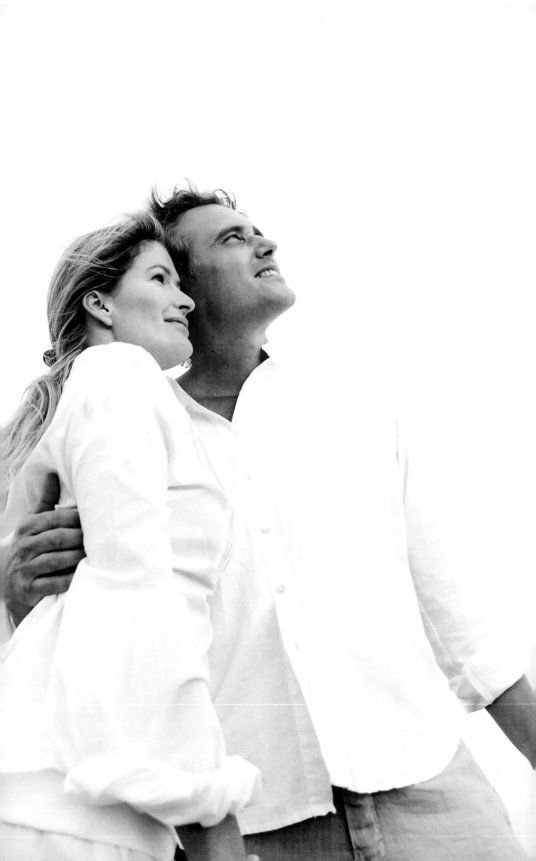

CHAPTER 20

Other options

If you're in the process of undergoing infertility treatment, you may have started out with an idea of how much time, energy and money you were willing to invest in trying to become pregnant. You may have even set limits on the amount of resources you were going to devote to your quest, hoping for a positive outcome long before then. But now as you approach or surpass your limits, it can be difficult to think about stopping your treatment or reconsidering your options.

Take heart in knowing that many others have been in your shoes and have emerged from their experiences with a renewed sense of purpose and promise. You may feel that you've reached the end of a long and painful road, but this can actually be the beginning of something new and exciting.

Adoption is one alternative to pregnancy that can bring fulfillment, meaning and pleasure to your life. And remember that not having your own children doesn't mean you still can't experience the joy of children.

WHEN TO CONSIDER ALTERNATIVES

For so long, what's kept you going is hope, but hope can be a barrier to knowing when it's time to stop fertility treatment. If you find yourself at this crossroads, it's a good idea to take a break from treatment and give yourself some room to breathe. It won't be easy, not when you've been single-mindedly pursuing parenthood. But you might be surprised to find that stopping treatment, even temporarily, lifts a weight off your shoulders. You can exhale, slow down, and reconnect with the person you were before you started on this path.

Before making any decisions, it's essential that you give yourself permission to grieve. Instead of feeling pressured to make a choice right away, let yourself fully experience feelings such as loss, disappointment and anger.

As you work through a range of emotions, you may find that you're also dealing with regret in the form of what if questions. What if I hadn't waited so long to start a family? What if I'd married sooner? Instead of replaying those past choices, strive to move forward and focus on the present. Seeking the guidance of a mental health professional who's knowledgeable about infertility issues can be invaluable. Individual and marriage counseling may also help you work through the grieving and decision-making processes.

Ultimately, your decision to stop infertility treatment will likely come down to the depletion of one or more of the following resources:

- *Biological.* You may no longer have any viable eggs or sperm, or your doctor may inform you that the chance of further treatment being successful is extremely low. Coming up against this wall can be painful, but it can also give you the freedom to let go and take your life in a new direction.
- *Emotional.* Dealing with the ups and downs that come with infertility is often all-consuming and emotionally draining. You may have reached the point where you've simply run out of steam. A voice in your head is telling you it's time to stop. Or you may be picking up on more subtle cues. You notice that you're having difficulty making your next doctor's appointment, or you're looking at a friend's recent adoption in a new light.
- *Physical.* In the process of trying to get pregnant, you may have undergone complex and even painful procedures. The physical strain of medications or surgery can lead to burnout. Your body is telling you it's time to stop or take a break.
- *Financial.* It's impossible to put a dollar amount on your desire to have a baby, but financial considerations are unavoidable. Your instinct may be to push those considerations aside and try for yet another treatment. At some point, though, the money will run out. Before that happens, give yourself a chance to re-examine your priorities. Will the cost of more treatments make it harder to pursue adoption, plan for retirement or attain other life goals? You don't want to look back later and wish you'd more carefully considered other wants and needs.

Deciding as a couple Before discussing this major life decision as a couple, take some time to explore your thoughts and feelings as individuals. You might find it helpful to separately write down the pros and cons of the choices in front of you. What are the positives and negatives of continuing with infertility treatment? What about stopping it? What are your feelings about other options, such as adoption or child-free living?

Once you've done your own soul searching, create a safe space to explore these issues openly and honestly as a couple. Thoughtful conversations can help you reach a decision that takes into account the feelings of both of you. Sometimes turning to a third party for guidance, such as a counselor or clergy person or even a trusted friend, can help you objectively evaluate your situation.

What if you disagree on what to do next? It's not uncommon for a man to be ready to stop treatment before a woman is, although the reverse also can be true. By the same token, one of you may wish to explore adoption while the other is uncomfortable with that option. This difference of opinion can lead to feelings of frustration, guilt and resentment. It's crucial to keep the dialogue between the two of you going and negotiate a plan you both can live with. Keep in mind that no decision needs to be permanent. It's

OK to test the waters. You may, for example, decide to stop pursuing infertility treatment and embrace a child-free life. That doesn't mean you can't later choose to give infertility treatment another try or pursue adoption.

ADOPTION

After devoting so much time, money and hope into having a baby, it can be daunting to change your mindset and embrace the idea of adoption. Often it's a process of realizing that becoming a parent matters more to you than getting pregnant. When you reach this point, adoption no longer feels like a last resort but rather an exciting opportunity. It can be a relief to finally move beyond infertility treatment and stride forward in this new direction.

Issues to consider Making the choice of whether to adopt and how to go about the process depends on a variety of factors and personal preferences. Here's a checklist of questions that can help you sort through some key issues:

- If you're a couple, are both of you open to adoption?
- Are you in a financial position to take on the cost of adoption?
- Do you desire an infant, or are you willing to adopt an older child? If so, how old?
- Are you willing to adopt siblings rather than one infant or child?
- Are you comfortable adopting a child of a different ethnicity or race than your own? If so, will that child be welcomed and nurtured by your extended family and community?
- Are you comfortable adopting a child from another country, or do you prefer to adopt domestically?

- Are you willing to adopt someone with special behavioral, medical or physical needs?
- Do you have a preference for a boy or a girl?
- Do you want the birth mother to know who you are and you and your child to know who she is? Or do you prefer an anonymous arrangement?
- If you prefer open knowledge of the birth mother, how involved do you want to be with her during and after the pregnancy?
- Are you prepared for outside parties to evaluate your marital and medical history, financial and employment status, and home life?
- Are you prepared to wait an indeterminate period of time before you are matched with an adoptee?

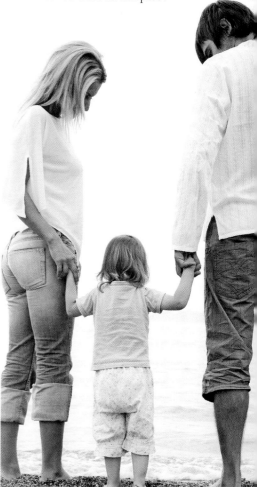

Selecting an adoption resource If you think adoption is something you want to explore further, talk to your family doctor or fertility specialist, religious leader, or friends who have adopted to find out what resources and agencies are available in your community. Local medical centers and religious organizations may also provide educational programs for prospective adoptive parents. Contacting adoption agencies directly is another option. Many agencies will send you information or provide free, no-obligation informational sessions that outline how the adoption process works.

As you explore adoption, you'll discover that there are a number of avenues to choose from:

 Public adoption agencies. These agencies are often part of a state's foster care system. They will match you with an infant or child who has been removed from his or her home.

 Licensed adoption agencies. Private adoption agencies include nonprofit and for-profit organizations. They're significantly more expensive than public agencies but are more likely to match you with a baby rather than an older child.

 Unlicensed private adoption agencies or facilitators. Unlike licensed private agencies, unlicensed private adoption services are unregulated and aren't required to adhere to state standards designed to protect adoptive and birth parents.

 Independent adoptions. Independent adoptions involve working with an adoption attorney who will help you identify prospective birth mothers in the United States and set up an adoption. Not all states allow this type of adoption.

 International adoptions. An international adoption means adopting an infant or child from another country to live with you in the United States. This type of adoption usually requires a lot of paperwork and some overseas travel. In addition, things can change quickly. A country may be open to foreign adoptions and then decide to not allow them. However, international adoptions can happen more quickly than private domestic options.

Along with choosing an adoption resource, you'll need to decide whether you want to pursue a closed or open adoption. A closed adoption is anonymous, involving no contact with the birth mother and no exchange of personal information. In contrast, an open adoption involves some sharing of personal information as well as some contact with the birth mother during and possibly after her pregnancy. Often, birth mothers in open private adoptions choose from among prospective adoptive parents.

According to a recent report, contact with the birth mother occurs in 68 percent of private domestic adoptions and 39 percent of public domestic options. The vast majority of international adoptions are closed adoptions.

How to begin the process Whether you plan to adopt domestically or internationally, you'll be required to undergo a home study. As part of this screening process, expect to share information regarding your background, finances, employment, and physical and mental health. A social worker will also conduct interviews with you and arrange for a home visit.

The purpose of the home study is twofold. It establishes that you're willing and able to create a supportive, loving and stable environment for a child. It also allows an adoption agency to get a clearer sense of who you are as people so that it can make the best match possible. Most adoption agencies are able to arrange a home study, or you can work with an independent home-study provider. The entire process can last anywhere from two to 10 months.

Many agencies also require that you take part in educational sessions before or during the home study. These sessions cover a range of issues related to adoption and help you determine the characteristics in a child that would best suit you as adoptive parents. Once the home study is complete, an agency can begin the process of matching you with a child.

Forums and support groups As you explore adoption, it can be beneficial to reach out to others who understand what you're going through. Many online adoption forums and support groups bring people together virtually to share information and offer guidance. Local support groups allow you to meet in person regularly with other pre-adoptive and adoptive parents. Sharing the joys and challenges of the adoption process with others can make the experience a lot less overwhelming.

CHILD-FREE LIVING

What if you've decided to stop infertility treatment, but you've also determined that adoption isn't the right choice for you? At this moment of transition, you may be feeling isolated and alone. The idea of not having children makes some couples feel outside the norm or set apart from the rest of society. Rest assured that neither is the case.

The number of adult women who are childless — whether by chance or by choice — has grown steadily. According to a 2010 Pew Research Center report, 1 in 5 women today end their chilbearing years without having children, compared with 1 in 10 in the 1970s. This trend extends to married couples, for whom being childless is becoming increasingly common.

Myths and facts about child-free living If you're considering not having children, you may be facing some fears about the road ahead. How will being childless affect your mental and emotional health? How will it affect your marriage? How will you redefine your life goals? What will it be like to grow old without children?

There are many inaccurate stereotypes about living without children. One of them is that you'll always be unhappy. Right now, you may still be recovering from the emotional and physical toll of undergoing infertility treatment, as well as the pressure to become a parent. As you let go of those expectations and embrace a new path, you'll likely experience a range of new, positive emotions and become more hopeful for the future.

Other myths about child-free living include:

▶ *People without children are selfish.* Studies on child-free adults negate this stereotype. In fact, a high percentage of people without children are dedicated to helping others as teachers, social workers and volunteers.

▶ *People without children have less meaningful lives.* It can take time to fully embrace life without children. People who are able to make that leap find that a child-free life is both satisfying and fulfilling. For some couples, pursuing new professional, educational or personal goals is important, but such changes aren't necessary.

▶ *Being around other people's children will always be painful.* There will be times throughout your life when you do experience moments of sadness over not having a child. A family member's announcement that she's pregnant or a co-worker's baby shower may bring back a pang of loss. Those twinges of sadness tend to decrease in frequency and intensity as time goes on so that spending time with children becomes a rewarding and joyful experience.

▸ *Child-free people who are middle-aged and older are lonely and unhappy.* This is another persistent myth that research does not bear out. In fact, studies show that older people without children do not experience greater loneliness, unhappiness or dissatisfaction with life than do their peers with children.

▸ *Child-free marriages are unhappy marriages.* Fighting infertility can cause a strain on any marriage, but once you're able to accept and embrace a child-free life, you may find that your marriage is actually stronger. Your shared experience of adversity has forged a closer bond, and you now have more time to invest in your relationship.

The benefits of child-free living

From where you stand right now, it may seem impossible to imagine any benefits to not having children. You've put a lot of energy into the dream of becoming a parent. Yet as you move through your grief and set your sights on the future, you may be surprised to feel a sense of gratitude for all that you have and all that is possible. Many paths lay before you, some of which wouldn't be an option with a child.

Not having children gives you the freedom to invest more deeply in other relationships. Child-free couples have more time to spend with each other, enriching and deepening their marriages. In the same way, you'll have more time to build and strengthen your relationships with family and friends.

A child-free life also opens up opportunities to invest more fully in your career. As a result, you may find that your income increases, opening up additional opportunities. You might choose to travel, pursue further education or immerse yourself in a creative pursuit. Having more time for political or social causes is another aspect of a child-free life.

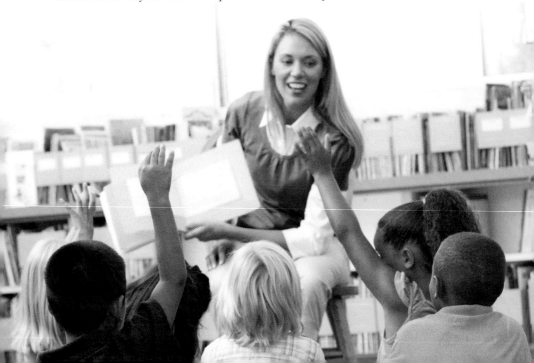

Other ways to get involved with children A child-free life doesn't mean a life without children. There are many ways that you can still interact and spend time with children — having a positive influence on their lives while at the same time fulfilling your nurturing instinct. Consider these options:

- Accept an offer to become a godparent to the child of a friend or family member.
- Spend time with nieces and nephews. If you wish, offer to establish college funds for them.
- Become a mentor to a child in need through an organization such as Big Brothers Big Sisters.
- Teach religious classes at your place of worship or engage in other child-related activities that it sponsors.
- Sign up to coach a sports team in your community.
- Tutor children at your local school, in an after-school program or through another community organization.
- Volunteer at a children's hospital.
- Help out at a homeless shelter or child care program that serves children and families in need.
- Explore the idea of becoming a short-term or longer term foster parent.

FINDING SUPPORT

As you consider the options ahead of you, it may help to reach out to others who are struggling with similar decisions or who have already embraced new paths. Online forums and support groups can be a source of comfort, feedback and shared knowledge. Organizations for couples struggling with infertility, such as Resolve.org (see page 274), also offer guidance and encouragement for those considering a child-free life. In addition, your local community might also have a support group dedicated to child-free couples and individuals.

Embarking on a new path may seem daunting, but it can reap rich rewards. Be kind to yourself as you work through what can be complex and conflicting emotions. Know that whatever route you choose, it's absolutely possible to reclaim a sense of purpose and excitement for the future.

Additional resources

American Fertility Organization
315 Madison Ave., Suite 901
New York, NY 10017
888-917-3777
www.theafa.org

American Pregnancy Association
1425 Greenway Drive, Suite 440
Irving, TX 75038
americanpregnancy.org

American Society for Reproductive Medicine
1209 Montgomery Highway
Birmingham, Alabama 35216-2809
205-978-5000
www.asrm.org

Centers for Disease Control and Prevention
1600 Clifton Road
Atlanta, GA 30333
800-232-4636
www.cdc.gov/art

Mayo Clinic Health Information
www.MayoClinic.org

Resolve: The National Infertility Association
1760 Old Meadow Road, Suite 500
McLean, VA 22102
703-556-7172
www.resolve.org

Society for Assisted Reproductive Technology
1209 Montgomery Highway
Birmingham, Alabama 35216-2809
205-978-5000, ext. 109
www.sart.org

Society for Reproductive Endocrinology and Infertility
1209 Montgomery Highway
Birmingham, AL 35216
205-978-5000
www.socrei.org

Index

invasive prenatal tests, 107
iron, 49
isotretinoin (Amnesteem, Claravis), 46
IUD (intrauterine device), 46
IVF. *See* in vitro fertilization
IVF cycle
  average cost, 216
  canceled, 204
  defined, 201
  number of embryos transferred, 210

J

Jane's story, 130–131
Japanese custom, miscarriage and, 115
journals, 245

K

Kallmann syndrome, 161, 188
Klinefelter syndrome, 126, 159, 163
known donors, 231–232, 233, 260
Kristen and Chris' story, 116–117

L

laparoscopy, 176, 179
lesbian couples, 262
letrozole (Femara), 186
leukocytospermia, 154
lifestyle
  adjusting, 15–31
  IVF success and, 200–201
  in medical history, 171
lightheadedness
  as emergency symptom, 102
  as pregnancy sign, 98
Lisa and Scott's story, 180–181
long-acting birth control, going off of, 46
low birth weight, IVF and, 212
low-density lipoprotein (LDL) cholesterol, 36
lubricants, 93
luteal phase, 78
luteal phase defect, 139–140
luteinizing hormone (LH), 16, 24
  in hormone production regulation, 120
  in ovulatory phase, 78
  production of, 70
  surge, 84, 173
  synthetic versions of, 137
  testing urine for, 82–83

M

male
  in baby's sex determination, 71
  infertility, 151–165
  partner history, 171
male fertility
  age and, 126–128
  age-related risks, 128
  evaluations, 152
  pregnancy rates and, 127
  See also sperm health
male problems, 151–165
  anejaculation, 161–163
  chromosome defects, 163–164
  ejaculation issues, 161–163
  evaluation of, 151–152
  hormone imbalances, 158–161
  hypospadias, 158
  infertility evaluation, 165
  leukocytospermia, 154
  retrograde ejaculation, 154–155, 161–163
  specialists and, 156–157
  sperm, 152–155
  sperm duct abnormalities, 156–158
  structural and anatomical issues, 155–158
  tumors, 158
  undescended testicles, 155–156
  varicoceles, 155
male reproductive organs, 68–69
mandrake root, 43
marijuana, 28
medications
  aromatase inhibitors, 186
  cancer and, 188, 248
  clomiphene (Clomid, Serophene), 30–31, 86, 116, 180, 185–186
  cost and, 184
  for erectile dysfunction, 163
  fertility, 184–188
  gonadotropins (Repronex, Menopur), 186–187
  human chorionic gonadotropin (HCG), 73, 99, 113, 187
  male infertility and, 160
  metformin (Glucophage), 187–188
  for oocyte maturation and release, 202–204
  for ovarian stimulation, 202
  preconception and, 46–48
  to prevent premature ovulation, 202
  for specific conditions, 188
  sperm health and, 65
men without female partner, 260–261

getting, 77
irregular, 135
late, 96
See also menstrual cycle
personal history, 170
PGD (preimplantation genetic diagnosis), 214–216
PGS (preimplantation genetic screening), 92, 214–216
physical exam, 171–172
PID (pelvic inflammatory disease), 112, 140
pituitary disorders
male infertility and, 161
tumors, 135
placenta, beginning formation of, 73
planning ahead, 89–90
plastics, chemicals in, 28–29
POI. *See* primary ovarian insufficiency
polycystic ovary syndrome (PCOS)
aromatase inhibitors and, 186
defined, 137
diagnosis, 137
symptoms, 137
treatment, 137–138
population-based screening, 54
positive self-talk, 23
postcoital testing, 179
post-ejaculation urinalysis, 156–157
preconception visit with doctor, 45, 89–90
preconception planning, 89–90
pregnancy
age effect on, 119–131
biochemical, 106
conception and, 73–74
ectopic, 103, 111, 112–114
heterotopic, 113–114
immunizations guide, 50–51
molar, 106
rates, 93
when to tell people, 100
pregnancy complications
age and, 124–126
IVF and, 212
pregnancy determination
care provider visit and, 101–103
early signs and symptoms, 97–98
fatigue, 97
food aversions/cravings, 98
headaches and dizziness, 98
increased urination, 98
mood swings, 98
nausea, 98

raised basal body temperature, 98
slight bleeding and cramping, 97
tender, swollen breasts, 97
tests, 98–101
pregnancy loss
as difficult experience, 114
emotional recovery, 114
physical recovery, 114–115
recurrent, 109–111
as risk factor, 124–125
See also miscarriages
pregnancy preparation
alcohol, tobacco, and other toxins and, 26–29
birth control and, 45–46
chronic medical conditions and, 52–53
diet and, 29
exercise and, 18–20
genetic tests, 53–55
immunizations, 49–52
lifestyle adjustments, 15–31
medications and supplements, 46–48
sleep and, 24–27
stress and, 20–23
vitamins, 48–49
weight and, 15–31
preimplantation genetic diagnosis (PGD), 214–216
preimplantation genetic screening (PGS), 92, 214–216
premature delivery, IVF and, 212
prenatal vitamins
birth weight and, 49
choosing, 48–49
importance of, 48–49
prescription vs. OTC, 49
primary hypogonadism, 159–161, 188
primary ovarian insufficiency (POI)
approach to, 138–139
causes of, 138
defined, 138
symptoms, 138
progesterone, 78, 206
progesterone blood levels, 84
progestin implants/injections, 46
progressive muscle relaxation, 23
prolactin, 135, 177
protein
legumes, 39
orientation toward, 37–39
plan, 38–39
requirements, 39
sources, 38
See also diet